Contents

Tables and Figures

Published by JR Publishers, Melbourne, 2023.
jgrogers@unimelb.edu.au and jro24161@bigpond.net.au

ISBN printed book 978-0-6458191-0-6
ISBN eBook 978-0-6458191-1-3

Edited by Jill Reid and Pauline Sanders
Designed by Creative United

Suggested citation. (Replace italicised text with details of relevant chapter).
Chapter Author, 2022. Chapter title. Chapter page numbers. In Rogers, J.G., & Robertson, J.A. *Looking Back Looking Forward Oral health in Victoria 1970 to 2022.* JR Publishers. Melbourne.

Foreword

As the Head of the Melbourne Dental School I am delighted to be able to introduce this important and timely book that traces the complex interactions of social, political and economic factors that have shaped the oral health of Victorians, and more broadly Australians, over the past five decades.

Oral health is vitally important to health and wellbeing and should not be seen as being separate from systemic health. The oral cavity can be a window to recognising more general health issues. During the past fifty years, whilst there have been improvements in oral health, there continues to be a large and unequal burden of preventable oral disease. Indeed, inequality has increased, and poor dental health is a key marker of disadvantage and social inequity. Public dental health services offer only a tattered safety net evidenced by unacceptably long waiting times for even basic dental care, thus allowing clinical problems for the patient to get steadily worse. The mouth has effectively been left out of the body.

Considering the prevalence and severity of oral diseases such as dental caries and periodontitis, the burden they impose on the quality of life of the individual and the cost to society, this is a shameful state that needs urgent and immediate focussed attention. It is my view that this is a challenge that all of us connected to the profession have responsibility to address.

In this, the first ever book on the history of Australian dental public health, John Rogers and Jamie Robertson provide a historic analysis of the development of the dental health system. The book details a roadmap of how we arrived at the current state of oral health and the present dental health system, as well as a compass indicating future trends and directions.

Their detailed research and insightful perspectives will enable public health professionals including academics and students; policy makers; oral health professionals; oral health advocates; health historians and sociologists; dental and general epidemiologists; political scientists; and inquisitive lay public to learn from the past and help to create a system that is more equitable for all. With a combined 100 years of experience in both the public and private dental health sectors John, who specialises in policy development and implementation, and Jamie, a noted historian of the dental profession, are perfectly positioned to describe the history of oral health and the development of the dental health system in our society.

This book deals with more than history though as the authors go onto make proposals for a world's best practice approach in line with the recently released WHO Global Strategy on Oral Health. Their comprehensive research and scholarly synthesis emphasises the need to listen closely to the echoes of public dental history if we are to avoid repeating the mistakes of the past. As the celebrated writer William Faulkner reminded us *The past is not dead, it is not even past*. It is important that we are aware of the lessons of the past to be able to plan a fairer future.

This is a highly recommended read.

Professor Alastair J Sloan

Head of Melbourne Dental School, The University of Melbourne

Preface

This book is the collaborative work of a Public Dental Health policy specialist (Rogers) and a clinician and historian of the dental profession (Robertson). Many of the areas which we cover have been studied by others but few have tried to capture the breadth of the social milieu in which policy is formed and debated while presenting quantitative analyses of the relevant health variables.

This history places the epidemiology of dentistry and dental health in the context of the overarching political and societal changes in which the distribution and determinants of oral health have occurred. There was a paucity of data about the dental health of Victoria's population in 1970, but by the 1980s questions were being asked not only about dental health status but also people's ability to access dental care due to cost and geography. In the 1990s political changes at state and national levels ensured dental care remained a prominent electoral issue, which, in turn, raised its importance to bureaucracies.

Public service bureaucracies concern themselves with who gets what, at what cost and under what circumstances. As more budgetary funds are channelled, even if haltingly, to public sector dental and general health agencies, there is a need to account for them. That fact has helped prompt administrative changes in the governance and regulation of all registered health professions. In this study we have used dentistry as an exemplar for the evolution of health profession governance.

To the best of our knowledge, no one has followed the twin tracks of dental health status and related legislative and societal changes over time. In the 50 years since 1970 the population has more than doubled and is living longer. While these decades have seen significant improvement in the dental health of the majority of Victorians, dental inequality in disadvantaged groups has increased. The saying that "a rising tide lifts all boats" is only true if the boats were all watertight in the first place.

From a time when false teeth were given as a wedding present and first teeth were routinely extracted, improvements have been achieved through disease prevention, a rise in health literacy among most of the population, and variable access to care when disease occurs. Diversification of the dental workforce and legislative changes have also facilitated improvements.

As a consequence of this success, most people are now retaining their own teeth but are more prone to gum disease and tooth decay. Greater understanding of biology and technological developments have afforded ever more options for the prevention and treatment of disorders – for those who can pay for it. Older, poorer people in particular are suffering from dental neglect.

Today, we know more about the adverse impact of oral disease on overall health, yet public dental waiting times average almost two years and dentistry remains excluded from Medicare. While there are many reasons for poor oral health, it is often a clear sign of social disadvantage. In terms of the public dental health system, the mouth has been left out of the body.

Governments pay for over 60% of general health care costs, but less than 20% of dental care costs. We argue that public dental health funding should be sufficient to at least allow disadvantaged groups to access the basic dental care needed for general health.

In this book we have brought together over 300 sources related to oral health epidemiology, legislation, finances, workforce, program reviews, reports and audits, supplemented by interviews with key players. We have used the WHO building blocks for health systems as a framework for our analyses and the principles in the 2022 WHO Global Strategy on Oral Health to chart a future in which better oral health is achievable for all.

While there is a particular focus on Victoria, the issues are common across all states and territories, and indeed internationally.

Improving oral health and reducing longstanding inequalities requires action at all levels of government and in all sectors of civil society. There is an urgent need for a national conversation about how the current situation can be remedied.

John Rogers and **Jamie Robertson**

Acknowledgements

Many colleagues have contributed to the writing of this book and have improved it significantly. Pauline Sanders has toiled long and hard to research, edit and advise. Tony McBride, Martin Hall, and Meredith Kefford have critically appraised endless drafts and have provided important insights to enhance the story. The University of Melbourne Dental Alumni Research Foundation provided a scholarship that significantly progressed the work.

We appreciate the input from many colleagues who have shared their experiences and commented on drafts. Contributors include Hanny Calache, Anne-Louise Carlton, Deb Cole, Martin Dooland, Loc Do, Pat Field, Shalika Hegde, Matt Hopcraft, Dan Hurley, Clare Lin, Mandy Leveratt, Janet McCalman, Rodrigo Marino, Rachael Martin, Roisin McGrath, Mike Morgan, Tan Nguyen, Lloyd O'Brien, Anil Raichur, Allison Ridge, Alistair Sandison, Julie Satur, Natalie Savin, Susanne Sofronoff, Rowan Story, Katy Theodore, Catherine Thompson, Tony Triado, Martin Whelan, Beth Wilson, Rebecca Wong, Clive Wright and Michael Wright.

Jill Reid through her editing and Francesca Carra with her design work, have considerably enhanced readability. Mihiri Silva, Stuart Dashper, Duncan Fardon and Chris Feik have been helpful in facilitating the process through to publication.

Thank you also to the following organisations for their financial support of this book: Australian Dental Association Victorian Branch, The University of Melbourne Dental Alumni Research Foundation and the Melbourne Dental School.[1]

We would especially like to thank our partners for their forbearance over the long journey.

1 Our funders did not influence our approach nor have editorial control.

About the authors

Our book does not include recognition of all the key people who advocated, planned and implemented the dental programs discussed. Some individuals are mentioned in chapters such as Chapter 8: Alliances and Advocacy and in the reference list, but proper acknowledgement of contributions is a task for future historians.

Jamie Robertson graduated as a Bachelor of Dental Surgery from the University of Glasgow in 1967 and then spent two years working for a medical mission in northern Canada. His first post in Australia was at the Royal Dental Hospital of Melbourne. After running his own private practice for 40 years, Jamie took up a clinical position with cohealth, a large community health centre in the western suburbs of Melbourne, where he worked for five years. Jamie has served as a director on the boards of the Royal Dental Hospital of Melbourne and Dental Health Services Victoria. While working in dentistry, he completed Arts and Public Health degrees at the University of Melbourne.

John Rogers has been a Principal Fellow at the University of Melbourne Dental School since 2017. He has more than 45 years' experience in management and policy development in public dental health and community health in Australia and overseas. He has worked in Papua New Guinea, Yemen, Vietnam, England and Australia. In 2007 he was a WHO dental public health consultant in Vietnam. After public health roles overseas, John managed the Peninsula Community Health Service in outer Melbourne from 1985–89. He then served as Principal Oral Health Policy Advisor in the Victorian Department of Health until 2019. A Fellow of the Public Health Association of Australia, John holds a Bachelor of Dental Science, a Master of Public Health and a PhD and is a registered specialist in public health dentistry.

Chapter 1
Introduction – The Journey

John Rogers and Jamie Robertson

The way we were

Like most aspects of life, the oral health of Victorians has changed markedly over the past 50 years. In 1970 the population of Victoria was 3.4 million with 2.4 million people living in the state capital, Melbourne. Melbourne's suburbs seemed to stretch forever even then, although the central business district was surprisingly small.

Australia's economy was, then as now, largely dependent on the primary industries of agriculture and minerals. A television cost about $500 and reception was in black and white until 1975. Telephones were connected by landline and the internet was a scarcely conceived notion of science fiction. Australia's global connections by air relied on Boeing 707s whose replacement, the 747, arrived in 1971. The 747 itself was retired only in 2020.

Although Victoria's population was burgeoning through high migration, its culture was predominantly Anglo-Saxon. Its main sporting interest was Australian Rules Football, then dominated by the Victorian Football League comprising only Victorian-based teams. Cricketers replaced footballers on the ovals in summer.

Since 1970 so much of Melbourne's visible and invisible infrastructure has changed, the Victorian population has almost doubled and its migrant proportion has grown enormously. According to the 2021 census, 29.8% of Australia's population in 2020 was born overseas. The figure for 1947 was 9.8%.[2] A television set, now boasting a flat screen and colour reception, costs little more than it did in 1970. There is a completely new lexicon of words describing computers, their functions and connectivity and these machines have changed every aspect of administration and access to entertainment forever.

By 2020 air-travel time to Europe had shrunk to about 24 hours and the price of a litre of petrol had risen from 25 cents to about $1.60, only to surge beyond two dollars in early 2022.

Oral health changes

In the same time frame, there have been dramatic changes in the extent of oral diseases and their treatment. In 1970 most children and adults had experienced tooth decay. Eighty percent of older people had no natural teeth. It was still common in some communities for a woman to be given a set of dentures as a 21st birthday or wedding present. Since then, the ability to prevent some disease, for example by fluoridation of water supplies, and an increase in the size and mix of the dental workforce have led to better oral health. In turn, these developments helped changed the mindset, still current in 1970, that tooth loss was inevitable and the only variable was the rate at which this occurred.

The current view is that good teeth are valuable functional, psychological and social assets that are worthy of care and maintenance. This attitude can only be maintained and reinforced when the majority can access affordable care that is atraumatic, aesthetic and durable. However, there is still a large and unequal burden of preventable oral disease among Victorians. While access to emergency dental care has improved since 1970, disadvantaged groups still have difficulty accessing dental care due to long public dental waiting times for general care.

2   <https://www.abs.gov.au/statistics/people/population/australias-population-country-birth/latest-release>. Accessed 29 August, 2022.

About this book - *Looking Back Looking Forward*

In 2000, just past the halfway mark of our history, country music icon Slim Dusty sang "Looking Forward Looking Back". Near the end of a career spanning almost seven decades, he sang of "making sense of what I've seen". This is what we attempt in this book. As was the case for Winston Churchill, through this process we have recognised that the further back you look, the further forward you can see. Our research emphasises the need to listen closely to the echoes of public dental health history if we are to avoid repeating the mistakes of the past. We agree with Mark Twain: while history may never repeat itself, "it does often rhyme".

The book describes the events, drivers and motives which have led to policy and legislative changes. It reviews successful and failed policies and programs, the stop–start nature of Australian government funding and changes in the dental system. To our knowledge, no one has followed the twin track of oral health and related legislative and societal change over the past 50 years.

This history traces oral health and disease alongside the complex interaction of social, political and economic factors that have shaped Victorians' oral health over the past five decades. It offers a road map of how we arrived at the current state of oral health and the present dental system, as well as a compass indicating future trends and possible directions. It delves into the past to propose a future where better oral health is available to all.

Method in the madness

Having presented our objectives, how have we proceeded?

We have adapted the World Health Organization's framework that describes health systems in terms of core components or "building blocks" (WHO, 2010) as our general framework. In this history of public dental health in Victoria, we focus on the building blocks of leadership and governance, workforce, financing, the service system and health information systems including research.

Dedicated chapters consider leadership and governance, workforce, the service system and financing follow, while health information systems and research are covered within the service system chapter. To complete our analysis, we have included a review of trends in the oral health of Victorians since 1970 and further chapters on prevention interventions, alliances and advocacy, and the evolution of clinical services.

Our scope covers the arena of dental public health: namely, "the science and practice of preventing oral diseases, promoting oral health, and improving quality of life through the organised efforts of society" (Daly et al., 2013).

Dental public health focuses on the oral health of populations. It is concerned with the distribution and determinants of oral disease (epidemiology) and evidence-based approaches to prevent disease and to promote social equity in access to dental care. Provision of dental care to disadvantaged groups is part of the broader focus to advocate to all levels of government for oral healthy environments for all.

Analysis of Victoria's oral health system over 50 years was indeed a broad scope and raised many questions. Some of those considered are outlined in Box 1.1.

Box 1.1 Questions arising

For whom is oral health better or worse – who are the winners and losers? What has happened to levels of inequity? How does Victorians' oral health compare nationally and internationally?

What changes have there been in oral health behaviours, expenditure on dental care, government funding and access to dental services?

What have been the barriers and enablers for developing good oral health policy? Which governments have supported and which governments have ignored dental programs?

What roles have legislation, workforce and research played in shaping the system?

Why do governments pay more than 60% of general health care costs but less than 20% of dental care costs? Why if you have a boil on your bum will Medicare cover the cost of treatment, but if you have a boil on your gum, it will not? Why has the mouth been left out of the body?

What interventions to prevent dental disease have been introduced and have these been successful?

We have interviewed key players, undertaken a literature review of published articles and sourced "grey literature". The latter included government and non-government reports, reviews, audits, budget documents, plans, annual reports and media articles. More than 300 documents have been sourced to help answer our questions. Importantly, many people have given their time to review drafts and comment on errors of omission and commission. We are most grateful for their efforts. Responsibility for inaccuracies rests with the authors.

> The health of each of us is more secure when health for all is assured.
> – Nancy Milio

Why bother?

But why bother to read our book? You no doubt have many other interests vying for your attention. Well, good oral health matters and, if we want a fairer society, more focus on good oral health for all is necessary (Box 1.2). Data are from Victoria unless stated as Australian and are referenced in chapters 9 and 10.

Box 1.2 Why bother about oral health?

A healthy mouth enables individuals to eat, speak and socialise without pain, discomfort and embarrassment. Oral disease affects both the individual through reduced general health and the community through health system and economic costs.

Some improvements in oral health have occurred over the past 50 years in Victoria. However, there continues to be a large and unequal burden of preventable oral disease. Poor oral health is a clear marker of disadvantage. The tooth gap between Health Care Card holders and non-card holders increased from three to six teeth in the 12 years to 2018.

Tooth decay is one of the most prevalent health problems and is the most expensive disease condition to treat. At $5 billion in 2018–19 in Australia, tooth decay was more costly to treat than falls.

The rate of hospitalisation of children with potentially preventable dental disease is the highest of all potentially preventable admissions.

More than a quarter of adults (28%), including half (51%) of people over 55 years, have gum disease. Understanding of this condition is poor. Only half of those with gum disease are aware they have this condition.

There has been an increase in reported oral health problems over the past 25 years. Problems include discomfort with appearance, avoiding certain foods and experiencing toothache.

Oral cancer is the tenth most common cancer.

Dental care is one of the most significant areas of health expenditure, totalling $10.6 billion in Australia and $3.2 billion in Victoria in 2018–19. Unlike most other forms of health care, individuals predominantly bear the cost: 71% compared with 20% for all other forms of health care in Victoria in 2018–19.

States with higher per capita public dental funding have better oral health. South Australian 12-year-olds have less than half the tooth decay experienced by Victorian children of the same age.

A range of health conditions are closely associated with oral disease. Advanced gum disease exacerbates diabetes by making it harder to manage sugar levels and is associated with adverse pregnancy outcomes and heart disease. Poor oral health can also lead to a poor diet, aspiration pneumonia and infective endocarditis.

Oral health is fundamental to overall heath, wellbeing and quality of life.

Public health measures

Public health initiatives, including those in oral health, have come about as leaders in society sought to remedy or ameliorate levels of disease or other health issues which were chronically or episodically present in the community. Interventions have generally been more successful when the causes of the problem were understood. Nonetheless, measures such as storing grain to protect against famine or quarantining against infection were practised for millennia before the causes of famine and infection were known. With the rise of scientific enquiry and statistical analysis over the past 150 years, causative agents, protective factors and mathematical probabilities have been discovered at accelerating rates, and these have enabled the introduction of evidence-based interventions which have benefitted humanity at both individual and societal levels.

Many of these interventions, such as reticulated clean water supplies, mandatory building regulations and sanitation, have been social. Others have been medical, for example, inoculations against contagious diseases including smallpox, polio and tuberculosis. Other interventions have been regulatory, such as road speed limits and the compulsory wearing of car seat belts which have reduced traffic accidents and deaths. Restrictions on smoking and the introduction of plain cigarette packaging have decreased smoking rates.

Australia has adopted all of these measures, in either compulsory or voluntary form. The compulsory route has been more effective in some cases. For example, optimal dietary folate levels have been known since the early 1990s and folate-fortified wheat flour became available within the decade. However, the number of neural tube defects such as spina bifida and non-syndromic cleft palates and lips fell dramatically only after its mandatory addition to all flours in 2009 (PHAA, 2018, p. 6).

On the other hand, triple antigen inoculation of infants remains optional, and vaccination hesitancy among parents has led to a resurgence of outbreaks of measles, which, in turn, has led to the exclusion of non-inoculated children from preschools and primary schools during outbreaks (NCIRS, 2021).

Over the past 50 years strong associations between oral health status and various systemic disorders have been well established. It is now recognised that to treat one without reference to the other will produce suboptimal outcomes for people. In future, the paradigm for preventing and treating disease and illness must be underpinned by much closer collaboration between the dental and medical professions. This has to be in addition to addressing the social and commercial determinants of health (see Chapter 6).

The winds of change

The ebb and flow of political changes at a state level have been augmented by international developments in relation to the duties of care and responsibilities of dental professionals; the declining influence of individual professions vis-a-vis governance bureaucracies; rising expectations of disease prevention to lessen the expensive treatment of its consequences; and encroaching corporatisation of health services in both the private and public sectors. These administrative "push" changes have been complemented by "pull" changes through which expectations for ever-improving health and wellbeing have continued to escalate.

At the level of treatment, if one excludes function, the quest for the perfect pearly white smile through dentures has given way to attaining the same goal through tooth bleaching, straightening and veneering. In 1970, the then recent invention of the water-cooled air turbine handpiece led to reclining dental chairs replacing the old upright ones to facilitate better vision and access and greater efficiency in restoring teeth. New capital equipment has been introduced and accelerated with computerised technology (though not without entering some blind alleys along the way). For those dental professionals adopting it, the array and cost of increasingly sophisticated health equipment keeps expanding in inverse proportion to its useful half-life. In comparison, the introduction of low-cost preventive measures, such as water fluoridation, has maintained more teeth in a healthy state than any number of well-equipped palaces (NHMRC, 2017).

In the following chapters we demonstrate that approaches to improving the oral health of Victorians over the past 50 years have reflected changing ideologies in the state's political economy as well as international trends in social thought. Events over this period may be categorised into approximate decades, as shown in Box 1.3.

> ' Those who control the past control the future and those who control the present control the past. '
> – George Orwell

Box 1.3 Approaches to the dental and oral health of Victorians over 50 years

1970s   Legislative response to demonstrated shortcomings in tackling dental disease (particularly community water fluoridation and workforce) towards the end of a "small government", conservative state government

Limited take-up by the Victorian governments of the progressive national government's school dental program

1980s   Release of pent-up enthusiasm for social change with the advent of a more socialistic government

Expansion of community dental clinics

1990s   Return of neo-liberal governments at a state- and, subsequently, national level with unanticipated consequences

Restructure of the public dental system

Brief flowering of Labor national government's adult dental program before its closure by subsequent neo-liberal national government

2000s   Consolidation of community control over the health professions

Additional funding for public dental and prevention programs from state government

Integration of school dental service into the community dental program

First national oral health plan

2010s   Adjustment to new regulatory requirements with mounting pressures on practice administration standards

Targeted national government funding of child and adult dental programs

Expansion of prevention initiatives

Resurrection of the school dental service as the Smile Squad

We now turn to our analysis of the past and a plan for a healthier future...

Appendix

Appendix 1 Timeline of significant National and Victorian dental public health reviews, audits, reports, and plans 1970 to 2022

Code: Victorian, National

Year	Dental public health initiative
1972	*Dentists Act 1972 (Vic)* and *Dental Technicians Act 1972 (Vic)*.
1973	*Health (Fluoridation) Act 1973 (Vic)*.
1977	Commencement of the water fluoridation of Melbourne.
1980	Report of the committee of inquiry into the fluoridation of Victorian water supplies for 1979–80 (Myers et al., 1980).
1982	Report of internal committee reviewing the Victorian school dental service. May 1982 (Health Commission of Victoria, 1982).
1986	*Ministerial review of dental services (MRODS). Final report* (Department of Health, 1986).
1988	Dental Health Strategy. Victorian Government response to MRODS, Including establishing the Community Dental Program.
1992	*Improving dental health in Australia. Background paper no. 9* (Dooland, 1992).
1993	Follow up report on audit of School Dental Health Service (Auditor-General of Victoria, 1993). *Impact of change in oral health status on dental education, workforce, practices and services in Australia* (NHMRC, 1993).
1995	*Future directions for dental health in Victoria* (DH&CS, 1995). Follow up report on audit of School Dental Health Service (Auditor-General of Victoria A-GV, 1995).
1996	*The Victorian school dental service child dental health promotion strategy 1995–2000* (DHS, 1996).
1998	Review of *Dentists Act 1972* and *Dental Technicians Act 1972* Final Report, July 1998 (Doyle, 1998). *Report on public dental services.* (Senate Community Affairs References Committee, 1998).
1999	*Promoting oral health 2000–2004. Strategic directions and framework for action* (DHS, 1999).
2001	*Oral health of Australians: National planning for oral health improvement. Final Report.* (AHMAC Steering Committee for National Planning for Oral Health, 2001).

Year	Dental public health initiative
2002	Victorian Auditor General audit of the Community Dental Program (A-GV, 2002).
2004	*Healthy mouths, healthy lives: Australia's national oral health plan 2004–2013* (AHMC, 2004).
2005	Community dental services follow up report (A-GV, 2005).
2007	*Improving Victoria's oral health* plan (DHS, 2007).
2009	*A healthier future for all Australians: Final report June 2009* (National Health and Hospitals Reform Commission, 2009).
2012	*Report of the National Advisory Council on Dental Health. 23 February 2012* (National Advisory Council on Dental Health, 2012).
2013	*National oral health promotion plan* (Wright, 2013). *Action plan for oral health promotion 2013–2017.* (Department of Health, 2013).
2015	*Healthy mouths, healthy lives: Australia's national oral health plan 2015–2024* (COAG Health Council, 2015). *Performance audit. Administration of the child dental benefits schedule.* Department of Health. Department of Human Services. ANAO Report No. 12 2015–16 (Auditor General-Australia, 2015).
2016	Review of access to public dental services in Victoria by (A-GV, 2016). *Introducing competition and informed user choice into human services: Identifying sectors for reform. Productivity Commission preliminary findings report overview. (Chapters 12 & 13)* (Productivity Commission, 2016).
2017	*Introducing competition and informed user choice into human services: Reforms to human services. Inquiry report* (Productivity Commission, 2017)
2019	Smile Squad school dental program commenced (Premier of Victoria, 2019). Follow up of access to public dental services in Victoria report (A-GV, 2019). *Filling the gap: A universal dental care scheme for Australia* (Duckett et al., 2019).
2020	*Victorian action plan to prevent oral disease 2020–30* (DHHS, 2020). *National oral health plan 2015–2024 performance monitoring report* (AIHW, 2020).
2022	Update of the oral health promotion evidence base (Rana et al., 2022).

References

Australian Health Ministers' Advisory Council (AHMAC) Steering Committee for National Planning for Oral Health. (2001). *Oral health of Australians: National planning for oral health improvement. Final report.* <https://www.aihw.gov.au/reports/dental-oral-health/national-planning-oral-health-improvement/contents/summary>

Australian Health Ministers' Conference. (AHMC). National Advisory Committee on Oral Health. & South Australia. Department of Health. (2004). *Healthy mouths, healthy lives: Australia's national oral health plan 2004–2013.* Adelaide: South Australian Department of Health. <https://catalogue.nla.gov.au/Record/3298219>

Australian Institute of Health and Welfare (AIHW). (2020). *National oral health plan 2015–2024: Performance monitoring report.* <https://www.aihw.gov.au/reports/dental-oral-health/national-oral-health-plan-2015-2024/contents/about>

Auditor General. (Australia). (2015). *Administration of the child dental benefits schedule. Department of Health. Department of Human Services. The Auditor-General ANAO Report No. 12 2015–16 Performance Audit.* <https://www.anao.gov.au/sites/default/files/ANAO_Report_2015-2016_12.pdf>

Auditor-General of Victoria. (A-GV). (1993). *Report on ministerial portfolios, May 1993.* <https://www.audit.vic.gov.au/sites/default/files/19930501-Ministerial-Portfolios-May-1993.pdf>

Auditor-General of Victoria. (A-GV). (1995). *Report on ministerial portfolios, May 1995.* <https://www.audit.vic.gov.au/sites/default/files/19950501-Report-on-Ministerial-Portfolios.pdf>

Auditor General Victoria. (A-GV). (2002). *Community dental services.* <https://www.audit.vic.gov.au/report/community-dental-services?section=.>

Auditor General Victoria. (A-GV). (2005). *Results of special reviews and other investigations. May 2005.* <https://www.audit.vic.gov.au/sites/default/files/20050504-Special-Reviews-and-other-Investigation-May2005.pdf>

Auditor General Victoria. (A-GV). (2016). *Access to public dental services in Victoria.* <https://www.audit.vic.gov.au/report/access-public-dental-services-victoria?section=32003--4-addressing-barriers-to-access#page-anchor.>

Auditor-General Victoria. (A-GV). (2019). *Follow up of access to public dental services in Victoria. November 2019. Independent assurance report to Parliament 2019–20:9.* <https://www.audit.vic.gov.au/report/follow-access-public-dental-services-victoria>

COAG Health Council. (2015). *Healthy mouths, healthy lives: Australia's national oral health plan 2015–2024.* <https://www.health.gov.au/resources/publications/healthy-mouths-healthy-lives-australias-national-oral-health-plan-2015-2024?language=en>

Daly, B., Batchelor, P., Treasure, E. T., & Watt, R. (2013). *Essential dental public health* (2nd ed.). Oxford: Oxford University Press.

Department of Health. Victoria. (DHV). (1986). *Ministerial review of dental services: Final report.* Melbourne: Department of Health.

Department of Health. Victoria. (DHV). (2013). *Action plan for oral health promotion 2013–2017.* Retrieved from <https://content.health.vic.gov.au/sites/default/files/migrated/files/collections/research-and-reports/1/1303009_htv_oral_health_web---pdf.pdf>

Department of Health and Community Services (DH&CS). Victoria. (1995). *Future directions for dental health in Victoria.* Melbourne: VGPS.

Department of Health and Human Services. (DHHS). (2020). *Victorian action plan to prevent oral disease 2020–30.* <https://www.health.vic.gov.au/sites/default/files/migrated/files/collections/research-and-reports/o/victorian-action-plan-to-prevent-oral-disease-2020.pdf>

Department of Human Services. Victoria. (DHS). (1996). *The Victorian school dental service child dental health promotion strategy 1995–2000.* Melbourne: DHS.

Department of Human Services. Victoria. (DHS). (1999). *Promoting oral health 2000–2004. Strategic directions and framework for action.* <https://www.vgls.vic.gov.au/client/en_AU/search/asset/1159746>

Department of Human Services. Victoria. (DHS). (2007). *Improving Victoria's oral health.* <https://vgls.sdp.sirsidynix.net.au/client/search/asset/1291900>

Dooland, M. (1992). *Improving dental health in Australia.* Background Paper No. 9. Melbourne: National Health Strategy.

Doyle, R. (chair). (1998). *Review of Dentists Act 1972 and Dental Technicians Act 1972. Final report, July 1998.* <http://ncp.ncc.gov.au/docs/Victorian%20review%20of%20Dentist%20Act%201972%20and%20Dental%20Technicians%20Act%201972%2C%20July%201998.pdf>

Duckett, S., Cowgill, M., & Swerrisen, H. (2019). *Filling the gap: A universal dental care scheme for Australia.* <https://grattan.edu.au/wp-content/uploads/2019/03/915-Filling-the-gap-A-universal-dental-scheme-for-Australia.pdf.>

Health Commission Victoria. (HCV). (1982). *Report of internal committee reviewing the Victorian School Dental Service. Unpublished.* 1982.

Lane, J. (1970). *Dental services for Australians. [Pamphlet 21].* Melbourne: Victorian Fabian Society.

Myers, D.M., Plueckhahn, V.D., & Rees, A.L.G. (1980). *Report of the committee of inquiry into the fluoridation of Victorian water supplies for 1979–80.* <https://vgls.sdp.sirsidynix.net.au/client/search/asset/1289094>

National Advisory Council on Dental Health. (NACDH). (2012). *Report of the National Advisory Council on Dental Health.* <https://catalogue.nla.gov.au/Record/5978887>

National Centre for Immunisation Research and Surveillance (NCIRS). (2021). *No jab no play, no jab no pay.* <https://www.ncirs.org.au/public/no-jab-no-play-no-jab-no-pay>

National Health and Hospitals Reform Commission. (NHHRC). (2009). *A healthier future for all Australians. Final report 2009.* Canberra: Commonwealth of Australia.

National Health and Medical Research Council. (NHMRC). (1993). *Impact of change in oral health status on dental education, workforce, practices and services in Australia.* Canberra: NHMRC.

National Health and Medical Research Council. (NHMRC). (2017). *Public statement 2017. Water fluoridation and human health.* <https://www.nhmrc.gov.au/about-us/publications/2017-public-statement-water-fluoridation-and-human-health>

Premier of Victoria. (2019). *The Smile Squad – Free dental vans to hit schools soon.* [Media release]. <https://www.premier.vic.gov.au/smile-squad-free-dental-vans-hit-schools-soon>

Productivity Commission. (2016). *Introducing competition and informed user choice into human services: Identifying sectors for reform. Productivity Commission preliminary findings report overview.* <https://www.pc.gov.au/inquiries/completed/human-services/identifying-reform/preliminary-findings>

Productivity Commission. (2017). *Introducing competition and informed user choice into human services: Reforms to human services. Productivity Commission inquiry report. No. 85, 27 October 2017.* <https://www.pc.gov.au/inquiries/completed/human-services/reforms/report/human-services-reforms.pdf>

Public Health Association of Australia. (PHAA). (2018). *Top ten public health successes over the last 20 years, PHAA Monograph series No. 2, Canberra.* <https://www.phaa.net.au/documents/item/3241>

Rana, K., Ekanayake, K., Chimoriya, R., Palu, E., Do, L., Silva, M., Tadakamadla, S., Bhole, S., Leshargie, CT., Wen, L.M., Ha, D., & Arora, A. (2022). *Effectiveness of oral health promotion interventions: an Evidence Check rapid review.* Sax Institute 2022. <https://www.health.vic.gov.au/preventive-health/oral-health-planning>

Senate Community Affairs References Committee. Australia. (1998). *Report on public dental services.* <https://www.aph.gov.au/parliamentary_business/committees/senate/community_affairs/completed_inquiries/1996-99/dental/report/index>

World Health Organization. (2010). *Monitoring the building blocks of health systems: A handbook of indicators and their measurement strategies.* World Health Organization. <https://apps.who.int/iris/handle/10665/258734>

Wright, F.A.C. (Ed). (2013). *National Oral Health Promotion Plan.* Commissioned by National Government. Canberra.

Chapter 2
Legislation and Governance – As ideas evolve so must legislation

Jamie Robertson

Introduction

This chapter looks at how the governance and regulation of dental care providers in Victoria have evolved since 1970 due to legislative processes. Initiatives were set in train by a combination of dissatisfaction or frustration expressed by the public to politicians and by the gradual absorption of changing concepts of social equity by receptive political and administrative actors. The concept of "protection of the public", which inspired the original dental legislation in Victoria and which for a long time simply meant exposing and prosecuting unqualified practitioners, has broadened to include promotion of access to care and its affordability. This has led to diversification of the dental workforce to fill gaps in care or lessen its expense.

For the latter half of the period of study, increasing layers of bureaucratisation accompanied increasing governmental outlays in the private and public sectors. In turn, all these factors have changed dental practices and attitudes to public dental health. For Victoria, Figure 2.1 provides a timeline of the major reviews and legislative changes that have shaped dental health care and the dental professions in Victoria over the past 50 years.

Figure 2.1 Timeline of Victorian Government Acts, regulations and reviews

1972	*Dentists Act 1972* *Dental Technicians Act 1972*
1973	*Health (Fluoridation) Act 1973*
1985–86	Ministerial Review of Dental Services, 1985–86
1989	Creation of Dental Hygienists by Regulation, 1989
1994–95	Dental Auxiliary Workforce Review Victoria, 1994–95
1998	Review of Dentists Act 1972 and Dental Technicians Act 1972, 1998
1999	*Dental Practice Act 1999.* End of Dental Board of Victoria and formation of Dental Practice Board of Victoria.
2005	*Health Professions Registration Act 2005*, forerunner of National Law in 2009
2009	*Health Practitioner Regulation National Law (Victoria) Act 2009*
2017	Drugs, Poisons and Controlled Substances Regulations 2017

The pressure for change

The first dental legislation in Victoria occurred in 1887 while it was still a British Crown colony. It was the end result of a private member's Bill which was strongly supported by a small group of proto-professional dentists. Its purpose was to create a register of dentists whose behaviour and credentials would be governed by a Dental Board of Victoria (DBV), thus protecting the people of Victoria. The board was also expected to authorise a course of study for those who wished to become dentists. Unfortunately, the first Act had many deficiencies and omissions, the most obvious of which were that registration was only voluntary and it was for life, and that the DBV was not granted the power to delegate the course of education to another body.

It took another 40 years and three more Dentists Acts to overcome the above deficiencies. By that time, 1927, there had been a Dental Faculty at the University of Melbourne for 22 years with a Bachelor of Dental Science as the qualifying degree. From 1928 onwards, registration had to be renewed each year, thus revealing for the first time the number of practising dentists, and no one could practise dentistry in the state without the Melbourne degree or an acceptable alternative. With this annual influx of registration fees and more power, the DBV was able to impose standards of ethical behaviour on dentists and to prosecute unregistered practitioners. Unfortunately, none of the Acts had placed on the DBV a reciprocal obligation to ensure that there were enough dentists to service the population; that was to be left to market forces.

Adam Smith's "guiding hand" might have worked in a steady state of population and prosperity, however, major economic and political upheavals and unequal prosperity upset any such calculus. The 1930s Depression, during which the number on the Dentists Register fell (DBV, 1993), followed by the Second World War and subsequent post-war immigration explosion all contributed to the worsening dentist-to-population ratio (Chapter 3). Among the many post-war immigrants were dentists whose degrees were not recognised and who were prosecuted by the DBV if they were found practising illegally. By the 1960s the political pressure on members of State Parliament by people unable to see a dentist was rising each year.

In a bid to fend off complaints from electors about long waiting times to see the inadequate number of dentists, Ronald Mack, the Victorian Minister of Health, set up a Dental Advisory Committee (DAC) in 1965 to investigate (State Government Victoria, 1965). A leisurely four years later, it reported its findings. Among its proposals were the graduation of one hundred dentists a year (more than double the then prevailing number), the fluoridation of Melbourne's water supplies and, only after all that, the possible introduction of dental auxiliaries to treat the damaged teeth of State school children (DAC, 1969).

There were two immediate problems with the recommendations: first, the State's well-entrenched Premier Sir Henry Bolte was strongly opposed to water fluoridation; and second, in order to produce more graduates, the University of Melbourne would require more academic staff and resources. Since university funding was a responsibility of the Australian Government, the State Government had neither the power nor the funds to increase university output.

The DAC's final proposal was contentious because for many years the dental profession had been opposed to the idea of allowing dental mechanics or technicians to make and provide dentures to patients directly. To allow auxiliaries to treat children would create a precedent and might breach the dam against encroaching dental mechanics. Nevertheless, the leaders of the dental profession could recognise the inevitability of permitting New Zealand-style dental nurses to treat school children, even if its rank and file could not. The dentist-to-population ratio kept deteriorating; a school-based dental service would quarantine the nurses from private practice, and the few dentists working in the existing school service were resigning in any case due to poor pay and conditions.

Using the DAC report as a cue, Melbourne dentist James Lane wrote a paper called, *Dental services for Australians*, which was published as a pamphlet by the Fabian Society in 1970 (Lane, 1970). Like the DAC report, Lane's proposals were to fluoridate Melbourne's water; provide dental health education to the community; create school dental therapists mainly to provide preventive measures; boost the output of graduate dentists; and set up a scheme for pensioners to receive treatment at private practices or public clinics at government expense. Lane's ideas all came to pass eventually but, as he was a socialist and the government was a Liberal/ Country Party coalition, his proposals played no part in governmental calculations.

By the time dental legislation was being drafted in 1970, there had been no changes to the *Dentists Act 1927* for 43 years. The status quo had suited the dental profession for most of this period. However, the combination of demographic pressures and increasing financial constraints on the DBV, whose scale of fees had been set in the Act, meant that the Board's financial woes outweighed its opposition to some weakening of professional autonomy. The DBV therefore had slightly different priorities to those of most practising dentists whose position was basically "Fluoride, yes: auxiliaries, no". The idea of increasing the number of dentists graduating from the University of Melbourne met no opposition from any quarter within Victoria, particularly as funding would have to come from the National Government, not the State.

A government dominated by the Liberal Party would usually have seen the dental profession as its natural ally, and vice versa, on most issues, but in 1971, when a Dental Bill was seriously debated, it found itself under pressure both from the electorate and from dental technicians who wanted to come in out of the proverbial garden shed and treat patients directly and legally. The Australian Labor Party (ALP) State Opposition vigorously promoted the technicians' cause, as did far too many voters for the comfort of dentists and Liberal politicians. In a parliamentary speech, Alan Lind, an Opposition MP, declared, "most honourable members have had more representations from the public on this measure (a Bill to change the Dental Act) than on any other" (Victoria, Legislative Assembly 1971, p. 2896). He also quoted a Gallup Poll which found that 69% of respondents supported the proposal to allow dental technicians to treat the public while only 17% opposed it (p. 2909). In the same debate, the junior coalition partner Country Party spokesman on Health, Thomas Mitchell said he was in favour of permitting both types of auxiliary workers – dental therapists and technicians (p. 2911).

Box 2.1 Sir Henry's denture

Tensions ran high in the 1970s as dentists representing the Australian Dental Association, and technicians from the Dental Technicians' Association hotly debated the wisdom or not of allowing dental technicians clinical rights to work directly with the public. The debate was passionate, protracted and publicised with intense lobbying of the State Government by both sides.

Whilst this was occurring, Sir Henry Bolte, Premier of Victoria, and Sir John Rossiter, Minister for Health, were meeting with members of the Dental Board of Victoria, Sir Benjamin Rank, representing the Medical Board of Victoria, and Professor Henry Atkinson of the Dental Faculty at the University of Melbourne, on how to best manage the proposal.

Sir Henry also did not wish for this contentious issue to influence a forthcoming by-election which was to be held in the marginal seat of Gisborne at that time.

The matter was settled unexpectedly! Sir Henry was visiting Ballarat when his denture broke. It was a weekend and he could not find a dentist to repair his denture. Eventually he was able to track down a dental technician who undertook the repair. Sir Henry was satisfied with the quality and timeliness of the work and became a supporter of the dental technicians' campaign to provide care directly to the public.

– *Anonymous.*

Meanwhile, a sub-plot featuring the Democratic Labor Party (DLP) had been brewing. The DLP, which had powerful leverage in marginal seats, strongly supported the dental technicians' case. It so happened that a by-election for the marginal Victorian seat of Gisborne was pending in late November 1971 and Premier Bolte's anointed candidate, Athol Guy, needed all the help he could get. The DLP offered to preference Guy in return for a pledge from the Coalition Government to permit the legalisation of technicians. Despite pleas to Bolte from the DBV and the Australian Dental Association (ADA) to stand firm, the pressure was too great. The contentious Bill was finally split into two parts with Health Minister, John Rossiter telling Parliament that a completely different Bill dealing with legislation for dental technicians would be soon introduced (Victoria, Legislative Assembly 1971, p. 2940). In May 1972, a Dentists Act was passed and in November the same year, a Dental Technicians Act was passed. While the dentists felt betrayed, they learned a hard lesson on the need to shape and harness public sentiment.

From the point of view of dental public health, the two Acts enabled the creation of two new categories of dental practitioners – dental therapists, who were only permitted to treat school- or pre-school children within the state school system[3] (Dentists Act 1972, s. 29(6)), and advanced dental technicians who could make full dentures for edentulous people. Dentists were unable to prevent a "grandfather" clause for some technicians but succeeded in limiting patient-treating powers to only those technicians who undertook further training. Over time, both newly created groups of providers decreased waiting times for treatment by siphoning off specific classes of patients. However, there was no mention of water fluoridation in the Dentists Act because of Henry Bolte's opposition to it, nor was there a means of increasing the number of dentists graduating from university.

Water fluoridation

Wherever it has been proposed, the fluoridation of community water supplies has been a vexed issue. Argument about the probable benefit to the many as opposed to the possible harm to some has never been resolved to the mutual satisfaction of pro- and anti-fluoridationists. Reasoned argument, alas, seldom changes or deflects deeply held belief. The strong case in favour of adjusting fluoride levels to approximately 0.7 parts per million in Victoria's water supplies had to wait until Henry Bolte departed from the political scene. He retired in August 1972 and a Bill was introduced under the premiership of Dick Hamer in the Spring session of Parliament the following year. It was debated at length and was passed on 11 December as the Health (Fluoridation) Act 1973. As with many other public health measures such as seat belt wearing and tobacco advertising, it was not tied to a specific medical or dental Act but required its own legislation.

The Public Records Office of Victoria holds a volume of newspaper clippings on water fluoridation dating from 1955 to 1982. It was compiled by an unnamed employee of the Melbourne Metropolitan Board of Works (MMBW). The MMBW archives also hold much correspondence on water fluoridation (PROV, VPRS 8609, unit 293, p 21). Articles and letters to newspaper editors cluster around times of parliamentary debates or suggestions to introduce fluoridation. The anti-fluoridationists may have been few in number but they were coordinated and tenacious; politicians and bureaucrats were kept busy responding to them.

The MMBW itself hastened slowly, taking more than three years to introduce the measures of the 1973 Act, and then only at the Silvan reservoir serving Melbourne's east, in 1977. There was an immediate flurry of reported symptoms but since then no more, even as fluoridated water supplies have spread across the state. If one accepts Bradford Hill's viewpoints on causation (Bradford Hill, 1965), then the more that people are exposed to an adverse variable, the more likely it is that side effects and symptoms would show themselves over time. Since 1977, Melbourne's population has more than doubled but in that time reports of fluoride-induced symptoms or effects have been noticeably absent in the media.

The three Victorian Government Acts of the 1970s created a more favourable environment for a reduction in the prevalence of dental disease through water fluoridation, and for an increase in the capacity of a broader dental workforce to treat existing disease. More actors were on the stage even though they might not have all been reading from the same script.

3 Dental Therapy Training Schools were established in Tasmania in 1966, South Australia in 1967, then NSW, Queensland and West Australia in 1974 thanks to grants from the Whitlam Government, and finally in Victoria in 1976.

Improving access and equity

Soon after the advent of the Dentists Act of 1972, one might say that a series of fortunate events occurred to enlarge and strengthen the Victorian School Dental Service. In an avowedly 'small government' environment, it was one thing to pass an Act but another to have recurrent funding to train and pay for the newly created dental therapists. Fortunately for Victoria, in Canberra Gough Whitlam's Labor Government in 1973 was at the height of its reforming zeal and it established and funded a national school dental service for all states (Commonwealth of Australia, 1973). Funding for this service was trimmed back by Malcolm Fraser's succeeding Liberal Government until it ceased in 1982 but it was enough to rapidly create and sustain a solid cohort of dental therapists before Victoria's budgetary constraints reduced the numbers trained in the 1980s (Biggs, 2008).

In 1982 the advent of an ALP government led by John Cain ended almost 30 years of Liberal Party dominated governments in Victoria. In that time, the state had changed greatly. More than one generation had known nothing but right-leaning governments while the population had almost doubled with most of that growth being in Melbourne. In 1955 Melbourne's population was about 1.6 million, or 60% of the total population of Victoria, and by 1982 the city's population had risen to 2.9 million or 72% of the state's total. In the same period, the number of registered dentists in Victoria had risen from 973 to 1900 (Australian Bureau of Statistics [ABS], 2019). While this was a dramatic rise, it simply meant that the dentist-to-population ratio had improved from 39 per 100,000 to 46 per 100,000 (Chapter 3). Neither ratio was adequate to overcome the incidence of unmet dental needs, let alone the underlying prevalence of dental disease.

In the early 1980s, the overwhelming majority of dental services were provided by the private sector. Public clinics were few and far between with the Royal Dental Hospital of Melbourne being almost alone in providing general dental care in Melbourne. Some regional hospitals also provided limited dental care (Chapter 4). Financial and geographic disadvantage for people who could not afford private care resulted in delayed and compromised treatment whenever it could be obtained. However, after a series of governments with an underlying political ideology of *laissez faire*, Victoria had elected a government more concerned with social equity and justice; two principles of the Alma-Ata Declaration of 1978 on Primary Health Care (WHO, 1978). These concerns were reinforced when the ALP led by Bob Hawke became the Australian Government in 1983. The arithmetic of output of graduates was still important but focus began to turn to access to care.

From its earliest days, the Cain Labor Government in Victoria began to develop a Social Justice Strategy for all aspects of the Victorian community (State Government Victoria & Cain, 1986). A well-publicised example of this was Cain's opposition to male-only membership of the Melbourne Cricket Club which happened to be on Crown Land. Membership was quickly changed to admit women as members without the sky falling in. The social justice lens also examined health care in the state and led to a range of other reviews.

Box 2.2 The birth of community dental clinics

Patients' rights and community participation in designing health services were not invented in the 1970s but were promulgated and promoted at an accelerated pace in that decade, especially in the Declaration of Alma-Ata (1978) and the Ottawa Charter (WHO, 1986). Not only was commerce becoming increasingly global; so too were ideas and social movements (Lewis, MJ, 2003).

Between 1985 and 1990, 16 District Health Councils (DHC) were set up in Victoria with the aim of supporting community involvement in health promotion and health planning, strengthening health system accountability, and educating people about factors which influenced their health (Legge & Sylvan, 1990). At the federal level, the Hawke Labor Government established a Consumers' Health Forum in 1987 (Short, 1998). Kensington Community Health Centre (KCHC) in Melbourne's inner west held three focus group meetings in 1987. The two most pressing concerns that emerged from these meetings were the need for better health care for older people and a reduction in waiting times to access public dental care.

Consequently, the KCHC and community members advocated for a dental clinic and shared their views with the Melbourne DHC. Further communication and collaboration led to a group of 80 community organisations including Brunswick Community Health and VCOSS. Representatives lobbied the State Minister for Health, David White, and the ALP Health and Social Welfare Committee as a Review of Dental Services was underway. Like new wine, new ideas generally have to mature before they are palatable. While the concept of accessible clinics in community-controlled health centres was only slowly being adopted in Victoria, the process had accelerated with the advent of the ALP government in 1982. Even though KCHC was an early advocate, it was not the first to establish a community dental clinic: that honour went to Brunswick Community Health Centre.

A Ministerial Review of Dental Services (MRODS) in Victoria was commissioned in September 1985 and reported in December 1986. It did not challenge the dental profession's autonomy as governed by the DBV, but it staked the significant claim that others had a valid interest in how public services, as opposed to private services, should be run. In justifying inquiries across many professions, the government was of the view that, "no longer can any profession conduct its own self-examination to the exclusion of other interested parties" (HDV, 1986, p. 19).

In spite of its broad title, MRODS did not distinguish between public and private sectors and the review was mainly limited to public sector dental services. It did, however, make recommendations for the training and deployment of the dental workforce based on a demonstrated improvement in dental health thanks to the fluoridation of reticulated water supplies. It even recommended the introduction of a new dental auxiliary, the dental hygienist, to augment oral health education and promotion across the private and public sectors. The DBV licensed the first of these in 1989 a mere 78 years after they first appeared in Connecticut.

Typically, many of the MRODS recommendations required increased funding which would have to come from the State Government. But MRODS was delivered into a world of economic uncertainty. Australian inflation in the 1980s was high and rising, with bank home-loan rates reaching 17% in 1989, while the global stock market crash of October 1987 had seen shares fall by 40%. All governments became cautious about spending money. Nevertheless, some of the review's recommendations required minimal funding, while others involved efficiency programs which could save money, for example, by employing more therapists than dentists for the School Dental Service. A pilot community dental clinic within the existing health centre at Brunswick was established.

In 1988 the government responded to MRODS with the Dental Health Strategy (Chapter 4). A further 29 public dental clinics were established under local management to create the Community Dental Program (CDP). The VDS was expanded, additional dental therapists employed to increase services to primary school children, and an intern scheme established for ten graduating dentists per annum.

Meanwhile, in 1987 the Australian ALP Government had found funding for Australia's first National Oral Health Survey which was completed in 1988 (Barnard, 1993). In terms of social justice, the survey found that poor people had worse oral health than richer people and could only afford episodic emergency care in the private sector. Furthermore, they had to wait long periods for free public care, and their situation would likely worsen over time as people were retaining teeth longer and the burden of disease would keep growing. A separate National Health Survey in 1990 (ABS, 1993) showed that, thanks to Medicare, people on low incomes could visit doctors and hospitals as easily as high-income earners, whereas this was not so in the largely private dental sector

(Dooland, 1992), which was not included in Medicare. This survey revealed once again the paucity of dental statistics in Australia and the pressing need for more data and good analyses to enable better planning and service delivery.

National Competition Policy

By 1992 the legislative upheavals of Victoria's dental Acts were 20 years in the past. A new status quo had been established, albeit in an economy in deep recession with high unemployment. In the election of that year, the State's ALP government was replaced by a Coalition government led by Jeff Kennett, who was elected on a platform of structural reform and dynamism. Some of that reform involved swingeing cuts to the education and health budgets. In addition, in 1992 the Council of Australian Governments (COAG), which was chaired by Prime Minister Paul Keating, set up a committee of inquiry, known as the Hilmer Committee, to inquire and advise on the need for a national competition policy (Hilmer, 1993). The underlying premise was that free-market forces tend to be more efficient than monopolistic or restrictive practices and that their employment of innovation and competition would promote community welfare.

The Kennett-led Liberal Party espoused minimal government intervention in the economy of the state and was intent on reviewing all legislation in order to remove any irrelevant and unnecessary statutes. Such thinking alarmed all registered professions as they pondered their fates in a future in which anyone could compete with them for clients, regardless of academic credentials. With the Hilmer Inquiry underway and endorsed by Kennett, the professions had reason to be fearful.

Fred Hilmer's committee of inquiry reported in August 1993, and by 1995 a National Competition Policy (NCP) was established. In Victoria, the Kennett Government used the NCP as a convenient justification to attack restrictive practices. The health professions worried that if any person with a stethoscope or dental handpiece could open a practice, why would anyone study at university for five or six years, and what would happen to existing practitioners? One caveat under the NCP that might help the professions was the principle that legislation should not restrict competition unless it could be demonstrated that the benefits of any restrictions outweighed the costs. Thus forewarned, the health professions set out to justify their existing status under the catch cry of "public safety"; an echo from the nineteenth century.

Although the Kennett Government was averse to initiating restrictive practice legislation, even before the release of the Hilmer report's recommendations, it was not opposed to acting on the basis of improving public health. After prompting by the DBV, in 1994 the government introduced a Dentists (Amendment) Bill to overcome deficiencies in the 1972 Act. These deficiencies concerned the lack of regulations and codes of practice for infection control, and a corresponding lack of power for the DBV to enforce them or enter dental premises to investigate suspected breaches (Victorian State Government, 1994). In 1972 no one had anticipated the AIDS epidemic of the 1980s and the consequent urgency to enforce dramatic improvements to infection control measures. In the years following the onset of the epidemic, the National Health and Medical Research Council (NHMRC) had produced codes of practice and guidelines for infection control but these could not be enforced because there was no means of adding regulations to the Victorian Act. Even though the ALP Opposition supported the Bill, it fell victim to the exigencies

of parliamentary time and was only reintroduced in April 1999 when a completely new Bill was drawn up.

At a national level in the early 1990s, armed with the results of national health and dental health surveys, ideas were germinating on how to improve health equity through better access and affordability. Federal Minister for Health, Brian Howe appointed Jenny Macklin as Director of the National Health Strategy. Macklin authorised a series of background papers on various health issues to furnish ideas and knowledge to policy makers and stakeholders. Paper No. 9, titled *Improving dental health in Australia* (Dooland, 1992), was a distillation of research and ideas. Its author, Martin Dooland was then Director of the South Australian Dental Service. The paper went so far as to put forward tentative proposals for national emergency and general dentistry schemes and it too was cellared within Canberra's bureaucracy. It did not, however, have long to mature as a national election was scheduled for 1993.

Rehearsal for a national dental health scheme

By 1993 the ALP Australian Government had been in power for 10 years and Paul Keating had replaced Bob Hawke as Prime Minister. The government had become unpopular and Australia's economy was faltering, although less so than in many other countries in a global downturn. The pre-election sentiment was that the ALP would lose power to the Opposition led by Liberal Party leader John Hewson. The ALP therefore put forward as many attractive promises as it could think of, one of which was a national dental treatment scheme; one it had "prepared earlier" as it were. Thanks to Hewson's promise to bring in a new Goods and Services Tax (GST), he lost the "unlosable election".

The ALP Government thus found that it had to polish schematic proposals into a functional program which it called the Commonwealth Dental Health Program (CDHP) (Biggs, 2008) (Chapter 4).

Although targeted at disadvantaged adults, the CDHP possessed some elements of a rehearsal for a national dental health scheme. In the program's short life, the Australian Government provided $240 million for service delivery and $5 million for administration and analysis. A condition of funding was that participating states were not allowed to reduce their pre-existing dental health funding. The aim was to reduce barriers, whether financial, geographic or attitudinal, and to care for Health Card holders and, later, for Seniors Card holders (Senate, 1998). The underlying objectives were to move people from episodic emergency care to routine services; to reduce rates of dental extractions and increase those of restorations; and to gradually move the focus from disease repair to its prevention.

With speed, an Emergency Dental Scheme started in January 1994 and a General Dental Scheme was added in July of that year (Biggs, 2008). The dental treatment could be provided by both private and public sectors and payment to providers was based on an existing Department of Veterans' Affairs fee schedule. In less than three years of operation, before it was wound up in December 1996, the CDHP saw a dramatic fall in waiting times in the public sector. There was indeed a reduction in extraction rates and a concomitant rise in restoration rates (Senate, 1998) (Chapter 4). Nevertheless, due to the huge reservoir of previously unmet needs, there was scarcely time to see a shift from disease repair to its prevention.

John Howard's Coalition Government, elected in March 1996, soon terminated the CDHP (Biggs, 2008). It became a victim of several cost-cutting moves by the new government whose philosophy was minimal governmental intervention in the economy. In some respects, the CDHP was a victim of its own success: waiting times had plummeted, more people were seen annually, people were happy with the quality of care, and the proportion of restorative care rose. For politicians the problem had been solved; time to move onto the next problem.

The demise of the program had many consequences, however. In the public sector, clinics' waiting lists ballooned and, consequently, treatment reverted to emergency care as opposed to planned routine restorative care (Senate, 1998, p. 35). In the private sector, many practices saw an income stream dry up. Some consequences were less obvious. For many patients, their experiences gave them an idea of what a dental service could and even should be and they were unimpressed at the CDHP's curtailment. In addition, Australian and State public servants also learned from the experience. They learned to implement, analyse and evaluate dental policies and their outcomes. At the national level the Senate committee report noted that "a better-informed environment emerged which could sustain more detailed dental health policy analysis, leading to improved service and better oral health" (Senate, 1998, p. 31). In other words, health bureaucrats began to see dental health policy as being more than just about dental workforce numbers and population ratios; oral health was on the policy agenda.

Successive reviews trigger change in Victoria

In the mid-1990s dental policy in Victoria continued to unfold without regard to the CDHP. It had been known for some years that public sector dentistry had been operating sub-optimally. Common complaints and recommendations had been aired through an internal review of the Victorian School Dental Service (HCV, 1982), the 1986 MRODS (HDV, 1986), and the 1989 On site analysis for change of dental health services (DHS, 1989). The SDS review spoke of poor coordination, low morale and lack of leadership and these sentiments were amplified in the other reports. The new-broom Kennett Government had the energy to drive change in the interests of access, efficiency, structure and morale. In July 1994 it set up another review, the Dental Auxiliary Workforce Review Victoria (DAWRV), chaired by Liberal MP Robert Doyle, to investigate the utility and efficiencies of the various occupations which had been created or modified over the previous 20 years.

Several recommendations were made. The most substantial were that advanced dental technicians should be called dental prosthetists who should be allowed to make partial dentures and whose training should be suspended for five years; that dental hygienists and dental therapists should have some common core training which still allowed clinical specialisation with prospects for a clinical pilot study permitting them to treat patients beyond the then legislated age groups; and that newly qualified dentists should have a twelve-month mentored internship (DH&CS, 1995). These recommendations lay dormant until taken up again in yet another review, chaired again by Doyle, the Victorian *Review of Dentists Act 1972* and *Dental Technicians Act 1972*, which was published in July 1998 (DHS, 1998).

Concurrently with the DAWRV inquiry, the Department of Health and Community Services (DH&CS) produced a policy document called *Future directions for dental health in Victoria* which presented a vision for 2010, including the structural reorganisation of public dental services and preventive health measures for the state (DH&CS, 1995a). The main outcome of the new policy was that in September 1995 a new coordinating and supervising agency, Dental Health Services Victoria (DHSV), was born (DH&CS, DAWRV, 1995b). The theory had been that the purchaser and supervisor of services should not be the same entity in order to permit quality control but, in fact, because the new body controlled the Royal Dental Hospital of Melbourne (RDHM), it turned out that DHSV became both purchaser and provider of services. All state funding for public dental services was channelled through DHSV and depended on meeting various performance indicators. In turn, DHSV made a series of agreements with regional clinics including the RDHM. This meant that, for the first time, statewide statistics could be gathered and analysed in a coordinated way. It also allowed the management of DHSV to think strategically for the first time about planning the form and extent of dental services into the future.

At a national level, the introduction of the NCP in 1995 prompted the initiation of various review panels to investigate whether certain social objectives, such as public safety, could override laissez-faire market forces (Hilmer, 1993). In Victoria before the NCP came into force, a State *Nurses Act 1993* and a *Medical Practice Act 1994* had been passed but a Dentists Amendment Bill was still to be reintroduced. An enforced delay caused by a state election meant that the dental profession became the first to have its whole regulatory apparatus viewed through the prism of the NCP. The Nurses Act and Medical Practice Act were each subsequently reviewed and amendment Acts for them were passed in March and May 2000, respectively.

In place of the limited amendments planned in the Dentists Bill in 1994, Victoria's Department of Human Services (DHS) instigated the review, mentioned above, "to examine the case for reform of legislative restrictions on competition contained in the *Dentists Act 1972*, the *Dental Technicians Act 1972* and associated regulations" (DHS, 1998). It became a root and branch review of the entire dental workforce, excepting dental assistants, who were not required to be registered.

The review commenced in April 1997, 86 separate submissions were received, and the final report was published in July 1998. In essence, the report recommended maintenance of registration for reasons of competency in treatment and infection control, not as a restriction on numbers practising. It also recommended that the three boards governing dentists, advanced dental technicians and therapists, respectively, should be collapsed into one.

When a new Bill, based on the report, was debated in 1999 there was rare bipartisan agreement on the need for it and the Bill's passage was swift (Victorian State Government, 1999a). A Newspoll had shown that over 80% of Victorians supported the maintenance of controls in the dental profession. Introducing the Bill, the Treasurer, Alan Stockdale said that its aims were to minimise community health risk in dentistry and to promote access to care (Victorian State Government, 1999b). He explained that much of the Act dealt with investigations of complaints by the public and for the first time it introduced the idea that professional misconduct could include unnecessary and unrequested treatment. The era of informed consent had been put into black-lettered law.

New millennium, new leadership, new actors

The Dental Practice Bill 1999 was among the last to be enacted by the Kennett Government because, to the surprise of many, the ALP became a minority government with the support of independents in the State election of September 1999. The dental profession and the State of Victoria entered the new millennium under new leadership. The governing bodies of dentists, advanced dental technicians (now called dental prosthetists) and dental therapists were fused into one body called the Dental Practice Board of Victoria (DPBV) (*Dental Practice Act 1999* (Vic)). The new board comprised 11 members of whom only five were permitted to be dentists. The others were two dental prosthetists, one dental auxiliary, two non-dental members of the public and one lawyer (*Dental Practice Act 1999, s. 70*). For dentists, it meant that the profession's governing body had gone from an all-dentist one of seven members, to a governing body of 11 in which dentists were a minority. For the people of Victoria, it was the first dental Act to enunciate the principle of access to dental care.

At the governing level, this permitted or, rather, forced a commonality of view when considering the dental needs of the community. However, a mutual lingering suspicion about the reforms remained at the level of frontline service delivery. As the new century dawned, another group of actors, the health bureaucrats, was becoming more involved and influential in the regulation of dental services.

Due to a series of events, health bureaucrats, politicians and their political advisors had been made more aware of the issues, complexities and pressure points in dentistry, its governance and workforce training. Key events included an internal review of the SDS in 1982; the MRODS in 1986; the birth of DHSV in 1995 to coordinate and administer public dental services; the birth, life and death of the CDHP in the nineties, and the recalibration of what it meant to have restricted entry professions in an era of the NCP. The fact that increasingly large sums of public money were being committed to dental services for which accountability was required necessitated monitoring and evaluation of what was being done, by whom and at what cost. Meanwhile, dental academics were playing their part in contributing to the debates and reviews. The whole concept of dental public health (DPH) as a discipline of study, as opposed to a state of dental wellbeing, had been gathering pace since the Acts of 1972.

Before the arrival of Clive Wright at the University of Melbourne's Dental Faculty in 1975, dental academics involved with DPH had been few and far between and their political involvement had been minimal. Certainly, Professor Arthur Amies' anti-fluoridation views had allowed Premier Henry Bolte a fig leaf of intellectual support for his own parliamentary delaying tactics, and progress had to wait until they both retired. On the other hand, Professor Elsdon Storey was a strong supporter of water fluoridation during the debates of the early 1970s. His brother, Haddon Storey, was Attorney General in the Hamer Government and together the brothers garnered support within the Liberal Party to facilitate the passage of the Health (Fluoridation) Act 1973 (Vic). While neither Amies nor Storey was interested in DPH as a separate field of study, Wright came with political commitment and, with the fresh eyes of an outsider, he set out to change things. As he has said, "In my years in Melbourne it was

clear that (DPH) required (an) understanding (of) the broader impact of social change and an appreciation of the political process in Australia" (F. A. C. Wright, personal communication, February, 2020).

In Australia about 80% of dental services are delivered through the private sector. Health professions as a whole prefer minimal governmental interference with their autonomy. However, when governments believe it to be in their own interests to intervene, then more complex relationships develop between the professions and the government. As DPH emerged as an academic discipline, it tended to highlight inequalities and the shortcomings and successes of dental care. This could not fail to affect the triangular relationship between the profession, the government and the community. This is especially true when "policy entrepreneurs", in the phrase of Jenny Lewis (Lewis, 1997, p. 17), identify social problems, supply their own solutions, and advocate for their implementation. Regardless of the worthiness of a cause, politicians' responses invariably boil down to "how much is too much, and can we afford it?" The ideological leanings of a government will dictate how much it is willing to spend, both overall and on any particular issue.

Neither the Whitlam Government in its design for Medibank nor the Hawke Government in its Medicare iteration felt that dental services were universally affordable. The problems in the British National Health Service provided a cautionary tale for the Keating Government which took these lessons on board when it introduced the CDHP for a targeted clientele with limitations on treatment (Chapter 4). Potential problems with the Australian Dental Association (ADA) were lessened when the Association realised that most CDHP candidates were not attending private practices anyway and that private practices could participate in the program.

National harmonisation

The new DPBV started in July 2000. However, it took until 2002 for a consensus on the scope of practice for prosthetists, dental therapists and dental hygienists to be published by the Board. Progress was slow, but it was progress, and the merged Victorian Board was forging a template for other states to follow. Even though the political complexion of Victoria's government had changed in 1999, the impetus for efficiency and administrative reform did not wane. To mark the start of a new era in administration and technology, online annual registration for all dental practitioners in Victoria began in 2001.

The logic of merging the different dental governance agencies extended to a desire to harmonise many procedures and investigatory powers in all registrable health disciplines. As one of the registrable health occupations, dentistry was numerically dwarfed by nurses and medical practitioners, but dentistry was a useful test case and it was rising to the challenge, even if many private dentists felt threatened by perceptions of encroaching bureaucratisation. The irresistible logic of harmonisation, if not the complete fusion of boards, led the Bracks ALP Government to pass the Health Professions Registration Act 2005 (Vic). Under this Act, each of the 11 existing registrable occupations, plus a new one of Medical Radiation Practitioner, would retain their own boards for administrative functions but all would subscribe to a uniform set of investigative powers.

The Act's main purpose was to "protect the public by providing for the registration of health practitioners and a common system of investigations into the professional conduct, professional performance and ability to practise of registered health professionals" (*Health Professions Registration Act 2005*, p. 1). This was the first Victorian Act involving dentistry whose stated purpose was to protect the public even though that had been implicit in all previous Acts. If the professions were going to use "public safety" as their *raison d'etre* for restricted entry, then they were going to be held accountable to it. There was also a clear intention that the professionals' behaviours, skill sets and their own health would be open to investigation and judgement. This was an example of the social contract between the professions and society whereby certain privileges are conferred in exchange for actions beneficial to society. These principles, earlier enunciated by Max Weber (Ritzer, 1975), had been laid out by the Parliament of Victoria in the new Act.

In anticipation of the 2005 Act and knowing that mandatory continuing professional education would be required of all practitioners, the DPBV in January 2005 introduced what they called continuing professional development (CPD) for all types of dental practitioner. What had been voluntary and attended only by the conscientious, became compulsory and a boutique industry suddenly mushroomed to cater for all. The objective was that the public would be served by a profession continuously refreshed and informed by new ideas and techniques. There has been no way to measure the success of this exercise even though the alternative, that of no requirement for continuing education, is unthinkable.

As the 21st century got underway – with the NCP in place and economic rationalism in ascendancy –, it became more plausible to think that national professional registration (as opposed to registration in each state and territory) would be a logical extension of the harmonisation begun in Victoria. It would eliminate much duplication of effort and reduce administrative overheads. It would facilitate the movement of workers from state to state; standardise regulations; and stop deregistered practitioners from starting again elsewhere. If all of the individual, autonomous registrable health occupations could be brought together under one regulatory umbrella, it would be much more efficient and smaller groups like the Podiatrists and Chinese Medicine practitioners would have their governing standards lifted. It was as though the health bureaucrats of Victoria had infected their interstate and Commonwealth counterparts.

At the national level, in June 2004, the COAG (COAG, 2004) asked the Productivity Commission, an independent advisory authority, to investigate all Australia's health workforce. Its brief was to investigate supply relative to current and expected demands, and to propose solutions to any problems found. Earlier workforce forecasts had predicted practitioner shortfalls in dentistry, nursing and medicine in future years (AIHW, 1998). One outcome from this forecast, already outdated by 2005, was that dentists and doctors were advertised as skill shortages at Australian embassies and high commissions overseas. It encouraged overseas trained dentists to apply for registration in Australia without any test as to whether they could readily be absorbed.

Specifically, the Productivity Commission was directed to inquire into "the context of the need for efficient and effective delivery of health services in an environment of demographic change, technological advances and rising health costs" (Productivity Commission, 2005). One observation was that the very independence of professions which had led to high-quality training and performance had also led to their uncoordinated administration and governance (Productivity Commission, 2005). The trick would be to retain high-quality practitioners at the delivery end, while reforming effectiveness and uniformity of administration at the governance end.

Box 2.3 AHPRA and "the National Law"

The primary role of AHPRA (Australian Health Practitioner Regulation Agency) is to protect the public and set standards and policies that all registered health practitioners must meet[A]. At its commencement in 2010, there were ten categories (16 in 2022) of health practitioner. Each of the 16 categories has its own national board. (To cover other health care workers who do not have to be registered, in 2015 COAG also established a National Code of Conduct).

All types of registrable dental worker come under the one category of dental practitioner governed by the Dental Board of Australia (DBA). Like all boards, the DBA is required to have a health profession agreement with AHPRA that sets out fees, budget and the range of services provided by AHPRA (now Ahpra) to regulate the profession. It is through such agreements with all boards that Ahpra administers the National Registration and Accreditation Scheme which is the practical manifestation of the National Law.

It was one thing to devise an entity called Ahpra but another thing to put it into practice as it grappled with the volume of registrants and set up procedures for dealing with notifications from the public. (A notification is a euphemism for a complaint in most cases). By staggering registration dates for different professions and improving investigative processes, its operations have become smoother in recent years, although the time taken to deal with notifications still lacks timeliness and transparency as Ahpra itself admits.

A See <https://www1.health.gov.au/internet/main/publishing. nsf/Content/work-nras> Accessed 23.2.2021.

The Productivity Commission report was completed in December 2005. It contained far-reaching recommendations for the planning, training and disposition of health professionals and it recommended a national system for the accreditation and registration of these professionals. In effect it proposed creating a national body to replicate many of the functions of the one created by the Victorian Health Professions Registration Act 2005.

At its 26 March 2008 meeting, COAG accepted the recommendations and a time frame for implementation (COAG, 2008). This set in-train a series of enabling Acts in each Australian state and territory legislature to create a Health Practitioner Regulation National Law (customarily called "the National Law") and effect an end to the existing Acts and governing bodies of their own jurisdictions. On 1 July 2010 the new world of national uniformity came into being as the National Registration and Accreditation Scheme established by state and territory governments through the introduction of consistent legislation in all jurisdictions. The registration and accreditation refer to individuals not institutions and their curricula, for which there is a separate body, the Australian Commission on Safety and Quality in Health Care (ACSQHC), which sets standards known as the National Safety and Quality in Health Care Standards (NSQHCS)[4].

As with the earlier Victorian scheme, each registrable health profession would be governed by an occupation-specific board, this time a national one, which would facilitate interstate movement of practitioners. The national boards would all sit under an umbrella body called the Australian Health Practitioner Regulation Agency (Ahpra) (AHWMC, 2009).

4 Please forgive this sudden dive into an alphabet soup of acronyms. The 21st century has seen an explosion of bureaucratic entities.

The formation of a national regulation agency (Ahpra) forced changes in how all registrable professions were governed. When many state-based separate agencies were collapsed into one large national one, settling-in problems could be anticipated and the delays in registration and re-registration in the first two years have been an example of this. Moving from a separate register for each profession in each state and territory to one large national register was a Herculean task. Online registration to a single register created an enormous data set which could help workforce planning, but to do that, other players would need to be involved, such as the Immigration Department and student-hungry universities, each with their own imperatives.

Governance and notifications in the new order

In recent years, while advances in technology, such as implant borne artificial crowns, have permitted more elaborate and adventurous courses of treatment, the risks for misadventure and mismatched expectations have grown as a result. In 1970 it was rare for a registered dentist to be reported, let alone be prosecuted, for a course of treatment; the DBV was more concerned with prosecuting non-registered operators. Equally, it was not unknown, but rare, for medical litigation to progress to court in Australia even though the status of "practitioner-as-god" was eroding even then. The loss of godlike status has accelerated since.

In 1982 the Australian Dental Association Victorian Branch (ADAVB) employed a part-time community relations officer (CRO), the first in Australia, to hear patients' grievances and help to resolve complaints against dentists.

The number of CROs and hours of work have grown ever since. This conciliation initiative took place six years ahead of the creation of the State Government's Office of the Health Services Commissioner (OHSC) in 1988[5] in the general trend towards patient empowerment during the 1980s.

At its establishment, the OHSC's role was "to receive, investigate and resolve complaints from users of health services" (HSC, 1999. p. 42). From the start, the HSC and the CROs of the ADAVB saw each other as colleagues and not rivals. This was formalised in 1999 when the HSC and ADAVB met to develop a protocol for facilitating the resolution of complaints about dentists (HSC, 1999). This was sensible as there was no fixed pathway for people to formalise a complaint and the agencies themselves guided complainants to the appropriate resolver of their problems. Through the Health Complaints Act of 2016, the OHSC became the Office of the Health Complaints Commissioner (OHCC or HCC) in February 2017.

Notwithstanding that the ADAVB CROs and the HCC continue to conciliate and interact with each other to reach amicable resolutions for most complainants at no or low cost, professional indemnity costs and premiums have kept rising to the extent that dentists who perform Orthodontics or implant procedures associated with Prosthodontics have to pay a premium surcharge. As with much else in life, greater rewards carry higher risk. It is notable that the conciliatory approach of the ADAVB and the resultant benefit of lower legal costs, have prompted the main professional indemnity insurer, Guild, to pay for the employment of the ADAVB's CROs.

5 Created through the powers of the *Health Services (Conciliation and Review) Act 1987.*

Dental practitioners who work in public sector clinics have been shielded from the rise in complaints and litigation partly because management has interceded to ameliorate the situation, partly because their clientele is less litigious, but most likely because the advanced clinical procedures requiring expensive componentry are not available within their clinics. Whereas dentists in private clinics largely self-select their scope of practice and thus their level of risk, those in community clinics are more circumscribed by scope of practice agreements with management and either a mandatory or prevailing ethos of concentration on primary care. An exception to the limitations on scope of treatment would be the specialist referral clinics at the RDHM, for which there are long waiting lists. Even here complaints are less likely because of the cautious and more transparent environment.

Since the establishment of Ahpra in 2010, in Victoria if people are unhappy with treatment or any aspect of their interaction with a registered health professional, they can now complain in five ways. The first and most direct is to the practitioner or practice owner or manager; the second is to the professional's association such as the ADA or AMA; the third is to the state-based Health Complaints Commissioner; the fourth is to Ahpra; and, finally, they can go directly to a lawyer. This is often the ascending scale when resolution is not achieved, although sometimes a practitioner is unaware of anything amiss until being contacted by any of the other four entities. There is no flow chart for patients or their agents to follow, which can add another level of frustration.

From a standing start, Ahpra's dealings with complaints, or notifications, from the public about practitioners and their care have struggled to develop a smooth and effective rhythm; the corporate knowledge of old state boards has had to be recreated. The more benign term "notification" is used by Ahpra because many of the queries can be resolved at first contact without reaching the level of a formal complaint. The timeliness and transparency of dealing with the notifications have been inadequate and high staff turnover has not helped.

Many complaints from most types of health practitioner about the slow and opaque processes led to an Australian Senate inquiry in 2016. Most of the 14 recommendations were accepted by the government with comments similar to a school teacher's "must try harder" on a report card (Australian Government, 2018). Ahpra itself acknowledged this in annual reports where difficulties were recorded. In its 2019–2020 report Aphra stated that each year it "makes changes to improve the notification process to improve its timeliness, quality and experience" (AHPRA, 2020).

One criticism of Ahpra has been that it is reactive rather than proactive; that it takes no action against practitioners unless a notification has been received. However, in its defence, Ahpra cannot be expected to know what is happening in every health practitioner's office. The only hint of a problem is through notifications; gossip is hardly a sound basis for legal action. One recurring criticism is that when investigations do take place, the investigator often has no background knowledge of the specific profession nor its customary standards (AMA, 2021).

Table 2.1 shows the number of notifications received and resolved by the Dental Board of Australia in the 10 years to 2021.

Table 2.1 Dental Board of Australia notifications by year, 2012–2021

Year	2012	2013	2014	2015	2016	2017	2018	2019	2020	2021
New notifications	476	586	582	428	497	526	539	749	784	710
Closed notifications	No mention	522	632	538	393	485	554	733	730	757

Source: Ahpra and DBA Annual Reports, 2012 to 2021.
Notes
1. Notifications exclude those for NSW, which has a different reporting system and body, the Health Professional Councils Authority (HPCA). In Queensland, the Office of the Health Ombudsman receives all complaints, filters them and passes on most to Ahpra.
2. Figures for years 2020 and 2021 were affected (probably reduced) by COVID-19 lockdown periods, especially in Victoria.
3. I have been unable to locate the number of closed notifications for the year 2011–12. Collation and classification changed during 2011–12.
4. The number of new notifications from 2013 to 2021 was 5,401, and the number closed was 5,344, suggesting near parity. However, that masks long delays for some more serious cases.

About 90% of DBA notifications concern dentists and about 6% concern prosthetists. Approximately two-thirds of the notifications concerned clinical care and a similar proportion lead to no further action beyond an initial enquiry. One reason for the early closure of notifications may be that the notifier (complainant) was referred to an agency better suited to deal with the case such as the Victorian Health Complaints Commissioner (HCC). This highlights a confusion: to whom should an aggrieved person complain? In theory, the different agencies – HCC, ADA Community Relations Officers and Ahpra – should consult and refer onwards for appropriate resolution, and generally they do so, but some people must get lost in the halting progress of their case. In its 2020–21 Annual Report, the HCC made an effort to differentiate between what it does and what Ahpra does (HCC, 2021).

In general, Ahpra was created to monitor the educational qualifications and professional conduct of health practitioners and not to settle arguments such as payment for an ill-fitting denture or lost filling. Both the ADAVB and HCC are more suited to such civil law examples. However, there is no common triage point to guide complainants; it all relies on interagency cooperation and this is where frustration mounts.

Notifications about dental and medical practitioners (about 4% and 5%, respectively, of their total numbers registered) are higher than for any of the other registrable health professions; for example, only about 0.5% of nurses are involved with notifications, although the actual number is highest of all because there are more nurses than any other type of health professional. The rate of notifications involving dentists and doctors may be associated with the fact that most are self-employed; or notifications may have more of a financial than a quality-of-service element.

As mentioned, Ahpra itself is aware of the need for timeliness and transparency in dealing with notifications but investigations can be slow and can prolong the torment for both notifier and the target of the notice. The COVID-19 pandemic induced a fall in notifications in 2021, which allowed some catch-up in the backlog of cases.

To put complaints about dental practitioners into context, in recent years the three complaint-handling agencies have each found against Victorian dentists fewer than 100 times a year. As a counterbalance, in the years 2013 to 2019 the ABS has consistently found that "patient experiences" of dental professionals (listening carefully to, showing respect to, and spending enough time with the patient) have been more positive than those of medical and nursing professionals (ABS, 2021).

Summary

Dental legislation began in Victoria with the Dentists Act of 1887. Its aim was to protect the public from untrained charlatans and promote a formal course of education for dentists. However, protecting public health was implicit, never explicit, in legislation. Throughout its 113 years of existence, the DBV was self-funded through fees and fines. Its interest in promoting the dental health of the public waxed and waned according to available funds but from the mid 1960s attitudes changed on several fronts. Through technological innovation and the advance of knowledge, the nature of dentistry itself changed from being one largely of tooth replacement to one of tooth restoration and aesthetic enhancement, and this created a greater public engagement with dentistry. Procedures became more complex for more people and took longer. This in turn required a larger and more diverse workforce.

Throughout the DBV's existence the dental workforce was never large enough, causing episodic pressure on politicians, who in turn put pressure back on the DBV and University of Melbourne Dental School. The drive to fluoridate water supplies was to reduce the prevalence of dental disease, thus reducing morbidity and therefore waiting times to see dentists. The gradual reduction in dental decay also helped to change public attitudes to undergoing treatment from an increasing range of dental specialties at one end of the spectrum and accepting the preventive measures and restorations of children's teeth by dental therapists at the other end. The rising tide of dental awareness was lifting all boats as the 21st century started.

After the DPBV started functioning in July 2000, it barely got through the typical stages of forming, storming, norming and performing before it was overtaken by the sweeping reforms of national uniform accreditation and governance for all health professions which ended it in 2010. Ten years have now passed since Ahpra and the Dental Board of Australia were formed. There is now a plethora of statistical data on workforce and accreditation but it is harder to ascertain data on better delivery of services and improvements to national dental health and wellbeing within that time frame. Better indices, such as the trend for lower tooth decay rates and more people retaining teeth for longer, had been noticed much earlier.

The State government has not completely abandoned the field of regulation since the national Act came into operation in 2010. One example of this has been that the Drugs, Poisons and Controlled Substances Regulations had to be amended in 2017 to permit oral hygienists and dental assistants with Certificate IV qualifications to handle and clinically use topical fluoride varnish, a Schedule 4 drug, both within dental clinics and in outreach settings. There will no doubt need to be amendments to other state Acts as practices and who performs them evolve.

In this chapter we have seen how legislation has been critical in helping to change the focus of the dental profession from being somewhat inward-looking to one which encompasses patient welfare and the need to be accountable to patients and regulators. Various legislative measures have facilitated changes in the ownership of private practices, such that non-dentists and third-party entities can own them, and the extension of public sector services. Publicly funded dental programs have also encouraged third parties to own practices. There has been a transition, with no end point in sight, from an era of cottage-industry practitioners to one of profit-orientated corporates and ever larger group practices, whether private or public. It is as well that the same legislative steps have broadened the scope and capacity for the public to seek redress for perceived wrongdoing through strengthened regulations of governance. The dental workforce has been augmented by a broader range of dental health professionals. The DBA now has a minority of dentists (five) although still a majority of dental practitioners (eight) in a board of twelve (Ahpra, 2020) rather than the pre-2000 DBV of seven dentists and no one else. Apart from external agencies like the Health Complaints Commission, notifications about dental professionals are investigated by Ahpra employees who report to the relevant board, namely, the DBA.

References

Australian Bureau of Statistics. (ABS) & Castles, I. (1993). 1989–90 *National health survey: Lifestyle and health, Australia*. Canberra: ABS.

Australian Bureau of Statistics. (ABS). (2019). *Historical population. A product containing a wide range of historical demographic data going back as far, where possible, to the beginnings of European colonisation.* (Reference period 2016) [Data set]. ABS. <https://www.abs.gov.au/statistics/people/population/historical-population/2016#data-download>

Australian Bureau of Statistics. (ABS). (2021). *Patient experiences in Australia: Summary of findings.* Reference period 2020–21 financial year. <https://www.abs.gov.au/statistics/health/health-services/patient-experiences-australia-summary-findings/2020-21>

Australian Health Practitioner Regulation Agency. (2020). Annual Report 2019/20 <https://www.ahpra.gov.au/Publications/Annual-reports/Annual-Report-2020/Notifications.aspx>

Australian Health Workforce Ministerial Council. (AHWMC). (2009). *Communiqué 8 May 2009. Design of new National Registration and Accreditation Scheme.* <https://www.ahpra.gov.au/About-Ahpra/Ministerial-Directives-and-Communiques.aspx>

Australian Government. (2018). *Australian Government response to the Senate Community Affairs Reference Committee report: Complaints mechanism administered under the Health Practitioner Regulation National Law, August 2018.* <https://www.health.gov.au/resources/publications/complaints-mechanism-administered-under-the-health-practitioner-regulation-national-law>

Australian Institute of Health and Welfare. (AIHW). (1998). *Australia's oral health and dental services. Dental Statistics and Research Unit.* Catalogue No. DEN 13, pp. 98–99. Canberra: AIHW.

Australian Medical Association. (AMA). (2021). *Submission to Senate Inquiry to the Health Practitioner Regulation Agency, 30 April 2021.* <https://www.aph.gov.au/Parliamentary_Business/Committees/Senate/Community_Affairs/AHPRA/Submissions>

Barnard, P. D., & Australia, Department of Health, Housing, Local Government and Social Services, (1993). *National oral health survey Australia 1987–88. A report of the first national oral health survey of Australia.* Canberra: AGPS.

Biggs, A. (2008). *Overview of Commonwealth involvement in funding dental care. Research paper no. 1 2008–09.* Parliament of Australia. <https://apo.org.au/node/2696>

Bradford Hill, A. (1965). Environment and disease: Association or causation. *JRSM, 58*(5), 295–300.

Commonwealth of Australia. (1973). *Budget papers. Payments to or for the states 1973–74.* Canberra: AGPS. <https://archive.budget.gov.au/1973-74/downloads/1973-74_Payments_to_or_for_the_States.pdf>

Council of Australian Governments. (COAG). (2004). *Council of Australian Governments' meeting communiqué, 25 June 2004.* Canberra: COAG. <http://ncp.ncc.gov.au/docs/Council%20of%20Australian%20Governments%20Meeting%20-%2025%20June%202004.pdf>

Council of Australian Governments. (COAG). (2008). *Council of Australian Governments' meeting communiqué, 26 March 2008.* Canberra: COAG. <http://ncp.ncc.gov.au/docs/COAG%20communique%2029%20Nov%202008.pdf>

Dental Advisory Committee. (1969). *Report of the Dental Advisory Committee to the Honourable the Minister of Health, 1969.* Melbourne: DAC.

Dental Board of Victoria. (DBV). (1993). *A history of its first hundred years.* Melbourne: DBV.

Dental Practice Act 1999 (Vic). <https://www.austlii.edu.au>

Dentists Act 1972 (Vic). <http://classic.austlii.edu.au/au/legis/vic/hist_act/da1972123>

Department of Health and Community Services. Victoria. (DH&CS). (1995a). *Future directions for dental health in Victoria.* Melbourne: VGPS.

Department of Health and Community Services. (DH&CS). (1995b). Dental Auxiliary Workforce Review Victoria (DAWRV). *Report to the Minister for Health. March 1995.* Melbourne: DHCS.

Department of Human Services. (DHS). (1989). On site analysis for change of dental health services. Unpublished manuscript. Melbourne. Victoria.

Department of Human Services. (DHS). (1998). *Review of Dentists Act and Dental Technicians Act 1972,* Final report July 1998. <http://ncp.ncc.gov.au/docs/Victorian%20review%20of%20Dentist%20Act%201972%20and%20Dental%20Technicians%20Act%201972%2C%20July%201998.pdf>

Dooland, M., & National Health Strategy. (1992). *Improving dental health in Australia. Background paper, National Health Strategy, No. 9.* Melbourne: National Health Strategy.

Health Commission Victoria. (HCV). (1982). *Report of internal committee reviewing the Victorian School Dental Service.* Unpublished manuscript. Melbourne. Victoria.

Health Complaints Commissioner. (2021). *Annual report 2020–21.* <https://hcc.vic.gov.au/sites/default/files/media-document/Health%20Complaints%20Commissioner%20%20Annual%20Report%202020-2021%20FINAL.pdf>

Health Department Victoria. (HDV). (1986). *Ministerial review of dental services. Final report.* Melbourne: HDV.

Health (Fluoridation) Act 1973 (Vic). <https://www.legislation.vic.gov.au/in-force/acts/health-fluoridation-act-1973/020>

Health Professions Registration Act 2005 (Vic). <https://www.legislation.vic.gov.au/as-made/acts/health-professions-registration-act-2005>

Health Services Commissioner. (HSC). (1999). *Annual Report 1998–99.* <https://vgls.sdp.sirsidynix.net.au/client/search/asset/1162637>

Hilmer, F. (1993). *National competition policy: Report by the Independent Committee of Inquiry.* Canberra: Commonwealth Govt. Printer. <https://www.australiancompetitionlaw.org/reports/1993hilmer.html>

Lane, J. (1970). *Dental services for Australians. [Pamphlet 21].* Melbourne: Victorian Fabian Society.

Legge, D., & Sylvan, L. (1990). Consumer participation in health: the Consumers' Health Forum and the Victorian District Health Council Program. In. A. Evers, W. Farrant & A. Trojan (Eds.), *Healthy public policy at the local level.* Boulder: Westview Press. Frankfurt am Main and Boulder Colorado, Campus Verlag and Westview Press, 176–198.

Lewis, J. (1997). *Interests, inequity and inertia: Dental health policy and politics in Australia.* [Unpublished doctoral dissertation]. University of Melbourne, Victoria.

Lewis, M. J. (2003). *The peoples' health: Public health in Australia 1950 to the present.* Santa Barbara: ABC-CLIO.

Productivity Commission. (2005). *Australia's health workforce. Research report.* Canberra. <https://www.pc.gov.au/inquiries/completed/health-workforce/report/healthworkforce.pdf>

Public Record Office Victoria (PROV). (n.d.). VPRS 6345/PO, Unit 257, 1134/P2 and VPRS 8609, Unit 293/P21.

Ritzer, G. (1975). Professionalisation, bureaucratisation and rationalisation. The views of Max Weber. *Social Forces, 53*(4), pp. 627–34.

Senate Community Affairs References Committee. Australia. (1998). *Report on public dental services.* <https://www.aph.gov.au/parliamentary_business/committees/senate/community_affairs/completed_inquiries/1996-99/dental/report/index>

Short, S. (1998). Community activism in the health policy process: The case of the Consumers' Health Forum of Australia, 1987–96. In A. Yeatman, (Ed.), *Activism and the policy process* (pp. 122–145). Routledge. <https://doi.org/10.4324/9781003114826>

State Government Victoria. (1965). *Victorian Government Gazette,* No. 31, May 5. <http://gazette.slv.vic.gov.au/images/1965/V/general/31.pdf>

State Government Victoria, & Premier Cain, J. (1986). *Social justice, the need for a strategic approach.* Melbourne: Government Printer.

Victorian State Government. (1971). *Victorian Parliamentary Debates, Legislative Assembly,* Vol. no. 305, 23 November, p. 2896.

Victorian State Government. (1994). *Victorian Parliamentary Debates, Legislative Assembly,* Vol. no. 419, 5 October, p. 569.

Victorian State Government. (1999a). *Victorian Parliamentary Debates, Legislative Assembly,* Vol. no. 443, 12 May, 1999, p. 972.

Victorian State Government. (1999b). *Victorian Parliamentary Debates, Legislative Assembly,* Vol. no. 442, May, 1999, p. 599.

World Health Organization. (WHO). (1978). *Declaration of Alma-Ata, 1978.* World Health Organization. (1978). Declaration of Alma-Ata. WHO Regional Office for Europe. <https://apps.who.int/iris/handle/10665/347879>

World Health Organization. (WHO). (1986). *Ottawa charter for health promotion.* <https://www.who.int/publications/i/item/ottawa-charter-for-health-promotion>

Chapter 3
Workforce – And then there were four

Jamie Robertson

Figure 3.1 Key developments in the non-dentist workforce, Victoria

Year	Event
1975	First advanced dental technicians registered (later known as prosthetists)
1977	First graduation of dental therapists to work in state schools
1989	Dental Board of Victoria (DVB) regulation to permit dental hygienists
2006	Second dental school opens at Latrobe University, Bendigo

Introduction

Knowledge of workforce numbers and their deployment in relation to the population is important for planning efficient and effective health services. From a public health perspective, however, medical and dental practitioners have historically been in chronic undersupply in Australia. This is because their training was either on a master–apprentice basis and therefore only suitable for a stable population size or, when training at tertiary level was introduced, little or no strategic workforce planning occurred. It remains the case today that the training of medical and dental professionals is not coupled with the demonstrated needs of society and there may be over- or under-production of new graduates from institutions with different imperatives, usually financial, from their host society and its government.

In 1970, at the start of our period of enquiry, only registered dentists could provide routine dental services, although a few dental mechanics were illegally making dentures for people from assorted premises. By 1975, advanced dental technicians and dental therapists had come into existence and dental hygienists were added to the dental team in 1989. While the numbers, training and scope of practice for the three additional practitioners have evolved over time, dentists still make up the great majority of the group of professionals collectively known as dental practitioners (Figure 3.1).

In this chapter we examine the division of labour among dental practitioners in Victoria which has been less a planned exercise in Taylorism, than a set of responses to political and occupational exigencies.

Dental schools

Victoria has two dental schools – at the University of Melbourne and La Trobe University (LTU) – and both are public institutions. Melbourne started teaching its dental Bachelor degree course in 1905 and LTU followed suit as recently as 2006. In 2008 the University of Melbourne introduced education reforms known as "the Melbourne Model". However, there was a delay of three years before the new Doctor of Dental Surgery (DDS) course could be introduced. This was to allow the first cohort of the new Bachelor of Biomedical Science to come through the system.

At the University of Melbourne, the new system meant graduate-level entry to the dental and medical schools in the Faculty of Medicine, Dentistry and Health Sciences thus extending the education to become a dentist to a minimum of seven years. The dental school at LTU continues to admit students straight from school and those studying to become a dental hygienist or oral health therapist gain a Bachelor of Oral Health after three years; for those eligible, two more years of study grants them an additional degree, Master of Dentistry.

Prior to the graduate-entry model of 2011, the University of Melbourne dental course was five years long and, until 1963 when the faculty and dental hospital moved to Grattan Street, its facilities at the Dental Hospital in Spring Street were too cramped to permit large intakes of students regardless of the state's population growth. Ironically, when the hospital and, later, the school moved again into new premises in Swanston Street in 2003, they moved into less space but with many more students. By 2020 the annual intake of Doctor of Dental Surgery students had risen to about 100.

Melbourne Dental School (MDS) also teaches a combined course in Oral Health Therapy and Dental Hygiene to a Bachelor of Oral Health (University of Melbourne, 2022) level, while prosthetists are trained at RMIT University in Melbourne.

Population growth

In 1970 Victoria's population was almost 3.5 million people. By 2020 it had nearly doubled to more than six million with the growth mostly in the city of Melbourne. Reflecting a global trend in urbanisation, the proportion of Victorians residing in the capital has kept on rising. In 1950 it was only 59%, but by 1970, due to high immigration rates, it was 71% and that rose to 77% in 2020 (Table 3.1). Some regional centres, such as Bendigo and Mildura, have grown but, overall, there has been relative rural depopulation over the past five decades.

Table 3.1 Examples of rapid population growth and urbanisation

Region	Population (millions)		
	1950	1970	2020
Canada	14.0	21.3	38.0
Australia	8.2	12.7	25.6
Victoria	2.2	3.4	6.5
Melbourne	1.3	2.4	5.0
M:V fraction[1]	0.59	0.71	0.77

1. Population residing in Melbourne (M) and Victoria (V).

The strong population growth shown above has been related to migration surges in the first and last 20 years of this 70-year period but, even during the middle 30 years, growth was still healthy. Victoria's population has also grown threefold and Melbourne's growth has been almost fourfold. Such growth rates have put strains on all forms of infrastructure and services, and their irregular nature has made strategic planning difficult. This has been true even when large rises in migration rates were anticipated; health, education and transport services were always playing catch-up.

Worldwide, professionals of all kinds have preferred to live and work in metropolitan centres, partly to retain family and friend networks and partly for occupational collegiality; this has exacerbated maldistribution of their services. Further, many remain city-bound because villages and small towns cannot sustain full-time practice or offer sufficient occupational and social amenities. From 1939 to 1963, rural Victoria suffered a net loss of 44 dentists causing the dentist-to-population ratio to drift from 1:4120 to 1:6589 (Melbourne Dental Hospital Council, July 1964, Appendix 5). At about the same time, in 1960, the overall State ratio was 1:2874 or 34.8 dentists per 100,000 population.

Table 3.2 shows increases in Victoria's population compared with the number of dentists in the seven decades to 2020.

Table 3.2 Rises in Victorian population and dentists, Victoria, 1950 to 2020

Year	Population	Rise (%)	Dentists (no.)	Rise (%)	Approx. ratio of dentists to population
1950	2,208,000		823		1:2683
1960	2,857,000	29.3	994	20.7	1:2874
1970	3,445,000	20.6	1,088	9.4	1:3166
1980	3,914,000	13.6	1,783	63.8	1:2195
1990	4,378,000	11.8	2,297	25.8	1:1906
2000	4,704,000	7.4	2,447	6.5	1:1922
2010	5,461,000	16.0	3,231	32.0	1:1690
2020	6,600,000	22.0	4,220	30.6	1:1564

Sources: Population from ABS, Dentists from DBV Registers 1950 to 2000, AHPRA Registers 2010 to 2020

Thanks to the Commonwealth Reconstruction Training Scheme (CRTS) for ex-servicemen which ran from 1944 until 1950, there was a surge of dental graduates through the 1950s (Powell & McIntyre, 2015). The scheme was created to give these young men the opportunity of university and vocational courses and to swell the ranks of so many depleted civilian occupations after World War II. It briefly led to a minor improvement in the dentist-to-population ratio but by 1970 the ratio had slipped back to 1:3166 (31.5 per 100,000). It was this observed slippage in the 1960s which had alarmed the Minister of Health, Ronald Mack and led him to establish a committee of inquiry into how to overcome ballooning waiting times to see a dentist. The pressure to "do something" was coming from all quarters. Jim Lane's Fabian Society paper of 1970 (Chapter 2) commented that the World Health Organization (WHO) was recommending a ratio of 1:2500 for developed countries (Lane, 1970).

Every five years from 1950 until 1975 Victoria's population grew by approximately 300,000. The rate subsequently decreased but since 2005 each five-year rise has been around half a million. The earlier growth spurt was largely from a migration wave comprising people from the United Kingdom and continental Europe who contributed to Australia's post-war industrialisation while the second spurt has been migration, especially from China and India, under a skilled migration program (Phillips & Simon-Davies, 2016). In each of these high-growth periods, migration has contributed more than 60% to population growth. Throughout the whole period there has also been a steady intake of refugees on a humanitarian basis.

High levels of migration have created large demographic changes in Australia, particularly in state capital cities. Many people arriving on a humanitarian basis have helped to repopulate some rural areas which were in decline. In turn, the dental needs and cultural preferences of migrants have helped to shape clinical and preventive dental services. For example, the non-English speaking Europeans arriving after World War II did not subscribe to the prevailing Anglo-Saxon view that most people should have all their teeth removed then have full dentures fitted while young so that no further toothache or treatment would occur. The old view based on a discredited focal sepsis theory, was yielding anyway but the migrants accelerated its demise. The steep rise in prospective patients overwhelmed the small number of existing dentists and increased the urgency to lower the burden of dental disease through preventive measures.

By the time of the second 20-year wave of high migration, the concept of "best practice" dentistry had shifted in favour of the conservation and restoration of dentitions, including the use of implants to support fixed prostheses. The change was largely underpinned by water fluoridation which had reduced dental decay in the population and which, thus, also influenced population's attitudes about the maintenance and even enhancement of their dentitions. Nevertheless, there still continued to be pockets of the population, particularly those in humanitarian resettlement programs, who had not had the benefit of fluoridation from birth and whose dental needs were great.

High-needs groups persisted in the local population including health- and age pension card holders, the homeless, the unemployed, Aboriginal Australians, and people with physical and intellectual difficulties. Most people in these groups rely on public sector dental services and therefore on adequately funded and geographically accessible clinics.

Arithmetic of the Registers

When the registration of dentists began in Victoria in 1888, it was voluntary and heavily grandfathered, meaning that medical practitioners, pharmacists and even a few rural blacksmiths were permitted to register. Moreover, until 1927 registration was for life or until a person gave notice of retiring. Only from 1928, with the introduction of annual registration fees, could the actual number of practising dentists in the state be ascertained. From 1928 until 1948, the number of dentists on the Register actually fell from 795 to 760 through a combination of the non-renewal of long-dead dentists, grandfathered doctors and pharmacists, or the very low output of graduates due to economic depression and war (DBV, 1993). During this time, particularly in the late 1940s, the state's population continued to grow under a Commonwealth government policy of mass immigration to boost the industrialisation of Australia.

By the mid-1950s the post-war bulge in graduates from the University of Melbourne subsided to an annual average of just 30. Even so, annual immigration continued at high levels throughout the 1950s and 60s and dentist-to-population ratios continued to deteriorate accordingly. The situation was made worse by the maldistribution of dentists across the state. Not only was there an undersupply of new graduates from Australian dental schools in the 1960s, but also many of them were attracted to the adventure of a lifetime by working in the British National Health Service and using that as a springboard to holidays in Europe. This too removed them from the pool of practitioners at home, but the adventure became more difficult after 1973 when Britain joined the European Economic Community and ceased completely when reciprocal recognition came to an end in 2000.

Available workforce data can only provide approximations of the numbers of clinicians practising at any given time. For a variety of reasons there will always be a number of practitioners who do not practise: for example, some work in administrative roles, are child rearing or are transitioning to retirement (AIHW, 1998; AIHW, 2012,).[6] An interesting spike in the non-practising group of dentists occurred in the late 1970s. After the reunification of Vietnam in 1975 many professionals in Malaysia, Singapore and Hong Kong feared further communist takeovers and sought the insurance of registration in Britain and Australia. Similarly, after the Soweto riots in 1976 many South African professionals did the same. At the time both groups enjoyed reciprocal registration with Australia but they had no wish to leave their homelands unless absolutely necessary and those on the Australian Dentists Registers remained so for a few years until the fear of civil strife passed and they stopped renewing their annual registrations here. These "phantom dentists", who numbered between 100 and 200, were never part of the Victorian workforce (DBV, 1993).

Since about 2000, young graduates have often only been able to find part-time work. Whether by necessity or by choice, part-time work compounds the uncertainty about the ratios. Nevertheless, the ratios still give an approximate guide to the dental workforce and to trends over time. Table 3.3 compares the size of Victoria's dentist workforce with that of other dental health professionals from 1970 to 2020.

---

6 Surveys by the Australian Institute of Health and Welfare's Australian Research Centre for Population Oral Health have shown this to be about 15% of the Register.

It can be seen that the total number of practitioners other than dentists has never been more than about 25% of the number of dentists. The proportion of treatment which they provided has been even less because many of them worked part-time.

Table 3.3 Fifty years of Victoria's population and dental workforce, 1970 to 2020

Category	1970	1980	1990	2000	2010	2020
Victorian population	3.44m	3.91m	4.38m	4.70m	5.46m	6.69m
Registered dentists	1,088	1,783	2,297	2,447	3,231	4,220
Dentists per 100,000 population	31.5	45	52.5	52	59	63
Dental therapist/OHT	n.a.	184	283	182	376	775
Prosthetists	n.a.	121	265	348	323	356
Dental hygienists	n.a.	n.a.	9	87	161	238

Sources: Workforce numbers from Registers or AHPRA from 2010 onwards
Notes:
Population in millions from Australian Bureau of Statistics, June each year
n.a. = not applicable

While the number of dentists has risen continuously from 823 in 1950 to 4,220 in 2020, the rate of increase has varied with two sharp rises in 1980 and 2010 (Table 3.3). The first spike was due in part to the "phantom" dentists described above and the second to a dramatic influx of overseas-trained dentists who passed the Australian Dental Council (ADC) qualifying exams. Since 1980 the total number of dental providers overall has been increased by dental therapists, prosthetists and, since 1990, dental hygienists.

From the table above, it can be seen that there has been a continuous rise in all types of practitioner with two brief exceptions. In the 1990s, the Kennett Government introduced a belt-tightening exercise on the number of public sector employees in the Health and Education Departments. Dental therapists were offered redundancy packages shortly before the School

Dental Service (SDS) was merged with the new entity of Dental Health Services Victoria (DHSV). Clearly, many therapists accepted the offer as we see that their numbers dropped from 283 in 1990 to 182 in 2000, before rising again to 376 in 2010. Other reasons for the fall in numbers include retirement due either to age or hesitancy about working in the new system, transfer to new roles within the public sector and the loss of an intake of students while the course transitioned from the school in St Kilda Road to the Royal Dental Hospital of Melbourne (RDHM) in 1996.

The other fall in dental workforce numbers was with the prosthetists whose number dropped from 348 in 2000 to 323 in 2010 before rising again to 356 in 2020. In the early 2000s, the training program for prosthetists was suspended for five years as recommended by the review into the Dentists Act 1972 and Dental Technicians Act 1972 (DHS, 1998).

Drivers of change

In 1963 the Melbourne Dental Hospital moved from cramped quarters to a new and larger building opposite the Royal Melbourne Hospital in Grattan Street.[7] Victorian politicians saw the relocation as a means to increase the number of practising dentists by increasing the output from the Melbourne dental faculty but the faculty retorted that, as staff numbers had not been increased and they were being asked to do more work, this was not possible. In fact, the faculty requested a reduced student quota (Atkinson, 1990); however, this request fell on deaf ears.

By 1970 when a Bill to address changes to the existing Dentists Act was before Parliament, the dentists tried to forestall the introduction of patient-treating therapists and technicians by arguing that this would be acceptable only after the effects of water fluoridation were seen and an annual output of 100 dental graduates was achieved (Robertson, 1989). As the prospect of such an increase in new dentists was remote, the politicians accepted the claim. They had nothing to lose as they knew that whatever extra funding was required to achieve this outcome would be coming from Commonwealth rather than State budgets.

Between 1970 and 1980 the number of dentists on the Victorian Register grew from 1,088 to 1,783, an amazing 63.8%. It increased further to 2,297 or another 28.8% by 1990. In the same period the first dental therapists and advanced dental technicians were entering the workforce.

Prior to 1982 it was tedious and almost impossible to glean demographic information from the Dentists Register but in December 1981 additional information began to be collected on a new computerised system. Computerisation (the very word was exciting at the time!) and the additional data it provided facilitated much richer and faster analysis of the composition and disposition of the dental workforce in Victoria.

The Ministerial Review of Dental Services

The Ministerial Review of Dental Services (MRODS) (HDV, 1986) was an early beneficiary of the Dental Board's decision to computerise its Register. In part the review was prompted by the understanding that the population of Melbourne was growing far beyond the capacity of a single institution – the RDHM – to provide timely services for all those people eligible to receive public care. Moreover, the situation was even worse in regional Victoria. The review was to provide information and an evidence-based argument for change.

During the period analysed for the review, 1981 to 1984, more than 20% of dentists on the Register were not providing clinical service in Victoria. This included the large number of "phantom" dentists from Singapore and South Africa which peaked at 196 in 1982 and declined to 173 by 1984 (Robertson, 1989). These two groups alone comprised about 9% of the Register and would skew any workforce planning if not omitted. Of the practising dentists, only 207 (13%) were in the public sector (Robertson, 1989) and of that 207, only 76 (36%) were in the peak productive age group of 31 to 50 years old. The hollowing out of the public sector workforce was due to the loss of younger dentists leaving to work in

---

7 Curiously, this was a return to their relationship in Lonsdale Street when these two institutions commenced in the 19th century.

the booming private sector accompanied by a compensatory rise in older dentists (mainly men) in the over-50 age groups returning from private practice, often after their health had deteriorated.[8] Among the public sector dentists, approximately one third worked in the RDHM with the rest either teaching, working in other hospitals or in the SDS (Robertson, 1989).[9]

The MRODS highlighted the discrepancy of dentist-to-population ratios between Victoria's regions and the metropolitan area. The regions averaged one general dentist to 4,063 people (1:4063), while Melbourne "enjoyed" a ratio of 1:2894. For access to specialist dentists of any kind, the situation was even worse. The ratios were 1:75188 in the regions and 1:20921 in Melbourne. There were also wide variations within the five rural and three metropolitan regions,[10] especially for specialists, who rarely ventured far from the city. For example, in Gippsland the specialist ratio was 1:20408 people, while the Central Highlands/Wimmera had 1:33898. In the Western Metropolitan region, containing Collins Street and the Dental Hospital, it was 1:7485, while the North-Eastern Metropolitan region, with its much bigger population, had a ratio of 1:74627 (Robertson, 1989).

Over the four years examined by MRODS, ratios of general dentists declined very slightly across Victoria but the ratios of specialists dramatically improved (Robertson, 1989). This is consistent with the fact that in 1978 a Specialist Register was created which permitted some dentists who restricted their practice to one area to be "grandfathered" as specialists. It also encouraged younger dentists to study further for better financial opportunities.

The MRODS final report was released in 1986. The Review is an example of Dental Public Health (DPH) as an academic discipline, a policy tool for the strategic planning of services, and an announcement that ad hoc measures more generally were no longer acceptable. Community health dentist John Spencer and political scientist Jenny Lewis were the Review's chief investigators and authors (HDV, 1986). They produced the first comprehensive DPH report in Victoria (Prof. H. Atkinson, personal communication, May, 1989). It examined the status of dental services and the workforce as they existed in the early 1980s and it heralded changes to come as a result of increased political interest in and scrutiny of the state's dental health and wellbeing. In contrast, the Dental Advisory Committee report of 1969 (DAC, 1969) had been less rigorous and the process certainly more rancorous.

---

8 In 1970–71, J. Robertson worked at RDHM with a large group of post-angina or post-cardiac arrest male dentists easing their way to retirement.

9 The Melbourne Dental Hospital gained a Royal Charter in 1969 and became the Royal Dental Hospital of Melbourne.

10 Rural: Barwon-South Western, Central-Highlands/Wimmera, Loddon-Campaspe/Mallee, Goulburn/North Eastern, Gippsland. Metropolitan: Western, North-Eastern, Southern

Among the rich mine of MRODS statistics was the fact that in the mid-1980s about 42% of private dentists were solo practitioners; the corporatisation of dentistry had not yet begun. A 1998 Australian Institute of Health and Welfare (AIHW) publication, based on 1992 data, showed that about 42% of dentists in Victoria were still solo practitioners (AIHW DSRU, 1998, Table 3.4). However, by 2013 this figure had dropped to 26% (AIHW, 2016, Table 9.6). The fall was due less to a rise in corporate practices and more to the cost pressures on solo practitioners, resulting in practices' decisions to merge or expand. The costs of the plant and equipment needed to deliver high-quality care were outstripping the practices' capacity to pay. Younger dentists were tending to form group practices to achieve economies of scale. Nevertheless, the proportion of corporate practices has been rising in the 21st century, both in Australia and internationally, as third parties have seen opportunities for profit making.

A discussion on that subject is beyond the scope of this study even though the trend has developed during the later stages of the period under review. Its significance and influence will continue to rise in years to come.

Reorganisation in a time of stress

The MRODS recommended the expansion of the public sector in order to broaden the accessibility and affordability of dental services (Chapter 2). Ten years later Australia's economy had gone from boom to bust with wild swings in unemployment levels. In 1986 and again in 1996, the unemployment level was 8%, but in between it had oscillated from 6% in 1988 to more than 11% 1991. These factors put greater strains on public sector dentistry while causing tightening in the private sector and a reduction in dental student numbers. As described in Chapters 2 and 4, the Commonwealth Dental Health Program, which was introduced in 1994 and had benefitted the private and public sectors alike, was terminated in 1996 by the incoming Howard Government. This resulted in even more strain on the public sector resources.

In the decade of 1990 to 1999 the rate of Victoria's population growth slowed to just seven per cent and there was near stasis in the number of registered dentists with the dentist to population ratio marking time. However, since 2000 the population has grown at an accelerated rate: 16% in the decade to 2009 and an amazing 22% from 2010 to 2019. Additions to the Dentists Register have increased even faster, so that the number of dentists per 100,000 population has risen from 52 in both 1990 and 2000, to 59 in 2010 and up to 63 in 2020.

These are theoretical ratios only because, as already noted, the number of dentists actually practising is always lower than that shown on the Register. For example, the AIHW has reported that about nine out of ten registered dentists actively practise but some are not clinicians or only work part-time. In its National Health Workforce data set for 2015, AIHW calculated that the number of full-time equivalent (FTE) dentists per 100,000 of the population was 53.4 for Victoria (AIHW, 2020, December 31). Nevertheless, comparing "like with like" over time suggests a trend even if it does not reveal an actual service capacity.

The AIHW's investigations and reports survey practising dentists only. As such, although irregular, they thus give a more accurate picture of those in clinical practice and the services being delivered than the Dentists Register would suggest. The AIHW's 2015 summary of oral health in Australia (AIHW, 2016) permitted comparison of theoretical and practical ratios. The study showed that there were 7.9 dentists per 100,000 in the public sector compared with 44.6 per 100,000 in the private sector. It also showed that Australia-wide 38% of dentists were women while the portion of dentists whose initial qualification was from an Australian university had fallen to 65%. This latter figure pointed to another demographic phenomenon in the dental workforce; the surge in skilled migration.

Sunset on dental colonialism

For most of the twentieth century, Australian states enjoyed reciprocal recognition of their medical and dental qualifications with Great Britain and its Dominions. When the Empire morphed into the Commonwealth this continued for a period. However, Australia was slow to recognise qualifications from other countries. This Britano-centric world view became indefensible and increasingly counterproductive during the immigration explosion in the 1950s and 1960s.

In order to take advantage of the increasingly diverse sources of immigration, the National Government established the Committee on Overseas Professional Qualifications (COPQ) in 1969. After several trial exams, the first exams for overseas dentists took place in Sydney in 1978. The exams had written and clinical parts and of the initial 29 candidates only two succeeded in passing the second exam (DBV, 1993).

As the name implies, the remit of COPQ was for professions in general. In the 1980s its functions regarding dentists were taken over by the Australian Dental Examining Council (ADEC) which in turn was replaced, as described below, by the Australian Dental Council (ADC) in 1992.

After many years of investigative inspections by members of the British General Dental Council (GDC) to Australian Dental Schools – for which the Australian hosts had to pay – a new national body called the Australian Dental Council was formed in 1992 to remove the resented vestige of colonialism. The irregular visits by British grandees were to ensure that Australian standards were high enough to allow reciprocal registration between the two countries. By the 1980s the GDC visits had become mere sinecures, possibly because Britain's priorities were focused on its fellow European Union members.

The ADC was modelled on the recently established Australian Medical Council and received encouragement, but no funding, from the Commonwealth government, so that for its first few years it was hosted at the Dental Board of Victoria's (DBV) offices in Jolimont and its first President, Dr Lloyd O'Brien, had to get used to multitasking because of the lack of support staff.

Dental workforce and population needs

The objectives of the ADC were to develop accreditation standards of dental education in Australian university dental schools and accreditation standards and procedures for assessing overseas-qualified dentists who wished to gain registration in Australia. In its early years, the annual number of such dentists was small and the pass rates were about 30%. This scarcely affected the total number on the Register of each state. By 2000 the number of candidates had crept up to 105, of whom 43 passed. Victoria gained about a quarter of them.[11] After that, numbers of candidates each year rose rapidly with the majority coming from India and China. From 2005 to 2010, of the 3,858 candidates who sat the final practical exams, 1,688 passed, which translated to an average of 281 new registrations per year (ADC, 2015; ADC, 2019). This was equivalent to the output from about five or six extra dental schools.

Over the past 20 years, in addition to the ADC "virtual" dental school increasing the supply of overseas-trained dentists, the output of domestic graduates has also increased. What began as a move to ward off a projected shortage of dentists (AIHW, 1998) has in recent years become a means to compete in the global market for international students and their fees. The increased output has been achieved by two means: firstly, through the creation of new dental schools and, secondly, through existing schools greatly increasing their intakes.[12] La Trobe University is in the first category and University of Melbourne Dental School is in the latter.

Melbourne Dental School has increased its intake of students to about 100 each year by accepting full-fee paying local and overseas students beyond the Commonwealth-supported place limit. Admittedly, the overseas quotient of between 20 and 30 places is supposed to return to their home country after graduation but some remain to work in Victoria. La Trobe University opened a dental school at its Bendigo campus in 2006.[13] The first intake was for oral health therapists only, but students of Dentistry were admitted in 2008 with the first cohort graduating in 2013. The underlying premise of training students in rural settings in expectation that they would stay there to practise was sound. Nevertheless, there has been some leakage of graduates back to Melbourne.

11 The ADC does not track state destinations of those who practise after passing their exams.

12 Before the 21st century there was one dental school in each state except Tasmania. Since then four more schools graduating dentists have opened and a further three graduating Oral Health Therapists.

13 Other dental schools have opened in Australia in recent years. In addition to LTU, Charles Sturt University and James Cook University have opened in regional centres at Wagga Wagga and Cairns, respectively, in order to attract rural students and encourage graduates to remain in rural areas. Griffith University opened its dental school at Gold Coast, which is at least a decentralised location.

The increasingly large annual additions of dentists to the Register have seen the numbers rise from 2,447 in 2000 to more than 4,350 in 2020; an increase of about 77%. By the end of 2022 the number had risen to 4,845. Over the same time, Victoria's population has risen by about 40% to 6.7 million. This has significantly improved the dentist-to-population ratio from 52 to 66 per 100,000, with the previously noted caveat that numbers of FTE practising dentists will be lower.

Throughout the rapid rise in numbers of all dental practitioners, the great majority of them continue to work in the private sector. In Victoria in 2021 the proportions were 89% of dentists, 73% of oral health therapists, 93% of hygienists and 87% of prosthetists. Only dental therapists with the older qualification had a slight majority of 51% working in the public sector. There are only small variations in percentages of each in the other Australian states (National Health Workforce Datasets, 2021).

The Grattan Institute report on dental services in 2018 supplied the ratios of dentists per 100,000 population in other countries; notably Norway (101), Germany (89) and Japan (81) (Duckett et al., 2019). However, these raw numbers should be viewed with caution as none of these countries has fluoridation of water supplies which obviates much reparative care, nor do they have the same levels of other types of dental practitioner.

The same Grattan Institute report observed that there has been a rise in the number of younger dentists working part-time during the last 20 years and that the rise has been more pronounced for dentists than any other health profession. Assuming these dentists share the same attitudes to work–leisure balance as their counterparts in other professions (Duckett et al., 2019), the reasons could be either lack of demand for treatment, lack of opportunity to obtain employment, or both. As most patients pay for treatment themselves and incomes have stagnated over the period, discretionary spending may have weakened. Further, as practice set-up costs and administrative burdens have increased, young graduates may have been deterred from opening their own practices.

Public sector changes in employment of clinicians

Meanwhile, public sector financial ceilings have not permitted a take-up of more dentists, even though the demand for public care is rising. If the dentist-to-population ratio is expressed in FTE numbers, then the increase in dentists is not so pronounced, reaching only about 60 per 100,000 in 2018 (Duckett et al., 2019).

There have been several variables at play in altering the proportions of practitioners in the public sector. Until 2007 dental therapists and oral health therapists working as clinicians were confined to working within the public sector (*Miscellaneous Acts [Health and Justice] Amendment Act 1995 (Vic)*.[14] In that year the SDS was closed down as a separate entity managed by DHSV, and integration of its staff began.[15] Most therapists transferred to community dental agencies where they would continue to practise within their scope including preschool children, although some had an extended scope to treat adults. The rationale was to better integrate child and adult dental services into community health services. Minister for Health Bronwyn Pike noted that "more integrated service delivery will provide a family-centred approach that also makes better use of expensive dental infrastructure" (DHS, 2007, p. iii).

14 This amended Section 29(6) of the Dentists Act and allowed therapists to work in the public sector.

15 Dental Health Services (DHS) was the name under which the School Dental Service (SDS) operated prior to the establishment of Dental Health Services Victoria (DHSV).

Table 3.4 shows a breakdown of FTE dental health practitioners
by occupational group for the financial years 2008 to June 2020.

Table 3.4 Average statewide clinical operators by full-time-equivalent (FTE), Victoria, 2007–08 to 2019–20

	Agencies[1]		RDHM[2]			School Dental[3]		Total	
Year	Dentist	DT/OHT	Dentist	Specialist	DT/OHT	Dentist	DT/OHT	Dentist (incl Specialist)	DT/OHT
2007/08	167	31	30	12	1	3	43	212	74
2008/09	175	77	30	11	2			216	79
2009/10	179	83	31	13	2			223	85
2010/11	187	93	34	14	2			235	95
2011/12	183	90	31	16	3			229	93
2012/13	180	87	31	16	3			227	90
2013/14	214	103	36	19	4			268	106
2014/15	200	111	31	18	5			249	116
2015/16	206	112	32	17	6			255	117
2016/17	193	108	34	17	6			244	114
2017/18	189	116	32	15	10			235	126
2018/19	181	119	31	15	8			227	127
2019/20	166	102	29	16	7			211	109

Notes:

1. Self-reported by agencies as clinicians not on DHSV payroll; FTE represents average of all months in the financial year.
2. From DHSV payroll.
3. From DHSV payroll. School Dental Service was integrated into Community Dental Agencies by the end of 2007/08. Therefore, FTE for staff from SDS was reported under agencies from 2008/09.

N.B. OHTs have a broader scope of practice than DTs and although they are now registered separately, prior to 2010 they were on a common register. Each year the number of DTs declines while that of OHTs grows.

It can be seen from Table 3.4 that the total number of general dentists has been almost the same in 2007 and 2020 whereas the number of therapists has risen by almost half (46%). In the same period of time, the number of specialist dentists at RDHM has risen by about a third (28%), albeit from a low base. It can also be seen that there was a dramatic expansion of clinicians in 2013 when the number of dentists and therapists rose by 18% and 29%, respectively. The increase in clinicians was due to extra funding to help reduce waiting lists through a National Partnership Agreement between the Australian government and State governments, announced in 2012 but only implemented in truncated form in 2015 (Chapter 4) (Biggs, 2015). Since that high point there has been a decline in the number of dentists employed but the number of therapists continued to rise until 2019.

Another change in 2007 was that dental hygienists became entitled to examine patients and make diagnoses before rather than after the patient had seen a dentist. This did not mean that they could practice independently but it facilitated their use in aged care and pre-school settings and improved the flow of treatment in clinical settings (DPBV, 2007).

There are a few reasons why the numbers of therapists employed have increased during the 21st century while the number of dentists has fallen back to a level below that prevailing when the SDS ended. In 2008 not all the state's public dental agencies could immediately accommodate the suddenly redundant therapists especially considering the addition of another graduating cohort of OHTs. In addition, it took some time for a new routine to be learned whereby parents had to take their children to agencies rather than simply letting the schools and the SDS organise appointments and treatment. It can be seen from the table that the number of therapists working in agencies tripled from 30 to over 90 between 2008 and 2011, which meant that additional therapists coming from interstate or through graduation from not one but two universities, LTU and Melbourne, were also employed.

Another reason for public agencies to employ more therapists was that they established more outreach services of oral health education and dental health checks to primary schools and pre-school centres. They not only replicated the previous SDS preventive program but also extended it. A third reason for employing more therapists has been that their scope of practice has been widened in both procedures and age range. Instead of therapists being limited to seeing children up to the age of 18, the age limit for invasive procedures has been raised to 25 years and for examinations, diagnostic procedures and emergency care, therapists can now treat all adults.

In many public dental agencies, dentists do not use their full scope of practice either because the remuneration to the agency does not justify the time and materials spent, or because the dentists perform the procedures so infrequently that their skill levels have not developed enough. These impediments reinforce each other. The result is that therapists can do most of the work done by dentists in these situations, and as therapists are less expensive to employ, there is a preference to employ them. While being a rational use of the workforce mix, this raises issues about the potential de-skilling of dentists in the public sector and the inability to employ them to their highest scope of practice.

Workforce planning challenges

The AIHW's projections, made in 1994, concerning the number of dentists in Australia and their gender balance by the year 2020 turned out to be wrong. Instead of rising from 7,493 in 1992 to 7,612 in 2021 (AIHW, 1998, Table 3.10), the number of dentists has risen to more than 18,100, while the percentage of female dentists has exceeded the projected 16.5% to reach approximately 43% (APHRA DBA, 2020). The AIHW's dire warning of a national undersupply of dentists was a major factor underpinning the dramatic increase in their numbers. Over much the same time, the number of dentists in Victoria grew from 2,297 in 1990 to 4,845 by December 2022 (DBA, APHRA, 2022).

Projections of future demand are traditionally based on historic trends. Typically, they make assumptions based on known variables but cannot account for unknown variables. At about the same time that the AIHW report was released, the University of Melbourne Dental School used a WHO-created software program to forecast the need for dental services and workforce requirements for the years 2000 and 2020. This modelling showed that the ratio of dentists-to-population for 2000, then only six years in the future, was nearly correct, namely, 1:1998 forecast versus 1:1922 actual. It was, however, inaccurate for 2020. The forecast ratio was 1:2165 but the actual ratio turned out to be 1:1483. The investigators noted that the software did not take into account changing political priorities, changes in workforce mix or advances in technology (Morgan et al., 1994).

More recently, Tennant and colleagues (Tennant et al., 2017) have pointed out several false assumptions made in workforce predictions in the 1990s. Among their criticisms were that, as the population lived longer, dentists were retiring later and, while patients were retaining more teeth, they also had complex dental needs necessitating more care. Moreover, patterns of past dental care could not take account of changes in dental policy or schemes for publicly funded treatment. The rapid rise in population through immigration and the attendant rise in foreign dentists wanting registration were also not foreseen. Some of these variables fall on either side of the ledger. For example, the increase in overseas-trained dentists has outpaced the rise in population, and the lessening of childhood dental decay due to water fluoridation has been counterbalanced by more dentate people living longer with attendant dental needs. While forecast modelling becomes ever more sophisticated, our human genius for unpredictability continues to thwart the best-laid plans.

In a 2020 article on oral health workforce planning, Stephen Birch and co-authors commented on the paucity and deficiencies of planning for a "fit-for-purpose" dental workforce (Birch et al., 2020). They noted that using existing levels of service delivery productivity as a basis to project needs for future population size simply "baked in" existing deficiencies. They have proposed a bottom-up needs-based approach that draws on the three independent elements of epidemiology: care, pathways and productivity. They argue that plans must be predicated on the answers to four questions: Who are we caring for; what are the expected levels of risk and oral health; what services do we plan to provide for which different groups; and how do we plan to provide those services?

Unfortunately, previous plans have underestimated variables such as the size of the influx of overseas graduates and changes in the population's perceptions of needs. The funding imperatives of universities are also poorly related to workforce projections and, in terms of needs, today's extravagance has a tendency to become tomorrow's basic requirement. The private sector, in particular, responds with greater alacrity to evolving expressed needs, while in the public sector changes in policy and practice are more difficult to achieve. In both sectors, the power imbalance between service provider and consumer has changed greatly over the past 50 years.

Since the advent of new types of registrable dental practitioner in the past 50 years any attempt to calculate a workforce commensurate with observed needs has become even more difficult. By 2010, while dentists comprised about 75% of the practitioners on the Dental Register (AHIW, 2014), they provided more than 75% of the total care due to longer annual hours of clinical work (AIHW, 2014). Before circa 1980, when the first trained advanced dental technicians and dental therapists were emerging, dentists supplied all clinical services. At the same time, they could never meet demand for services due to their insufficient numbers and the geographic and financial-access barriers to care.

Private dental practices which provide about 80% of the clinical treatment in Victoria are also business enterprises which can only exist in an area of population size and density which allows them to be economically viable. Similarly, public sector clinics can only exist where the population density allows recruitment of staff and justifies spending public money on capital and recurrent expenses. These reasons mean that people who live in remote areas either have to travel long distances for services, or some form of outreach service needs to be provided by the private or public sector.

Bree Graham and colleagues have mapped private practices Australia-wide and correlated them with Statistical Areas Level 2 (SA2). These areas are the size of urban suburbs or larger rural areas and there are 428 in Victoria (Graham et al., 2019). Graham and her co-researchers have shown that only about a fifth of Victoria's SA2s do not have a private practice within their boundaries, and this is the smallest proportion for any state in Australia (Graham et al., 2019). Their analysis used the Index of Relative Socioeconomic Disadvantage (IRSD) and showed that Victoria has the smallest difference in practice-to-population ratios between the richest 20% and the poorest 20% of its population (Graham et al., 2019). This relatively egalitarian distribution of private practices is due to Victoria's compact size compared to other mainland states. In turn, this means that population nodes or hubs do not leave too many people isolated by great distances, and professional service providers who have branch practices do not have to be separated from their urban cultural or social networks for too long.

The new dental practitioners

The fourfold increase in the number of other dental practitioners since 1980 – from 305 to 1,364 – has broadened the reach of the dental workforce and altered the scope of practice of them all. Originally dental therapists were trained for, and their practice limited to, the SDS. Since that service stopped operating independently in 2008, about two thirds now work in public sector community health agencies (Teusner et al., 2016) and their patient age limit has been raised to 25 years if the dental therapists have studied to extend their scope of practice. Most of their patients are still primary school children and regardless of whether they practice in the public or private sector, their work is mainly restorative dentistry.

Tertiary-trained Bachelor of Oral Health graduates or oral health therapists (OHTs) with degrees mainly from LTU or the University of Melbourne, are gradually superseding dental therapists in the workforce. Their average age is younger and two thirds of them are in the private sector (Teusner et al., 2016), where their main duties are preventive. This is the opposite of the older dental therapists. Those OHTs who are in the public sector have the same orientation to restorative dentistry as dental therapists (Teusner et al., 2016).

Dental hygienists' tertiary training is delivered together with oral health therapists for part of their course of study. Originally, they were introduced to provide preventive services and oral health education. Now more than 95% work in the private sector (Teusner et al., 2016) with most employed in larger general practices and some in specialist practices. In general, they augment the services of the private or public clinics where they work and do not compete with dentists for patients.

Like dental hygienists, most prosthetists work in the private sector where they often have separate denture clinics. In both public and private sectors, dental prosthetists now make the overwhelming majority of removable dental prostheses or dentures. In Victoria they gained the right to make partial dentures under the Kirner ALP Government in 1991. Ironically, after the bitter struggle to stop technicians (prosthetists) treating patients for most of the 20th century (Chapter 2), most dentists would now not want to, and probably would also not be able to, construct dentures for patients by themselves.

The roles and scope of practice of the new types of dental practitioners have evolved to be broader than originally conceived. Formerly called dental auxiliaries, like the dentists, they too have been known as "dental practitioners" since the creation of the Dental Practice Board of Victoria in 2000. All types of practitioners share in the governance of the profession. Although dentists retain the broadest scope of practice, there is no implication that any occupational group is inferior. In Victoria, all of the dental practitioner workforces have grown in response to population growth and demand for improved dental health. As people are living longer[16] and retaining their teeth for much longer (Crocombe & Slade, 2007), the total potential pool of teeth requiring maintenance or treatment has grown enormously. Further, people's levels of self-perception in social appearance and dental wellbeing have risen over time, as they compare themselves with peers and they are exposed to mass advertising and social media propaganda.

Two other groups in the dental workforce are often overlooked and underappreciated: the dental assistants and dental technicians. Neither group requires registration because they do not treat patients directly by themselves. However, training courses for both groups have led to an expanded scope of practice based on higher levels of attainment.

Dental assistants (DAs) were formerly known as dental nurses, a term still in common use. Without them, dental practice would almost come to a halt, as any dentist confronted by their sudden absence would attest. For the restorative and surgical aspects of dentistry their contributions are virtually indispensable. In common with the situation in general nursing, the more that services develop in terms of technological sophistication, the more the DAs are required. For example, the advent of the high-speed, water-cooled drill in 1957 made DAs increasingly necessary as part of an operating team.

16 Life expectancy in Australia in 1970 was 71 years and in 2020 is 83.4 years. Data sourced from ABS Year books 1970 to 2010 and ABS *National, state and territory population data* released 17 June 2021.

The RDHM offered a three-year training course for dental nurses from at least the mid-1950s. In 1963 it moved to a spacious building opposite the Royal Melbourne Hospital in Grattan Street where it became possible and necessary to have larger yearly intakes. Moreover, attrition rates were high, as a career generally ended when a dental nurse got married. In the Victorian Public Service this was a mandatory ruling (though not solely targeting dental hospital nurses), while in the private sector it was more an unofficial rite of passage. Now women marry at an older age and enjoy a longer career in their occupations of whatever kind. In dentistry this has resulted in a more settled and better-trained workforce.

In its early years, private dentists viewed the RDHM dental assistant course as too long and impractical. In the late 1970s the Australian Dental Association Victorian Branch started a one-year course to supplement in-practice training for the great majority of dental nurses working in the private sector. After DHSV was created in 1995, and before RDHM moved to new premises in 2003, the Royal Melbourne Institute of Technology (RMIT) took over the training of DAs for the private and public dental sectors.

While training courses for DAs have not been mandatory, graduates gain greater theoretical and practical understanding of oral health, especially relating to infection control measures. Since the advent of voluntary practice accreditation of private and public dental clinics in July 2012, this has become increasingly important. Accreditation covers all the clinical and management aspects of a practice. It was an outcome of national regulation of all health professions in 2010, at which time the Australian Commission on Safety and Quality in Healthcare set national standards for eight areas of activity, six of which are relevant to dentistry (ACSQH, 2019).[17] As DAs are intimately involved across all six areas, their training and responsibilities have grown. Formal training has the added bonus of higher pay rates, commensurate with the level of attainment.

Courses up to Certificate IV level are now run by RMIT University and other TAFE colleges. Level IV certification in radiography or oral health education offers a possibility for a limited degree of independent patient contact within the context of a clinic. When administrative roles and training are added to clinical ones, there is now a much more structured career path for DAs than existed in 1970. Further developments in certification and scope of practice may in future lead to recognition by registration.

Dental technicians whose main activity was construction of dentures were generally called dental mechanics until the Dental Technicians Act 1972 (Vic) came into effect. The Act introduced licences after a three-year apprenticeship and dental technicians' names were placed on a roll, not a register. Those who wished to treat patients underwent further training to became advanced dental technicians (now prosthetists) and were part of a separate register. However, many technicians who made fixed prostheses of crowns and bridges chose to remain in dental laboratories, either their own or in larger commercial combines, and to work to the prescription of a dentist. As the population increasingly retained teeth, technician training had to follow that trend by continually upgrading skills for crown and bridge construction and the artistry of ceramic restorations. Technological advancement in CAD/CAM porcelain milling

17 NSQHS eight standards: Clinical Governance, Partnering with Consumers, Preventing and Controlling Healthcare-associated Infections, Medication Safety, Comprehensive Care, Communicating for Safety, Blood Management, and Recognising and Responding to Acute Deterioration. Dentistry omits the last two.

and an ever-increasing demand for better aesthetic appearance have meant that some ceramicists have become more celebrated than the dentists with whom they work. Meanwhile, many people still require removable dentures. As the dental technician role covers a broader range of tasks than a single person would wish to attempt, a de facto specialisation exists, mirroring what has happened in dentistry.

The dental team comprising a mix of practitioners still has a long way to go in terms of the coordination of planning and delivery of services to Victorians. To some extent this is a historical legacy of a cottage-industry approach in dentistry, but it is also due to a failure of collective leadership in forging a new best practice model. Since 1996, when the training of dental therapists moved into the RDHM, the opportunity for a more holistic management of dental patients has been available. Yet apart from minimal efforts, the training of dentists and therapists has remained siloed. Without early integration, even if only in theory rather than practice, it is hardly surprising that services continue to be relatively compartmentalised.

Corporatisation in the private sector is growing in the 21st century and is creating new models of care but these are more business models based on optimising – or is that maximising? – profit. It is unlikely that the owner-practitioner practice will disappear though because in the long run, good dentistry is based on a relationship and on trust. Corporate-earnings targets and high staff turnover do not enhance either of these.

In the public sector, DHSV introduced a new "value-based" model of care in 2018 but it is still too early to evaluate it. The new person-centred model focuses on prevention, early identification and minimal intervention, which supports clients to self-manage their own oral health (DHSV, 2019, p. 10) (Chapter 6).

A profit motive and a value basis are not necessarily mutually exclusive and perhaps other permutations may arise. Even now, there are enlightened clinics in the public and private sectors inventing their own new pathways but they are still few in number and are more like lighthouses than general street lighting. We are still a work in progress.

References

Atkinson, H. F. (1990). *In defence of ivory towers. The history of the Royal Dental Hospital of Melbourne.* Melbourne: H. F. Atkinson private publication.

Australian Bureau of Statistics (ABS). (2020). *National, state and territory population.* Reference period December 2020. <https://www.abs.gov.au/statistics/people/population/national-state-and-territory-population/dec-2020>

Australian Commission on Safety and Quality in Healthcare. (ACSQH). (2019). *The NSQHS standards.* <https://www.safetyandquality.gov.au/standards/nsqhs-standards>

Australian Dental Council. (ADC). (2015). *Annual report July 2014 – June 2015.* Melbourne: ADC Ltd.

Australian Dental Council. (ADC). (2019). *Annual report 2018/19.* <https://adc.org.au/files/corporate/annual-reports/2019_ADC_Annual_Report.pdf>

Australian Health Practitioner Regulation Authority, Dental Board of Australia (AHPRA DBA). (2020). *Annual report 2019/20. Ten years of your national scheme for safer health care.* <https://www.ahpra.gov.au/Publications/Annual-reports/Annual-Report-2020.aspx>

Australian Institute of Health and Welfare. (AIHW). (1998). *Australian oral health and dental services, p.72.* <https://www.aihw.gov.au/getmedia/195dc54a-7013-443f-95a6-b8c006967f89/ausoralhealth.pdf.aspx?inline=true>

Australian Institute of Health and Welfare. (AIHW). (2014). *Dental workforce 2012. National Health Workforce Series No. 7, Cat. no. HWL 53.* <https://www.aihw.gov.au/reports/workforce/dental-workforce-2012/summary>

Australian Institute of Health and Welfare. (AIHW). (2020, December 31). *Oral health and dental care in Australia.* <https://www.aihw.gov.au/reports/dental-oral-health/oral-health-and-dental-care-in-australia-2015/contents/about>

Australian Institute of Health and Welfare. (AIHW) and Chrisopoulos, S., Harford, J. E., & Ellershaw, A. (2016). *Oral health and dental care in Australia. Key facts and figures 2015.* <https://www.aihw.gov.au/reports/dental-oral-health/oral-health-dental-care-2015-key-facts-figures/summary>

Australian Institute of Health and Welfare Dental Statistics and Research Unit. (AIHW DSRU). (1998). *Australia's oral health and dental services.* The University of Adelaide. DSRU Series No. 18. Cat. no. DEN 13. <https://www.aihw.gov.au/getmedia/195dc54a-7013-443f-95a6-b8c006967f89/ausoralhealth.pdf.aspx?inline=true>

Biggs, A. (2015). *Dental health. Budget review 2015–16 index.* <https://www.aph.gov.au/About_Parliament/Parliamentary_Departments/Parliamentary_Library/pubs/rp/BudgetReview201516/Dental>

Birch, S., Ahern, S., Brocklehurst, P., Chikte, U., Gallagher, G., Stefan Listl, S., & Woods, N. (2020). Planning the oral health workforce: Time for innovation. *Community Dent Oral Epidemiol, 49*(1), 17–22. <doi.org/10.1111/cdoe.12604>

Crocombe, L., & Slade, G. (2007). Decline of the edentulism epidemic in Australia. *Aust Dent J, 52*(2), 154–156. <https://onlinelibrary.wiley.com/doi/10.1111/j.1834-7819.2007.tb00482.x>

Dental Advisory Committee. (DAC). (1969). *Report of the Dental Advisory Committee to the Honorable the Minister of Health, 1969.* Melbourne: DAC.

Dental Board of Victoria. (DBV). (1993). *A history of its first hundred years.* Melbourne: DBV.

Dental Board of Australia AHPRA. (DBV AHPRA). (2022). *Registrant data October 2022 to December 2022.*

Dental Health Services Victoria. (DHSV). (2019). *Annual report 2018–19.* <https://www.dhsv.org.au/__data/assets/pdf_file/0010/158635/DHSV-Annual-Report-2018-19.pdf>

Dental Practice Board of Victoria. (DPBV). (2007). *Practice of Dentistry by Dental Hygienists and Dental Therapists Code of Practice No: C002 [July 2007]*

Department of Human Services (DHS). (1998). *Review of Dentists Act and Dental Technicians Act 1972. Final report July 1998.* <http://ncp.ncc.gov.au/docs/Victorian%20review%20of%20Dentist%20Act%201972%20and%20Dental%20Technicians%20Act%201972%2C%20July%201998.pdf>

Department of Human Services (DHS). (2007). *Improving Victoria's oral health.* <https://vgls.sdp.sirsidynix.net.au/client/search/asset/1291900>

Duckett, S., Cowgill, M., & Swerissen, H. (2019). *Filling the gap. A universal dental scheme for Australia.* Melbourne: Grattan Institute. <https://grattan.edu.au/wp-content/uploads/2019/03/915-Filling-the-gap-A-universal-dental-scheme-for-Australia.pdf>

Graham, B., Tennant, M., Shiikha, Y., & Kruger, E. (2019). Distribution of Australian private dental practices. Contributing underlining sociodemographics in the maldistribution of the dental workforce. *Aust. J. Prim. Health, 25*(1), pp. 54–59. <https://www.publish.csiro.au/py/py17177>

Health Department of Victoria. (HDV). (1986). *Ministerial review of dental services. Final report.* Melbourne: HDV.

Lane, J. (1970). *Dental Services for Australians.* Victorian Fabian Society, Pamphlet 21.

Melbourne Dental Hospital Council (1964, July). *Appendix 5. Minutes of Melbourne Dental Hospital Council.* [Unpublished statement]. Melbourne: University of Melbourne Archives.

Miscellaneous Acts (Health and Justice) Amendment Act 1995 (Vic).

Morgan, M. V., Wright. F. A., Lawrence. A. J., Laslett, A. M., (1994). Workforce predictions. A situational analysis and critique of the World Health Organisation (sic) model. *Int Dent J, 44*(1), pp. 27–32.

National Health Workforce Datasets (2021). <https://hwd.health.gov.au/resources/information/nhwds.html>

Phillips, J., & Simon-Davies, J. *Migration – Australian migration flows and population.* <https://www.aph.gov.au/About_Parliament/Parliamentary_Departments/Parliamentary_Library/pubs/BriefingBook45p/MigrationFlows>

Powell, G., & Mcintyre, S. (2015). *Land of opportunity. Australia's post-war reconstruction. Research guide.* <https://www.naa.gov.au/sites/default/files/2020-06/research-guide-land-of-opportunity.pdf>

Robertson, J. (1989). *Dentistry for the masses?* [Unpublished Master's thesis]. Carlton, Victoria: University of Melbourne.

Tennant, M., Kruger, E., Walsh, L., & Brostek, A. (2017). Predicting the dental workforce. Flood, famine, hysteria or hysteresis? *Faculty Dental Journal, 8*(2), 82–86. <doi.org/10.1308/rcsfdj.2017.82>, Faculty of Dental Surgery, Royal College of Surgeons, England.

Teusner, D. N., Amarasena, N., Satur, J., Chrisopoulos, S., & Brennan, D. S. (2016). Dental service provision by oral health therapists, dental hygienists and dental therapists in Australia. Implications for workforce modelling. *Community Dent Health, 33*(1), pp. 15–22.

University of Melbourne. (2022, June 13). *Bachelor of oral health. Study.* <https://study.unimelb.edu.au/find/courses/undergraduate/bachelor-of-oral-health>

Chapter 4
The Oral Health System
– Plans, programs and politics

John Rogers

Introduction

The history of dental public health in Victoria and Australia over the past five decades unfortunately cannot testify to continual progress towards ever better oral health. Gains have been made, but major problems remain (Chapter 10). Dental diseases are still among the most expensive of all diseases to treat and, in contrast to medical care, individuals pay most of the costs (Chapter 9). The largest share of the burden of preventable oral disease continues to fall on disadvantaged populations.

While national governments have made some investments in dental public health since 1970, most have been short term. Victorian governments have also contributed spasmodically. By 2020 about 400,000 Victorians were able to access public dental care each year, representing less than 20% of eligible people (Chapter 5). While emergency care was more readily available by 2020, the wait for general dental care was almost two years.

This chapter reviews the evolution of the Victorian and Australian oral health systems since 1970. To understand why developments in public dental programs occurred at certain times – and how successful they were – we review funded dental programs and consider the drivers and the enablers that have occasionally elevated and kept dental health on the crowded policy agenda.

We examine the barriers that have restrained the political profile of dental health and how public dental programs have been shaped by the leanings of the government of the day and by the 32 significant dental public health audits, reports and plans undertaken over the past 50 years. Drivers for funding to dental public health programs are further examined through three case studies. It is hoped that our findings provide insights for more effective oral health policy in the future.

Victoria's oral health system

In Victoria, as in the rest of Australia, dental care is mainly provided in private practice, with the public dental sector providing around 15–20% of all dental services. In the main, public dental care for adults has been provided as a safety net to disadvantaged groups and is not included in the universal public health care program of Medicare (Box 4.1). Provision of public school dental services (SDS) has varied over the last 50 years as outlined in Chapter 5.

The public share of expenditure on dental services in Australia since 1970 has fluctuated between 10–20% (Chapter 9). By comparison, public expenditure has equated to around 75% in Japan, 35–40% in Sweden, and less than 10% in the USA and Canada (Canadian Academy of Health Sciences, 2014). As such, Victoria's dental system is more similar to the USA's predominantly private sector model than to those in Scandinavia and Japan, which, in keeping with stronger redistributive and universal welfare policies, allocate more public funding for dental care.

In Victoria, public dental care is provided at the Royal Dental Hospital of Melbourne (RDHM) and by community dental clinics. Care is targeted to children and adults on lower incomes (eligible groups are listed at Appendix 4.1). Private dentists work primarily in solo or small group practices, although the private sector is also involved in providing publicly funded dental services under certain Victorian and national government programs.

The dominant dental public health service in Victoria in 1970 was the RDHM, which was established in 1890. From 1983 to 1996 it was governed by a committee of management appointed by the Health Minister. A SDS managed by the Department of Health was established in 1921. Unlike those of other Australian states, it did not employ dental therapists, and only treated children from a small number of primary schools in lower socioeconomic suburbs.

There were fewer than ten dental clinics in general hospitals providing public dental care to the community and these were governed by the hospital boards. In addition, about 20 local governments had established pre-school dental clinics as part of their Maternal and Child Health Services. These were partially subsidised by the Victorian Department of Health and did not provide a full-time service (DH&CS, 1995).

Since 1970 the number of public dental clinics in Victoria has almost tripled from about 35 to 94, while the Victorian population has approximately doubled (Chapter 1). These are managed by 51 organisations – 26 community health services and 25 hospitals. A peak dental public health agency, Dental Health Services Victoria (DHSV), established in 1996 after the merger of the RDHM and the SDS, purchases dental care from public dental clinics on behalf of the Department of Health. Local government pre-school dental clinics have been integrated into community clinics. In 2019 the SDS was re-established as the Smile Squad and is building up a fleet of vans for examination and the provision of dental care for children in government schools (Chapter 5).

The best laid plans, reviews, reports and research

As an indication of an increasing focus on dental public health, most of the 32 significant dental public health reviews, reports and plans published between 1970 and 2020 have been undertaken since 2000 (17), with ten in the past decade and only four prior to 1990 (Appendix 1.1). There have been 17 Victorian and 15 significant national documents.

Implementation of plans and reports has varied. While some sank without trace, they have generally helped to raise the profile of oral health problems and put forward possible solutions. The importance of specific reviews, reports and plans will be explored in the discussion of enablers of the major dental initiatives in the next section. The impact of Victorian oral health plans and reviews is considered in Chapter 5.

Comprehensive national oral health planning only began in 1999 under the aegis of the Australian Health Ministers' Advisory Council (AHMAC). The first national oral health plan, *Healthy mouths, healthy lives: Australia's national oral health plan 2004–2013*, was endorsed by all state Health Ministers in 2004 (AHMAC, 2004). The second national plan, covering 2015–2024, is an extension of the first plan and was endorsed by the Council of Australian Governments Health Council in 2015 (COAG Health Council, 2015). Both plans have been general in nature and do not identify funding requirements or allocate responsibility for actions.

Some progress has been made in implementing the recommendations of the two national plans. Extension of water fluoridation has occurred in all jurisdictions except Queensland; there have been positive workforce developments; and governance has been democratised with broad representation on the Australian Dental Board of the oral health professions as well as consumers. However, limited access to public dental services and a limited prevention focus remain major issues across Australia.

The Australian Institute of Health and Welfare (AIHW) released the first monitoring report for the 2015–2024 oral health plan in 2020 (AIHW, 2020). Of the 31 key performance indicators, the report noted favourable trends in relation to seven indicators, unfavourable trends in nine, no change in a further nine, and no or insufficient data in six instances.

Dental research is predominantly undertaken in the universities that train undergraduate and postgraduate dental students. Dental practice-based research in Victoria also occurs through the eviDent Foundation, a partnership between the University of Melbourne Dental School and the Victorian branch of the Australian Dental Association (ADAVB). Australian government funding for dental research is minimal. Between 2017 and 2021, oral health research received only 0.23% of the National Health and Medical Research Centre (NHMRC) funding (Ghanbarzadegan, 2023).

'No human being is constituted to know the truth, the whole truth and nothing but the truth; and even the best of men must be content with fragments, with partial glimpses, never the full fruition.'

– William Osler

Public dental health programs 1970 to 2022 – Government focus and enablers for support

Funded initiatives

Government recognition of dental public health as a priority has occurred in cycles. A timeline of major public dental health programs set in train by Victorian and Australian national governments over the past five decades is presented in Figure 4.1.

Figure 4.1 Australia and Victorian government dental health funded initiative, 1970 to 2022

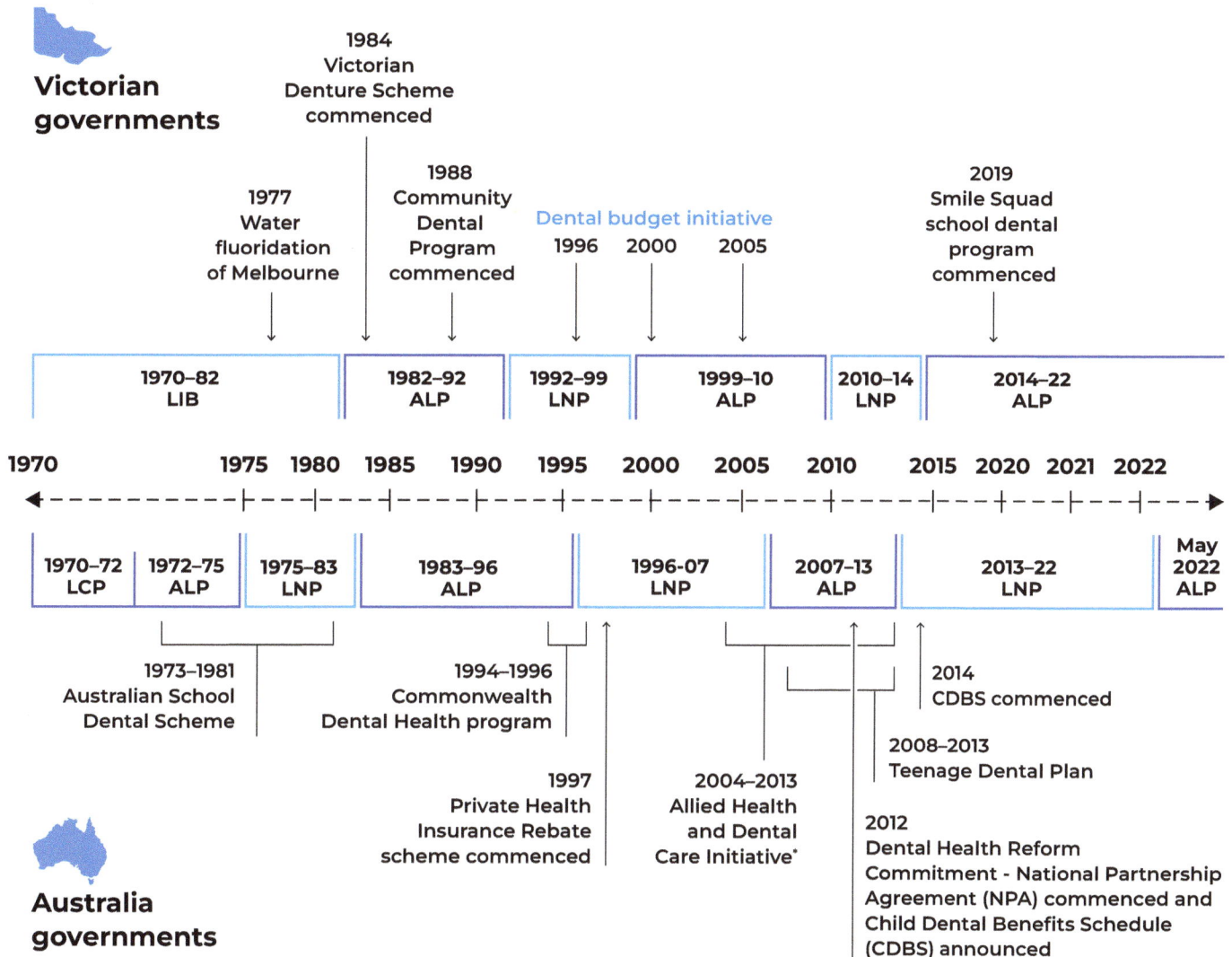

Victorian governments

1984
Victorian Denture Scheme commenced

1988
Community Dental Program commenced

1977
Water fluoridation of Melbourne

2019
Smile Squad school dental program commenced

Dental budget initiative
1996   2000   2005

| 1970–82 LIB | 1982–92 ALP | 1992–99 LNP | 1999–10 ALP | 2010–14 LNP | 2014–22 ALP |

1970   1975 1980   1985   1990   1995   2000   2005   2010   2015 2020 2021 2022

| 1970–72 LCP | 1972–75 ALP | 1975–83 LNP | 1983–96 ALP | 1996-07 LNP | 2007–13 ALP | 2013–22 LNP | May 2022 ALP |

1973–1981
Australian School Dental Scheme

1994–1996
Commonwealth Dental Health program

2014
CDBS commenced

1997
Private Health Insurance Rebate scheme commenced

2004–2013
Allied Health and Dental Care Initiative*

2008–2013
Teenage Dental Plan

2012
Dental Health Reform Commitment - National Partnership Agreement (NPA) commenced and Child Dental Benefits Schedule (CDBS) announced

Australia governments

Legend

ALP	Australian Labor Party		
CDBS	Child Dental Benefits Scheme	LNP	Liberal National Party Coalition
LCP	Liberal Country Party Coalition	NPA	National Partnership Agreements

Notes:
*Became the Medicare Chronic Disease Dental Scheme
1. The National Partnership Agreement (NPA) became the Federation Funding Agreement (FFA) in 2021-22 and 2022-23.
2. The Victorian government dental budget initiatives shown occurred in the financial years 1996-97, 1999-2000, 2004-05.

Fourteen significant government-funded dental initiatives have occurred between 1970 and 2022 – seven national, and seven Victorian government programs.

Larger national government programs have been established approximately every 20 years namely the:

- Australian School Dental Scheme (ASDS) 1973-1981
- Commonwealth Dental Health Program (CDHP) 1994–1996
- Private Health Insurance Rebate (PHIR) scheme from 1997
- Allied Health and Dental Care initiative in 2004 that became the Medicare Chronic Disease Dental Scheme (CDDS) 2007–2013
- National Partnership Agreement (NPA) from 2012-13 and the
- Commonwealth Child Dental Benefits Schedule (CDBS) from 2014.

In Victoria, significant new funding for public dental programs has occurred every 10 to 15 years namely the:

- Fluoridation of Melbourne 1977,
- Community Dental Program (CDP) 1989,
- Creation of Dental Health Services Victoria (DHSV) and a dental health budget initiative 1996
- Budget initiative 2004-05
- Smile Squad school dental program 2019.

Smaller funding allocations were provided in 1984 for the Victorian Denture Scheme, and in 1999–2000 for public dental clinics. The overall goal of these initiatives was to enhance access to public dental care and to prevent dental disease.

National government funding has been erratic over the past 52 years, with only three of the seven programs still operating in 2022. Over this period, the average duration of national government programs has been six years, and new governments have most often ceased the previous government's initiatives. All of the seven Victorian government initiatives remain active.

Political party approaches

Political ideologies have shaped dental programs markedly. Labor governments have more actively fostered a wider public health and social welfare public dental network than Coalition governments, which have focused more on supporting access to the private dental sector. Most of the 14 significant initiatives during the period under examination were Labor government programs: five of the seven Victorian programs, and five of the seven national programs. Coalition governments introduced two programs in Victoria and two nationally and have continued two Labor-initiated programs.

But which parties were in power and able to act? In the half century covered in our review, Coalition governments have been in power nationally for 30 years and Labor governments for 23 years (Figure 4.2). In Victoria the opposite has been the case; Labor has governed for 30 years and the Coalition for 23.

Figure 4.2 Governments and time in office, Victoria and Australia, 1970–2022. Years and (terms of office)

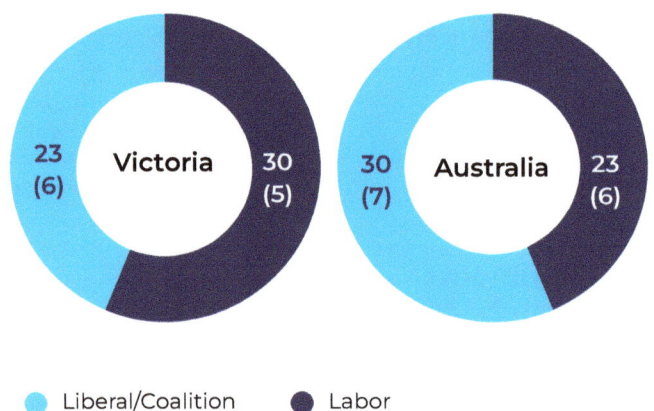

Victoria: 23 (6), 30 (5)
Australia: 30 (7), 23 (6)

● Liberal/Coalition ● Labor

Sources: Figures calculated using data from Australian Prime Ministers Centre (n.d.); McCann, 2016; National Museum of Australia (n.d.); and Parliament of Victoria, 2017.

While duration in power provided opportunities for reform, political ideology has been more important in shaping the dental public health policies of the two major parties.

Nationally, Labor governments have had an interest in redressing disadvantage by expanding public dental services; notably, the 1973 ASDS; the 1994 CDHP for adults; and the 2012 NPA. Coalition governments have focused more on efficiency, enhancing private provision, and support for individuals to meet the costs of dental care. Major Coalition programs have been the 2007 PHIR, and subsidised dental care for adults through public and private dentists such as the Allied Health and Dental Care Initiative in 2004 that became the Medicare CDDS in 2007. Organised dentistry has generally supported this approach, which involves fee-for-service payments to private practitioners rather than employment of more public dental professionals.

Notwithstanding their different political priorities in relation to dental health, governments of both political persuasions have not always used their incumbency to deliver dental health initiatives. Several national governments – namely, the Gorton (later McMahon) Coalition 1970–1972; the Fraser Coalition 1975–1983, and the Hawke Labor Government of 1983–1991 before Keating became Prime Minister – failed to introduce any significant dental programs. In the 1970s and 1980s these governments reflected a view that dental care was either primarily a state responsibility, or a lesser priority in the quest for fiscal balance (Duckett et al., 2019). More recently, the Morrison Coalition Government failed to support a senior's dental care scheme proposed by the Labor Opposition during the 2019 election campaign. This suggests that the Coalition favoured personal responsibility in health care and was reluctant to pay for state dental schemes (Daly, 2021).

A current challenge for the Albanese Labor Government is to implement the oral health recommendations in the final report of the Royal Commission into Aged Care Quality and Safety (RCACQ&S, 2021). The Commission found the need to improve the oral health of nursing home residents through improved diet, oral hygiene support and enhanced access to dental care through introducing a Medicare Seniors Dental Benefit Scheme.

Figures 4.3 and 4.4 show significant funded dental programs, legislation, plans and prevention programs put in place by the 14 national and Victorian governments in power between 1970 and 2022. Also shown are the key policy drivers that propelled dental public health higher on the policy agenda during these years.

National governments

Australian governments have varied in the levels of attention they have paid to dental public health (Figure 4.3).

Figure 4.3 Significant National Government dental health initiatives in Australia, 1970 to 2022

National Government	Significant dental Initiatives	Policy drivers
1970–72 Gorton, McMahon Coalitions		
1972–75 Whitlam Labor	**Australian School Dental Scheme (ASDS)*** 1973–81 ASDS was called the School Dental Service (SDS) in Victoria	School dental scheme was included in a social reform platform[1] but dental care was not included in Medibank.
1975–1983 Fraser Coalition	Abolished ASDS 1981	School dental scheme was included in a social reform platform[1] but dental care was not included in Medibank.
1983–1996 Hawke, Keating Labor	• National Health Strategy, Improving Dental Health in Australia 1992 • **Commonwealth Dental Health Program (CDHP)** 1994–1996	Financial difficulty with access to dental care;[2] inequality in oral health; and long public dental waiting times.[3] No opposition from organised dentistry. Supportive Minister for Health and need for an election sweetener that would stimulate the economy.
1996–2007 Howard Coalition	• Abolished CDHP 1997 • **Private Health Insurance Rebate scheme (PHIR)** 2007 – ongoing • Allied Health & Dental Care Initiative 2004 became **Medicare Chronic Disease Dental Scheme (CDDS)** 2007–2013	Coalition stated that the CDHP had done its job by reducing waiting times.[4] Dental insurance included within broader Private Health Insurance Rebate scheme. Dental care included in broader allied health initiative requiring a GP referral to a dentist.

National Government	Significant dental Initiatives	Policy drivers
2007–2013 **Rudd, Gillard,** **Rudd Labor**	• Continuation of PHIR • **Medicare Teen Dental Plan** 2008–13 • National Health and Hospitals Reform Commission (NHHRC) Final Report 2009[5] • Report of the National Advisory Council on Dental Health 2012[6] • Dental Health Reform 2012 – **National Partnership on Public Dental Services for adults (NPA)** commenced **& Commonwealth Child Dental Benefits Schedule (CDBS)** announced • National Oral Health Promotion Plan 2013.[8]	Coalition stated that the CDHP had done its job by reducing waiting times.[4] Dental insurance included within broader Private Health Insurance Rebate scheme. Dental care included in broader allied health initiative requiring a GP referral to a dentist.
2013–2022 **Abbott, Turnbull,** **Morrison Coalitions**	• Continuation of PHIR & NPA • **CDBS** introduced in 2014 • Senate blocked proposed Coalition closure of CDBS & NPA, 2015	Long public dental waiting times; inequity in oral health highlighted in National Health and Hospitals Commission Final Report[5] and Report of the National Advisory Council on Dental Health.[6] Dental reform was a condition for the Greens Party to form an alliance with Labor in 2012.[7]
2022–ongoing **Albanese Labor**	• Continuation of PHIR, CDBS and NPA	

*Note: Funded programs, as distinct to other types of initiatives, are shown in bold text.

Sources:

1. Department of Health, Australia (DOHA). (1973). Annual Report of the Director-General of Health. <https://nla.gov.au/nla.obj-1745801827/view?sectionId=nla.obj-1847550851&partId=nla.obj-1751321551>
2. McClennand, A. (1991) *In fair health? Equity and the health system.* Background paper No. 3. Melbourne: National Health Strategy.
3. Dooland, M. (1992). *Improving dental health in Australia.* Background Paper No. 9. Melbourne: National Health Strategy.
4. Costello, P. (1996). CPD HR No. 7, 20 August 1996:3274.
5. National Health and Hospitals Reform Commission. (NHHRC). (2009). A *healthier future for all Australians. Final Report 2009.* Commonwealth of Australia.
6. National Advisory Council on Dental Health. (NACDH). (2012). Report of the National Advisory Council on Dental Health. 23 February 2012.
7. Metherall, M. (2012)
8. Wright, F. (2013). National Oral Health Promotion Plan.

National Labor

The first critical initiative in public dental funding since 1970 came from the national level under the socially progressive Whitlam Labor Government in 1973. The two subsequent Labor governments also introduced dental programs. School dental services (ASDS) were included in Labor's ambitious social reform platform of 1972 (DOHA, 1973), which included universal health insurance but did not cover dental care (Box 4.1). While the Keating Labor Government's CDHP of 1994–96 had a considerable impact on public dental waiting times, it was short-lived as it did not survive under the incoming Howard Government.

The Hawke (later Keating) Government of 1983–1996 did not initiate a significant dental program until Keating had defeated Hawke as leader in late 1991. Keating took the promise of the CDHP to the 1993 election because the National Health Strategy had highlighted inequality in oral health outcomes and financial difficulty with access to dental care (Dooland, 1992). Further drivers were support from the Minister of Health, Brian Howe, and the need for an election sweetener that would stimulate the economy. Details are outlined in the following case studies.

Soon after the Rudd Labor Government came to power in 2007, means-tested Medicare benefits for preventive dental health checks for teenagers were introduced (Biggs, 2008). Known as the Medicare Teen Dental Plan, it had limited reach, privileged better-off families (Duckett et al., 2019), and was criticised for not providing funding for dental treatment (Hopcraft, 2023). The Plan was closed in 2013 and replaced by the CDBS in 2014.

The Gillard Labor Government's $4 billion dental reform package of 2012 was a condition for the Greens Party support for her minority Labor government (Plibersek, 2012; Metherell, 2012). Long public dental waiting times and inequity in oral health were highlighted in two Labor initiated reports: the National Health and Hospitals Reform Commission Final Report (NHHRC, 2009) commissioned by Minister Roxon and the Report of the National Advisory Council on Dental Health (NACDH, 2012) commissioned by Minister Plibersek. The Dental Reform Package included the CDBS and the NPA. The latter commenced in 2012, while the CDBS commenced in 2014 under the Abbott Coalition Government after it won the September 2013 election. The 2019 review of the CDBS determined that the utilisation rate of the approximately three million eligible children, increased from 30% in 2014 to 38% in 2018 (Commonwealth of Australia, 2019).

Dental reforms through oral health promotion were also considered. In 2012 Minister Plibersek established a National Oral Health Promotion Plan Advisory Committee to write a promotion plan. The committee was chaired by Professor Wright and completed a draft plan in April 2013 which was not publicly released (Wright, 2013). The Abbott Government did not proceed with this initiative.

National Coalitions

Of the four national Coalition governments since 1970, the first two did not initiate dental programs; the third focused on support for individuals to meet the cost of dental care, while the fourth continued Labor programs. Neither the Gorton/McMahon (1970–72) nor Fraser coalitions (1975–83) introduced programs. Fraser closed Whitlam's school dental scheme (ASDS), and the Howard Coalition (1996–2007) closed the Keating Labor CDHP in 1996, because it had done its job of "cutting public dental waiting times" (Costello, 1996). The Abbott Coalition attempted to close Labor Prime Minister Gillard's 2012 dental reforms (CDBS and NPA) in 2015, but the Bill failed to pass in the Senate, which the Coalition did not control.

The Howard Government introduced two dental programs that were extensions of existing primary health initiatives. In 1997 the PHIR which provided subsidies to premium holders was extended to include dental insurance (Biggs, 2008). Then, in 2004, when dental care was included in the allied health initiative, community-based dentistry attracted Medicare benefits for the first time. The PHIR now accounts for almost half of national government funding for dental public health and flows mainly to people on high incomes (Chapter 9).

In 2007 the Allied Health and Dental Care program morphed into the Medicare CDDS. The scheme covered a comprehensive range of dental services for people with chronic and complex conditions on referral from a general practitioner. Claims of over-servicing and rorting were made and the scheme was poorly targeted (Duckett et al., 2019). At the peak of the scheme, annual per person funding was $99 in New South Wales, $67 in Victoria, and $26 in the Northern Territory (AIHW, 2020). The program was closed down as part of the Gillard Labor Government's $4 billion dental reform package of 2012 (Plibersek, 2012).

Victorian governments

Victorian governments have also paid varying levels of attention to dental public health, in accordance with their political ideologies. Significant initiatives and policy drivers over the study period are shown in Figure 4.4 with funded initiatives in bold text.

Figure 4.4 Significant Victorian government dental health initiatives, 1970 to 2022

Victorian Government	Significant dental Initiatives	Policy drivers
1970–1982 Bolte, Hamer, Thomson Coalitions	• *Dentists Act 1972, Dental Technicians Act 1972* • *Health (Fluoridation) Act 1973* • **Fluoridation of Melbourne water** 1977	Shortage of dentists; high tooth decay rates in children; advocacy from dental technicians for rights to treat patients; advocacy from ADAVB and dental public health workers for fluoridation.
1982–1992 Cain, Kirner Labor	• **Victorian Denture Scheme (VDS)** 1983 • Ministerial Review of Dental Services (MRODS) 1986 • **Community Dental Program (CDP)** 1989 as part of the Dental Health Strategy 1988	Long public dental waiting times and inequity in oral health;[1] advocacy from health and social welfare organisations (Molar Energy Campaign, Chapter 8: Alliances and Advocacy).
1992–1999 Kennett Coalition	• Health budget cut of 10% in 1993 • Future Directions for Dental Health in Victoria plan 1995 • Reorganisation of public dental services with creation of DHSV 1996 • **Oral health budget initiative 1996** • *Dental Practice Act 1999*	Economic rationalist "new public management" approach for smaller governments.[2] "Restructure and improve the public dental health system to ensure the provision of effective, efficient, quality and consumer friendly services".[3] Dental Practice Act 1999 as a response to national efforts to reduce red tape as recommended by Hilmer.[4]
1999–2010 Bracks, Brumby Labor	• **Oral health budget initiatives** 1999–2000, 2004–05 • Extension of water fluoridation to rural areas • Promoting oral health plan 2000–2004 • Improving Victoria's oral health plan 2007 • Integration of the School Dental Service (SDS) into the CDP	"Increasingly low levels of effective access to public dental services";[5] funding available under the Fairer Victoria policy; advocacy from health and social welfare organisations.

Victorian Government	Significant dental Initiatives	Policy drivers
2010–14 Baillieu, Napthine Coalition	• Victorian action plan for oral health promotion 2013–2017, 2014 • Healthy Families, Healthy Smiles program 2014	Long public dental waiting times; focus on prevention of oral disease.
2014–present Andrews Labor	• Smokefree Smiles & Oral Cancer Prevention programs • **Smile Squad** SDS 2019 • Victorian action plan to prevent oral disease 2020–30, 2020	Cost of living pressures and long commuting times for working families. Long public dental waiting times and pressure to introduce a more preventive approach in public dental services (A-GV, 2015).

Sources:

1. Department of Health. Victoria. (DHV). (1986). *Ministerial review of dental services: Final report.*
2. Carter, J. (2020, October 7). *Ideological tide swamped state. The Age.*
3. DH&CS. (1995). *Future directions for dental health in Victoria,* p. 4. Melbourne.
4. Hilmer, F. (1993). *National competition policy: Report by the Independent Committee of Inquiry.* Canberra: Commonwealth Govt. Printer.
5. Auditor-General Victoria. (A-GV). (2002). *Community dental services.* Melbourne: Victorian Auditor-General's Office, p. 52.

While most of the State's dental funding initiatives of the past five decades have been Labor government schemes (1982, 1988, 2000, 2005, 2019), Coalition governments have been active in planning (1995, 2014), legislation (1972, 1973, 1999), the restructure of dental public health services (1995) and prevention (1977, 2014).

Victorian Labor

After a period of almost 27 years of conservative governments, the Cain (later Kirner) Labor Government (1982–1992) was elected on a platform of social reform. The VDS was established in 1984, allowing Health Care Card holders to receive subsidised dentures from participating private dentists and prosthetists. A comprehensive ministerial review of dental services (MRODS) was established to, "assess and make recommendations on dental services in Victoria" (DHV, 1986). The major goals, recommendations and outcomes of this review are presented in Chapter 5, Appendix 5.2.

The Government responded to the ministerial review in 1988 with a Dental Health Strategy, providing additional resources to establish 29 public dental clinics, located mainly in community health services.[18] Clinics were predominantly integrated into locally managed community health centres in under-serviced areas of metropolitan Melbourne. This Community Dental Program (CDP) initiative was part of a commitment to "health for all" through provision of primary health care "for the people by the people", as articulated by the World Health Organization in the Alma Alta declaration (WHO, 1978). There was a degree of concern about this move from the ADAVB, which considered that the boards of community health centres lacked the expertise to manage dental care.

Among the drivers for the new dental health strategy were a community advocacy campaign, the Molar Energy Campaign (Chapter 8); the upcoming 1989 State election; the State health plan which proposed establishing dental health services in community health centres, and the Government's Social Justice Strategy (DPC, 1988).

When the Bracks (later Brumby) Labor Government (1999–2010) rather unexpectedly won the 1999 state election, public dental waiting times stood at 21 months for general dental care and 25 months for dentures (Treasury Victoria, 2000). The new government provided dental public health funding in the 1999–2000 (Treasury, Victoria, 2000) and 2004–05 Budgets (Treasury & Finance Victoria, 2004); extended community water fluoridation into rural areas; and developed dental care programs for young children. The *Improving Victoria's oral health plan,* released in 2007, announced the integration of the SDS into the CDP (DHS, 2007). Consequently, the SDS would no longer exist as a statewide service managed by DHSV (Chapter 5).

The Andrews Labor Government (2014–present) initiated the $321.9 million Smile Squad school dental program in 2019 (Premier of Victoria, 2019). This program provides free dental care for all children at government primary and secondary schools (Chapter 5). The Government has outlined its prevention agenda in the *Victorian action plan to prevent oral disease 2020–30* (DHHS, 2020) (Appendix 5.2). Its main features are to improve the oral health of children through the Smile Squad program; to promote healthy environments; improve oral health literacy, oral health promotion, screening, early detection; and prevention services.

---

18 The 1988 Dental Health Strategy included establishment of new services under local management; the progressive decentralisation of general practice resources away from the RDHM; the expansion of the VDS; employment of more dental therapists to increase services to primary school children; and establishment of an intern scheme for ten graduating dentists per annum.

Victorian Coalitions

Among the first of the three Victorian Coalition governments during the study period, the Bolte, (later Hamer and Thompson) Government (1970–82) passed significant dental workforce legislation (Chapter 2). The Kennett Government (1992–99) also introduced legislation, and cut, restructured, and then expanded dental public health services. The Baillieu (later Napthine) Government (2010–2014) released a prevention action plan (Chapter 5) and implemented the *Healthy Families Healthy Smiles* early childhood program in 2012 (DHSV, 2023) (Chapter 6).

Bolte's 1972 dental workforce legislation was important because it allowed dental therapists to provide dental care to children and advanced dental technicians to provide dentures direct to the public (Chapter 2). When Hamer – a supporter of community water fluoridation – replaced Bolte, the Coalition commenced fluoridation of Melbourne's drinking water in 1977. This occurred later than in all the other Australian capital cities, except Darwin and Brisbane (Appendix 4.2).

There was no political divide in introducing water fluoridation in Australia – both Liberal and Labor governments made decisions to proceed. Hobart and Canberra were the first to be fluoridated in 1964. Appendix 4.2 outlines the dates and governments in office when capital cities were fluoridated.

The Kennett Government (1992–99) oversaw a decade of activity in relation to dental public health. Faced with a budget crisis, his government cut the health budget, including the public dental budget, by 10% in 1993, but later increased dental funding in 1996. As a supporter of neoliberal notions of "New Public Management" and smaller governments (Carter, 2020), and to "Restructure and improve the public dental health system to ensure the provision of effective, efficient, quality and consumer friendly services" (DH&CS, 1995), Kennett merged the SDS with the RDHM to form a new lead public dental organisation – DHSV (Chapter 2).

In addition, the Kennett Government allocated $44 million to build a new RDHM, and released two dental plans – *Future directions for dental health in Victoria* in 1995 and *Promoting oral health 2000–2004* in 1999 (DH&CS, 1995; DHS, 1999). Kennett's dental legislation of 1999 was in keeping with the national Howard Government's mood for deregulation (Hilmer, 1993) and for broadening the representative base of the dental board.

By comparison with the Kennett Government, the Baillieu (later Napthine) Coalition's (2010–2014) contributions to dental public health were subdued. In 2012 the *Healthy families, healthy smiles* preschool program commenced and the *Victorian Action plan for oral health promotion 2013–2017* was released (DHSV, 2023; DHV, 2013). These initiatives had a prevention focus. *Healthy families, healthy smiles* is discussed in Chapter 6, section 2.1 and the action plan is summarised in Appendix 5.2.

Victoria slow to benefit

Victorians have not always benefited fully from national government dental programs, largely because Victorian governments have been slow to implement programs such as the SDS of the 1970s (Chapter 5), or eligible families have not participated in programs such as the CDBS (Chapter 9). In the mid 1970s Victoria's Coalition Government was slower than those of other jurisdictions to engage with the growth phase of Whitlam's SDS. This left Victoria with national government funding of less than $5 per primary school child per annum, compared with South Australia and Western Australia which received more than $20 per child (Government bureaucrat, personal communication, 2006).

Lack of national dental health program

One public dental program that has never been implemented is the inclusion of dental care in Medicare. Box 4.1 outlines the background to the decision to "leave the body without a mouth".

Box 4.1 Dentistry and Medicare – Why leave the body without a mouth?

Our history tells the story of what has happened over 50 years, but there's one thing that has not happened. A reader of this history might wonder why when two versions of a national health insurance scheme have been introduced, in 1974 and 1984, neither has covered dental services.

There had nearly been a national dental insurance scheme in 1949 as the Chifley Government's *National Health Services Act 1948* included dentistry. The provisions of the Act had not been finalised at its proclamation and, in any case, it perished with the Chifley Government at the general election of 1949 when a Menzies Coalition Government was returned. Successive Coalition governments espoused small government and claimed that dental services were a state responsibility.

Under the Whitlam Labor Government, the subject of a national health plan was revisited in 1973 but given the level of opposition by the medical profession to national insurance, Whitlam chose not to take on the dentists as well (Menadue, 2021). Further, he was less interested in creating a salaried medical service than in subsidising people to access the existing private medical system through universal health insurance (Scotton, 1977; Boxall & Gillespie, 2013). As the main argument was about health insurance and there was almost no dental insurance at that time, the Government had little incentive to include dentistry. Anecdotally, it was also apparent by 1973 that the UK's National Health Service (NHS) dental services were haemorrhaging money.

Although the Medibank universal health insurance scheme came into being in 1974, it was gradually defunded after the Fraser Government came to power in 1975 (Scotton, 2000). This is consistent with what Jenny Lewis has called "a residual view of the role of the state" on the part of non-Labor governments (Lewis, 2000, p. 69).

In 1983 the Australian Labor Party (ALP) won government from the Coalition and R. J. Hawke became Prime Minister. Health insurance reform was a priority and a new version of Medibank, called Medicare, was created in February 1984.

It was largely similar to the original, with universal insurance cover and free public hospital care partly funded by a levy on income tax (Biggs, 2004). Once more there was no mention of dentistry or dental health but in July that year, the Minister for Health, Neal Blewett, established a Medicare Benefits Review Committee chaired by Justice Robyn Layton (Layton, 1986). One of the Committee's terms of reference was to assess the possibility of extending Medicare to other types of health practitioner (Commonwealth, 1985, p. 4025).

Although the Layton Committee found that dentistry met all the essential criteria for public funding, it was judged as not meeting the objectives of Medicare (Layton, 1986, p. 204). Dental academic, John Spencer, found the reasoning flawed (Spencer, 1998). However, regardless of what the Layton report said, no dental services were added to Medicare for fear of adding unknown and likely high costs at a time of both budgetary stricture and fierce opposition from the dental profession via the Australian Dental Association (ADA) (Layton, 1986 p. 202).

Several major health reviews, including the Health and Hospitals Reform Commission, have since recommended that the national government introduce a universal scheme for access to basic dental services (NHHRC, 2009). Public support for the concept of a national scheme within or beside Medicare has been constant, even among Coalition voters (Cresswell, 2011). More recently, the Grattan Institute published a proposal for just such a national dental scheme (Duckett et al., 2019). The ALP took a commitment for the first phase of this initiative to the 2019 Federal Election with the support of the ADA. The Morrison Coalition Government was returned and showed no interest in the scheme.

As far as national government funding is concerned, the mouth has not been put back into the body.

Policy enablers for dental programs – Three case studies of policy processes

The 14 funded dental public dental health initiatives identified in Figures 4.1, 4.2 and 4.3 were established in varied circumstances. (Chapters 2 and 3 provide background to the origins of these initiatives). In this section, we present three case studies in which we identify and analyse enablers for the establishment of funded dental health programs using Kingdon's multiple streams theory (Kingdon, 2010).

The case studies are the:

1. 1994–96 Commonwealth Dental Health Program (CDHP),
2. 2004–05 Victorian dental budget initiative,
3. 2019 Victorian school dental program, known as the Smile Squad.

Kingdon's multiple streams theory, developed in the 1980s, holds that policy change comes about when three streams – problems, proposals and politics – connect, and there is a policy window (Figure 4.5). The theory has been employed internationally in many policy areas and is considered valid (Rawat & Morris, 2016).

Figure 4.5. Kingdon's Multiple Streams Theory

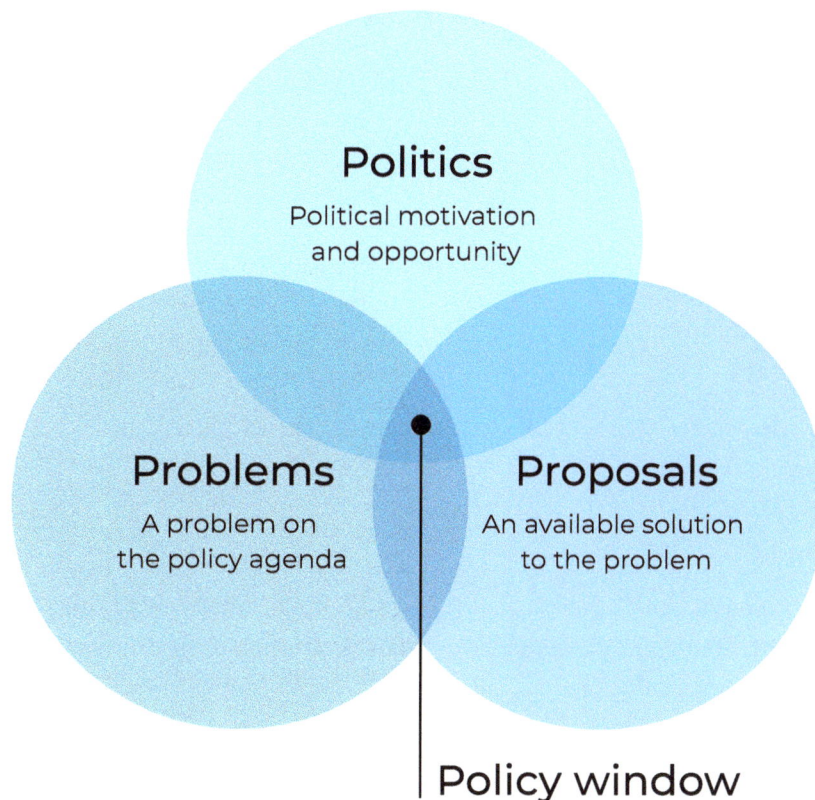

Based on Kingdon, 2010

1 Commonwealth Dental Health Program (CDHP) 1994–96

The objective of the CDHP was to improve the dental health of financially disadvantaged Australians; in particular, to shift the dental care provided to Health Care Card holders from emergency treatment to general dental care and prevention (SCARC, 1998). The Commonwealth provided a total of $245 million over the life of the CDHP, before it ceased funding and the states resumed full responsibility for public dentistry.

2 2004–05 Victorian Budget dental health initiative

This initiative provided a major boost for dental health services, investing $96 million over four years to significantly increase the number of people treated in the public sector, reduce waiting times, extend community water fluoridation in rural areas, and ensure pre-schoolers and primary school students had regular access to high-quality dental care (Treasury & Finance, 2004).

3 Smile Squad

The 2019–20 Victorian State Budget announced $321.9 million in funding over four years for the Smile Squad school dental program. Smile Squad dental teams visit schools to provide annual oral health packs, dental health examinations and follow-up treatment, as needed, at no cost to families (Premier of Victoria, 2019; DHV, 2023a).

Problems

In each of the three cases the problem was well defined and perceived as serious.

CDHP 1994–96: The issue of dental care made its way onto the policy agenda in the early 1990s through research undertaken by the *National health strategy* (NHS) initiative. This major policy inquiry, directed by Jenny Macklin, was tasked with reviewing Australia's existing health system. Among a series of background papers and issues papers delivered by the NHS, dental health research identified financial difficulty with access to dental care (McClelland, 1991), inequality in oral health and long public dental waiting times (Dooland, 1992).

Victorian Budget initiative 2004–05: A key enabler for the 2004–05 dental budget initiative was the Victorian Auditor-General's review of community dental services in 2002 (Auditor-General Victoria, 2002). Public dental waiting times had reached 22 months and the Victorian Government was spending less per capita on dental public health than most other states and territories (Chapter 9). A major recommendation of the Auditor-General's review was that the Government address the "increasingly low levels of effective access to public dental services" (Auditor-General Victoria, 2002, p. 52).

Smile Squad 2019: This school dental program was a response to both the problems of cost-of-living pressures (Premier of Victoria, 2019) and long commuting times for working families living in Melbourne's outer suburbs. Pressure had also built for the Government to respond to the 2016 Victorian Auditor-General's audit which called for the introduction of a more preventive approach in public dental services (Auditor-General Victoria, 2016).

Proposals

Proposed solutions were available for each of the three problems. The CDHP proposal clearly outlined a public dental program for adults (Dooland, 1992). The 2004–05 Victorian Budget rationale was to introduce additional services to decrease waiting times in the short term, allied with prevention initiatives (such as extending community water fluoridation) to reduce demand in the mid- to longer term. The Smile Squad would offer free dental care to children at government schools. Resources, such as dental chairs in community dental clinics previously used for treating school children, would be freed up to provide care for adults (Premier of Victoria, 2019).

All three proposals met the policy requirements of scientific plausibility (Nutbeam, 2003); technical feasibility (Kingdon, 2010); compatibility with government values and vision (Kingdon, 2010; Nutbeam, 2003), and reasonable cost (Kingdon, 2010).

Politics

Political motivation and opportunity were evident on relation to each initiative.

Prior to the establishment of the CDHP, a lack of opposition from organised dentistry to the proposal was important, as were the efforts of consumer and advocacy groups who were lobbying strongly for action (Lewis, 2000). In the lead up to the 1993 election, the national government was behind in the opinion polls and thought a major public dental announcement would boost its appeal. Several politicians were advocating strongly for an expansion of public dental services because of personal experiences of the impact of poor dental health. Further drivers were strong support from the Minister of Health and Social Security and the need for an election sweetener that would stimulate the economy.

The 2004–05 Victorian Budget dental initiative involved lobbying by Labor politicians in response to community advocacy. More than 100 Members of Parliament sent letters to the Minister for Health. Articulate, influential champions within the Minister's office and in government departments also advocated for the initiative. There was also a need to respond to the 2002 Victorian Auditor-General's review which had highlighted long public dental waiting times.

Political enablers of the Smile Squad proposal included the desire to address cost-of-living and time pressures on families by offering free and convenient dental care at schools. The benefits of investing in lifetime oral health for children were promoted, and the construction of the necessary vans was framed as positive for employment in rural Victoria.

In view of competing demands, politicians generally need to hear a loud community voice before supporting a particular program. In the case of the Smile Squad, the voice may have come mainly from families in Melbourne's outer suburbs who were facing cost-of-living pressures and were time poor because of long commuting times to their employment. In contrast, oral health advocates such as the Victorian Oral Health Alliance (VOHA) were campaigning for additional funding to reduce public dental waiting times, rather than for the return of the SDS. This notwithstanding, as a consequence of the Smile Squad program, public dental waiting times for adults are likely to decrease as resources previously used for treating school children will be freed up for adult care.

The politics in each of the three cases met the test of perceived political advantage, namely, by appealing to the public (Kingdon, 2010) and favouring the balance of interests (Nutbeam, 2003).

Policy window

In addition to the congruence of the problem, proposal and politics streams, elections provided the policy windows for the CDHP (1993 federal election) and the Smile Squad (2018 Victorian election). The 2004–05 Victorian Government Budget itself served as the policy window for the Victorian budget initiative of that year, and funding available under the Fairer Victoria policy was an enabler (DPC, 2005).

Each case study is considered under Kingdon's categories with the enablers or drivers outlined in Figure 4.6

Figure 4.6 Drivers for public dental initiatives

Kingdon policy stream	Commonwealth Dental Health Program, 1994	2004–05 Victorian Budget initiative	Victorian School Dental Program, Smile Squad, 2019
Problem Well-defined problem perceived as serious	• Financial difficulty with access to dental care [1] • Long public dental waiting times [2] • Inequity in oral health [1]	Long public dental waiting times [3] Victorian spending on dental public health lower than other states and territories [4]	Cost of living pressures on families [5] Time pressures on parents because of long commuting times for those living in outer suburbs [5] Tooth decay is the leading cause of preventable hospitalisation in children aged under 10 [7] Need to shift to a more preventive approach in public dental services [6]
Proposal Scientifically plausible; technically feasible; acceptable to government values, and reasonable in cost	Clearly outlined public dental program for adults [2]	Three pillar proposal: • Increase in public dental services • Prevention, including extension of fluoridation • Support for public dental workforce	Free dental care for children at government schools Resources previously used for treating school children to be used to provide care for adults

Kingdon policy stream	Commonwealth Dental Health Program, 1994	2004–05 Victorian Budget initiative	Victorian School Dental Program, Smile Squad, 2019
Politics Perceived political advantage (appealing to the public, favoured by balance of interests), and budget available	Lobbying from health and welfare advocacy groups No opposition from organised dentistry National government behind in 1993 election opinion polls Supportive Minister for Health with personal experience of the impact of poor dental health	Lobbying from Labor politicians responding to community members advocacy Victorian Auditor-General review of community dental services 2002 Articulate, influential champions within the Minister's office and in government departments	Desire to address cost of living pressures on families and convenient for families[6] Manufacture of vans in rural Victoria Investment in children for lifetime oral health Advocacy from Victorian Oral Health Alliance to reduce public dental waiting times National government CDBS funding to defray some costs
Policy window Government elections or budgets	1993 Federal election	Victorian budget 2004–05 Available funding under the Fairer Victoria policy	2018 election

Sources:

1. McClennand, A. (1991) *In fair health? Equity and the health system*. Background paper No. 3. Melbourne: National Health Strategy.
2. Dooland, M. (1992). *Improving dental health in Australia. Background paper (National Health Strategy, Australia), No. 9.* Melbourne: National Health Strategy.
3. Auditor-General Victoria. (A-GV). (2002). *Community dental services*. Melbourne: Victorian Auditor-General's Office.
4. Chapter 9, Financing of Dental Services.
5. Premier of Victoria. (2019, May 26). *The Smile Squad – Free dental vans to hit schools soon*. [Media release].
6. Auditor-General Victoria. (A-GV). (2016). *Access to public dental services in Victoria*. Melbourne: Victorian Auditor-General's Office.
7. Rogers et al., 2018.

Policy barriers

When formulating policy, it is also necessary to consider barriers to change. The perception that oral health has a low political profile has been a key barrier to reform in the past 50 years. This may be because oral disease is not usually life-threatening and not as "appealing" as other health concerns such as cancer in children. Moreover, oral conditions are predominantly episodic, and most people are usually only concerned when they have pain or discomfort.

Lack of political will on the part of some governments has resulted in policy inaction. Policy makers may not have been aware of the adverse impact that poor oral health can have on general health. Those not in contact with the disadvantaged groups who bear most of the burden of oral disease, may also not have been aware of the extent of poor oral health. The lack of a persistent, well-organised consumer voice, the high cost of dental care, and the isolation of dentistry from other health programs have arguably also been barriers to significant policy change.

Policy factors

The Kingdon model of the "4 Ps" is a useful theory to explain oral health policy successes, but myriad factors influence policy making. These include the factors outlined in Figure 4.7 such as the political context; key players (a coalition of community advocacy groups, media and oral health champions [Chapter 8]); system structures and capacity (Chapters 2 and 3); resources (Chapter 9); timing; and policy makers' evidence and judgement. The last factor can be influenced by the decision maker's personal interest in an issue. As a previous Victorian Minister for Health declared, "a personal connection does engender passion for an issue" (Personal communication, 2022). Another former federal minister has emphasised that using stories from everyday lives is powerful, noting that "anecdotes work" (Personal communication, 2022).

A positive outcome for good oral health policy requires key factors coming together – colloquially speaking, for "the stars to be aligned".

Figure 4.7 Policy factors

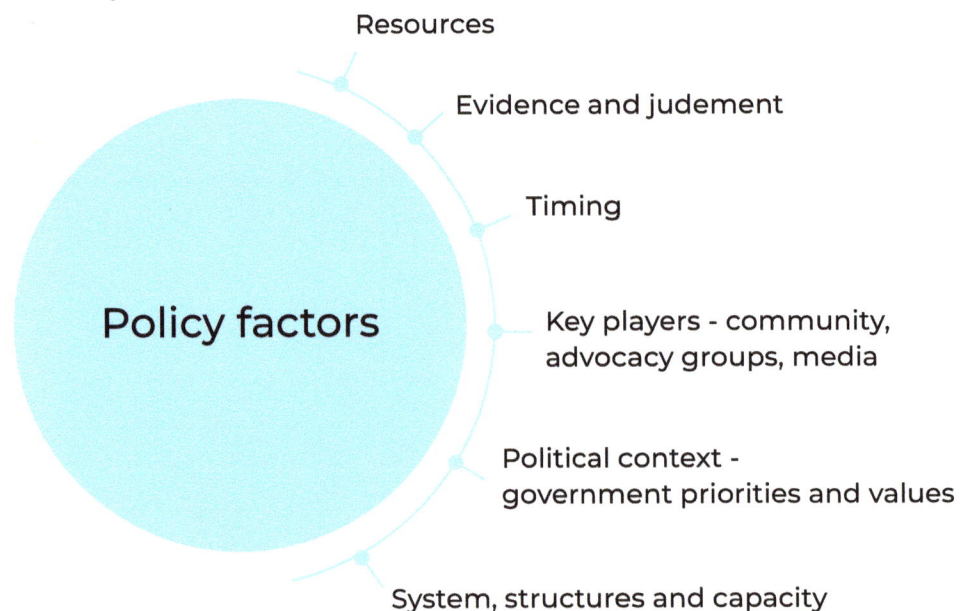

Resources

Evidence and judement

Timing

Policy factors

Key players - community, advocacy groups, media

Political context - government priorities and values

System, structures and capacity

Summary

Most dental services are provided in the private sector, with public dental services contributing up to 20% of total services. Since 1970 the number of public dental clinics in Victoria has almost tripled, from about 35 to 94, while the Victorian population has doubled (Chapter 1). Performance of the public sector to meet the dental need of eligible people has fluctuated, depending on available government funding (Chapter 5).

Since 1970 at least 32 significant reviews, reports and plans have examined dental public health at state and national levels, with most of these happening in the past 20 years. And yet, a national oral health plan was not developed until 2004. Dental issues have also been considered in broader plans and enquiries such as the Royal Commission into Aged Care Quality and Safety (RCACQ&S, 2021).

Results in achieving the oral health goals set out in national and Victorian oral health plans have been mixed. Most recently, the 2020 implementation report of the 2015–2024 national plan identified favourable trends against seven of the key performance indicators; unfavourable trends in nine; no change in nine; and no or insufficient data in six.

The prominence of dental health on the crowded policy agenda has fluctuated since 1970. The 14 significant government-funded initiatives implemented in that period have occurred infrequently in cycles – every 20 to 25 years for national programs, and every 10 to 15 years for Victorian government programs. While support for community water fluoridation has generally been bipartisan, political ideologies have shaped other dental programs. Labor governments have been more active in fostering public health and a social welfare network, while Coalition governments have concentrated on supporting individuals to meet the costs of dental care in the private sector.

Australian government funding has followed a roller coaster trajectory, with many programs initiated but not maintained. Most of the 14 significant public dental health initiatives during the period under examination have been Labor government programs. One program that has never been implemented is the inclusion of dental care in Medicare. The body has been left without a mouth.

Our case analyses found that oral health moved up the policy agenda and oral health policy changes occurred when Kingdon's three policy streams – problem, proposal, and politics – connected, and a "policy window", or favourable confluence of events, brought increased attention to dental health issues (Kingdon, 2010).

In each case, the proposal was compatible with government values and vision, plausible, technically feasible, and the cost was reasonable. Political motivation and opportunity were evident, and decision makers heard a loud community voice. From time to time, barriers to policy change have been overcome, in large part because oral health advocates have continued to carefully articulate the problems and put forward proposals to fix them. They have managed the politics, while waiting for a policy window.

Among the myriad influential factors, our analysis also suggests that good fortune in timing and favourable budget circumstances are also essential for policy success in dental public health.

Appendices

Appendix 4.1 Eligibility for public dental care in Victoria

Public dental services are provided through the Royal Dental Hospital Melbourne (RDHM) and over 50 integrated and registered community health services across Victoria.

Victorians who are eligible for public dental care

The following people are eligible for public dental care:

- All children aged 0–12 years
- Young people aged 13–17 years who hold a healthcare or pensioner concession card, or who are dependants of concession card holders
- People aged 18 years and over, who are health care or pensioner concession card holders or dependants of concession card holders
- All children and young people in out-of-home care provided by the Department of Families, Fairness and Housing (DFFH), up to 18 years of age (including kinship and foster care)
- All people in youth justice custodial care
- All Aboriginal and Torres Strait Islander people
- All refugees and asylum seekers

About priority access

Victorians who have priority access to dental care are offered the next available appointment for general care. They are not placed on the General Waiting List. If the person has denture care needs, then they will be offered the next available appointment for denture care or placed on the Priority Denture Waiting List.

People who have priority access

The following people have priority access to public dental services:

- Aboriginal and Torres Strait Islander people
- Children and young people
- People who are homeless or at risk of homelessness
- Pregnant women
- Refugees and asylum seekers
- People registered with mental health or disability services, who have a letter of recommendation from their case manager or a special developmental school

All other people seeking routine dental or denture care need to place their name on a waiting list.

Source: DHV, 2023b

Appendix 4.2 Australian capital city drinking water fluoridation by date and government in office, 1964 to 2008

Year	Capital city	State government
1964	Canberra (ACT)	Administered by federal government before 1989
	Hobart (Tasmania)	Labor Party
1968	Perth (West Australia)	Liberal Party
	Sydney (NSW)	Liberal Party
1971	Adelaide (South Australia)	Labor Party
1977	Melbourne (Victoria)	Liberal Party
1992	Darwin (Northern Territory)	Country Liberal Party
2008	Brisbane (Queensland)	Labor

Source: <https://en.wikipedia.org/wiki/Water_fluoridation_in_Australia>

References

Australian Health Ministers' Conference. (AHMAC). (2004). National Advisory Committee on Oral Health. & South Australia. Department of Health. *Healthy mouths, healthy lives: Australia's national oral health plan 2004–2013*. Adelaide: South Australian Department of Health.

Australian Institute of Health and Welfare. (AIHW). (2020). *National oral health plan 2015–2024: Performance monitoring report.* <https://www.aihw.gov.au/reports/dental-oral-health/national-oral-health-plan-2015-2024>

Auditor-General Victoria. (A-GV). (2002). *Community dental services.* <https://www.audit.vic.gov.au/report/community-dental-services?section=.>

Auditor-General Victoria. (A-GV). (2016). *Access to public dental services in Victoria.* <https://www.audit.vic.gov.au/report/access-public-dental-services-victoria?section=32003--4-addressing-barriers-to-access#page-anchor>

Australian Prime Ministers Centre (n.d.). Prime Ministers. <https://primeministers.moadoph.gov.au/prime-ministers>

Biggs, A. (2004). *Medicare – Background brief.* <https://parlinfo.aph.gov.au/parlInfo/search/display/display.w3p;adv=yes;orderBy=customrank;page=0;query=Content%3ABiggs%20Content%3A%22Medicare%20Background%20brief%22%20Date%3A01%2F01%2F2004%20%3E%3E%2031%2F12%2F2004%20Dataset%3Aprspub,jrnart,jrnart88;rec=0;resCount=Default>

Biggs, A. (2008). *Overview of Commonwealth involvement in funding dental care.* <https://parlinfo.aph.gov.au/parlInfo/search/display/display.w3p;adv=yes;orderBy=customrank;page=0;query=Content%3ABiggs%20Content%3A%22Overview%20of%20Commonwealth%20involvement%20in%20funding%20dental%20care%22%20Date%3A01%2F01%2F2008%20%3E%3E%2031%2F12%2F2008%20Dataset%3Aprspub,jrnart,jrnart88;rec=1;resCount=Default>

Boxall, A-M., & Gillespie, J. (2013). *Making Medicare: The politics of universal health care in Australia.* Sydney: UNSW Press.

Canadian Academy of Health Sciences. (2014). *Improving access to oral care for vulnerable people living in Canada.* <https://cahs-acss.ca/wp-content/uploads/2015/07/Access_to_Oral_Care_FINAL_REPORT_EN.pdf>

Carter, J. (2020, October 7). *Ideological tide swamped state. The Age.*

COAG Health Council. (2015). *Healthy mouths, healthy lives: Australia's national oral health plan 2015–2024.* <https://www.health.gov.au/resources/publications/healthy-mouths-healthy-lives-australias-national-oral-health-plan-2015-2024?language=en>

Commonwealth. *Parliamentary debates.* House of Representatives, 29 November 1985, p. 4,024.

Commonwealth of Australia. (2019). *Report on the Fourth Review of the Dental Benefits Act 2008.* <https://www.health.gov.au/sites/default/files/documents/2022/04/report-on-the-fourth-review-of-the-dental-benefits-act-2008.pdf>

Costello, P. (1996). CPD HR No. 7, 20 August 1996:3274.

Cresswell, A. (2011, August 20–21). Health of the nation (chart), *Weekend Australian*, p. 6.

Daly, J. (2021). *Gridlock: Removing barriers to policy reform.* Grattan Institute. <https://grattan.edu.au/wp-content/uploads/2021/07/Gridlock-Grattan-Report.pdf>

Dental Health Services Victoria. (2023) *Healthy families, healthy smiles.* <https://www.dhsv.org.au/oral-health-programs/hfhs>

Department of Health, Australia (DOHA). (1973). *Annual Report of the Director-General of Health.* <https://nla.gov.au/nla.obj-1745801827/view?sectionId=nla.obj-1847550851&partId=nla.obj-1751321551>

Department of Health. Victoria. (DHV). (1986). *Ministerial review of dental services: Final report.* Melbourne: Department of Health: Victoria.

Department of Health. Victoria. (DHV). (2013). *Action plan for oral health promotion 2013–2017.* <https://content.health.vic.gov.au/sites/default/files/migrated/files/collections/research-and-reports/1/1303009_htv_oral_health_web---pdf.pdf>

Department of Health. Victoria. (DHV). (2023a). *Free dental for all Victorian public school students.* Smile Squad. State Government of Victoria. <https://www.health.vic.gov.au/smile-squad>

Department of Health. Victoria. (DHV). (2023b). *Access to Victoria's public dental care services.* <https://www.health.vic.gov.au/dental-health/access-to-victorias-public-dental-care-services>

Department of Health and Community Services. Victoria. (DH&CS). (1995). *Future directions for dental health in Victoria.* Melbourne: VGPS.

Department of Health and Human Services. (DHHS). (2020). *Victorian action plan to prevent oral disease 2020–30.* <https://www.health.vic.gov.au/sites/default/files/migrated/files/collections/research-and-reports/o/victorian-action-plan-to-prevent-oral-disease-2020.pdf>

Department of Human Services. Victoria. (DHS). (1999). *Promoting oral health 2000–2004. Strategic directions and framework for action.* <https://www.vgls.vic.gov.au/client/en_AU/search/asset/1159746>

Department of Human Services. Victoria. (DHS). (2007). *Improving Victoria's oral health.* <https://vgls.sdp.sirsidynix.net.au/client/search/asset/1291900>

Department of Premier and Cabinet. Victoria. (DPC). (1988). *Social justice strategy.* Melbourne: DPC.

Department of Premier and Cabinet. Victoria. (DPC). (2005). *A fairer Victoria: Creating opportunity and addressing disadvantage.* Melbourne: DPC.

Dooland, M. (1992). *Improving dental health in Australia.* Background Paper No. 9. Melbourne: National Health Strategy.

Duckett, S., Cowgill, M., & Swerrisen, H. (2019). *Filling the gap: A universal dental care scheme for Australia.* <https://grattan.edu.au/wp-content/uploads/2019/03/915-Filling-the-gap-A-universal-dental-scheme-for-Australia.pdf>

Ghanbarzadegan, A., Ivanovski, S., Sloan, A. J., & Spallek, H. (2023). Oral health research funding in relation to disease burden in Australia. *Australian Dental Journal, 68*(1), 42-47.

Hilmer, F. (1993). *National competition policy: Report by the Independent Committee of Inquiry.* Canberra: Commonwealth Govt. Printer. <http://ncp.ncc.gov.au/docs/National%20Competition%20Policy%20Review%20report,%20The%20Hilmer%20Report,%20August%201993.pdf.>

Hopcraft, M. (2023). *How is public dental care funded in Australia?* Dental as Anything. <https://matthopcraft.substack.com/p/how-is-public-dental-care-funded>

Kingdon, J.W. (2010). *Agendas, alternatives, and public policies.* (Updated edition, with an epilogue on health care). New York: Longman.

Layton, R. (chair), & Department of Health. Australia (1986). *Medicare benefits review committee: Second report.* Canberra: AGPS.

Lewis, J. (2000). From 'Fightback to biteback': The rise and fall of a national dental program. *Australian Journal of Public Administration, 59*(1), pp. 60–72.

McCann, J. (2016). *Traits and trends of Australia's prime ministers, 1901 to 2015: A quick guide.* <https://www.aph.gov.au/About_Parliament/Parliamentary_Departments/Parliamentary_Library/pubs/rp/rp1516/Quick_Guides/AustPM>

McClelland, A. (1991) *In fair health? Equity and the health system.* Background paper No. 3. Melbourne: National Health Strategy.

Menadue, J. (2021). *Why dental care was excluded from Medicare and why it should now be included (an edited repost).* <https://johnmenadue.com/why-dental-care-was-excluded-from-medicare-and-why-it-should-now-be-included-an-edited-repost>

Metherell, M. (2012). Gillard's $4 billion dental fix. *The Age,* August 29 2012. <https://www.smh.com.au/politics/federal/gillards-4-billion-dental-fix-20120829-24zo4.html>

National Advisory Council on Dental Health. (NACDH). (2012). *Report of the National Advisory Council on Dental Health. 23 February 2012.* <https://apo.org.au/node/28453>

National Health and Hospitals Reform Commission. (NHHRC). (2009). *A healthier future for all Australians. Final report 2009.* Canberra: Commonwealth of Australia.

Nutbeam, D. (2003) How does evidence influence public health policy? Tackling health inequalities in England. *Health Promotion Journal of Australia 14*(3), 154–58.

Plibersek, T. (2012). *$4 billion dental spend on children, low income adults and the bush.* [Media release]. August 29 2012. <https://parlinfo.aph.gov.au/parlInfo/search/display/display.w3p;query=Id%3A%22media%2Fpressrel%2F1882137%22;src1=sm1>

Premier of Victoria. (2019, May 26). *The Smile Squad – Free dental vans to hit schools soon.* [Media release]. <https://www.premier.vic.gov.au/smile-squad-free-dental-vans-hit-schools-soon>

Rawat, R., & Morris, J.C. (2016). Kingdon's "Streams" model at thirty: Still relevant in the 21st century? *Politics & Policy, 44*(4), 608–38.

Rogers, J., Delany, C., Wright, C., Roberts-Thomson, K., & Morgan, M. (2018). What factors are associated with dental general anaesthetics for Australian children and what are the policy implications? A qualitative study. *BMC Oral Health, 18*(1), 1-12.

Royal Commission into Aged Care Quality and Safety. (RCACQ&S). (2021). *Final report.* <https://agedcare. royalcommission.gov.au/sites/default/files/2021-03/final-report-volume-1_0.pdf>

Senate Community Affairs References Committee. Australia. (SCARC). (1998). *Report on public dental services, May 1998.* <https://www.aph.gov.au/ parliamentary_business/committees/senate/ community_affairs/completed_inquiries/1996-99/ dental/report/index>

Scotton, R.B. (1977). Medibank 1976. *The Australian Economic Review, (10)*1, 23–35. <https://onlinelibrary. wiley.com/doi/10.1111/j.1467-8462.1977.tb00703.x>

Scotton, R.B. (2000). Milestones on the road to Medibank and Medicare. *Medical Journal of Australia, 173*(1), 5–8.

Spencer, A.J. (1998). *Responsibility for dental care and reflections on the CDHP.* National Seminar on the Role of the Commonwealth in the provision of dental services to the disadvantaged. 16 January 1998. Melbourne. Unpublished presentation.

Treasury, Victoria. (2000). *Budget estimates 2000-21. Budget paper No. 3.* p. 69. <https://www.dtf.vic. gov.au/sites/default/files/document/2000-01-BP3-BudgetEstimates.pdf>

Treasury & Finance, Victoria. (2004). *Service delivery 2004–05. Budget paper No. 3.* <https://www.dtf.vic.gov. au/previous-budgets/2004-05-state-budget>

World Health Organization. (1978). *Primary health care: report of the international conference on primary health care Alma Ata, USSR, 6–12 September 1978. Geneva, Switzerland, 1978.* <https://www.who.int/ publications/i/item/9241800011>

Wright F.A.C. (Ed). (2013). *National oral health promotion plan.* Unpublished manuscript. Commissioned by Australian Government. Canberra.

Chapter 5
The Victorian Public Oral Health Care Sector – Performance and the school dental program

John Rogers

Introduction

In line with the ebb and flow of budget allocations, most markedly in Australian government funding, the performance of Victoria's dental public sector has fluctuated considerably since 1970.

In this chapter we present a general picture of system performance and consider key indicators of success over the past five decades: waiting times for public dental care, the numbers of people treated and attendances, and the proportion of eligible people treated.

We draw predominantly on output measures and also on the limited data available on outcome measures such as changes in oral health status. Data have been sourced from government budget papers, public dental agencies' annual reports, findings of three Victorian Auditor-General's reports, and from public sector performance reviews and plans published during the period of study.

The mixed results in achieving the oral health goals outlined in plans and audits will be examined, alongside the history of the Victorian School Dental Service (SDS) – its rise, decline and resurrection.

5.1 Dental public sector performance

Waiting times – Months not days

Over the past five decades, eligible Victorians have had better access to emergency care than to general dental care at public dental clinics. The most recent data show that 91% of eligible people accessing clinics who were classified as the highest priority (Dental Emergency Triage Category 1) were treated within 24 hours. This was against a target of 90% (DHSV, 2022). In contrast, waiting times for general dental care have varied from 10 months to five years (Figure 5.1).

Figure 5.1 highlights the relationship between waiting times for public dental care and funding allocations. It indicates that dental health could be improved by sustained public funding at levels adequate to provide the recommended care.

> ' It is much more important to know what sort of a patient has a disease than what sort of a disease a patient has.
>
> – William Osler

Figure 5.1 Average waiting times for general dental care, Victoria, 1985 to 2022 (months)

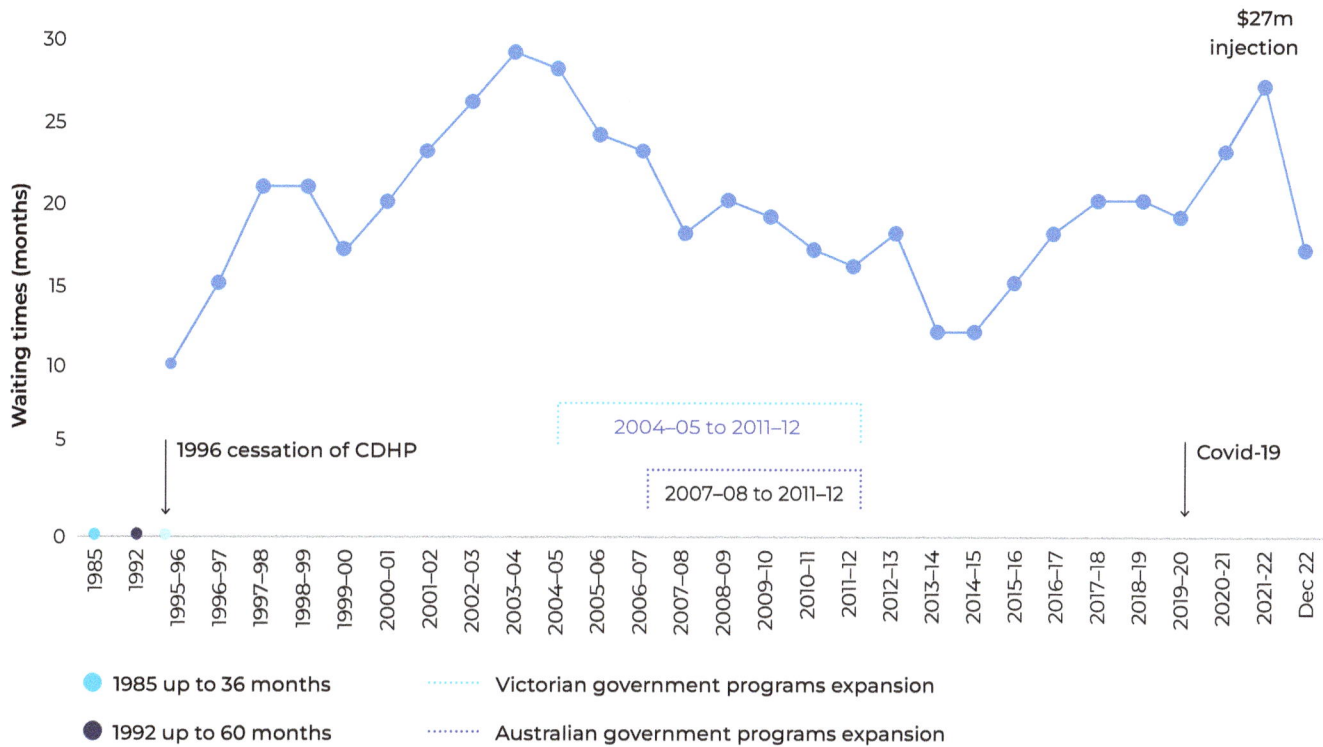

Note: The first case COVID-19 was reported in Victoria on 25 January 2020 (Storen & Corrigan, 2020).

Sources: 1985 and 1994 data were compiled from DHS, 1996 and DH&CS, 1995; 2022 data from ADAVB, 2023. Other data are from DHSV annual reports.

Certain population groups are eligible for priority access to public dental services and thus do not need to go on waiting lists. These groups are shown in Appendix 4.1.

In the 1980s waiting times for general public dental care were up to three years (DHV, 1986). By the early 1990s the wait had increased to five years in some public clinics (DHSV, 1997). The Commonwealth Dental Health Program (CDHP), which operated between 1994 and 1996, significantly decreased waiting times to 10 months, doubling the proportion of Victorians who had had a public-funded dental visit in the previous 12 months (Brennan et al., 1997). When the program was closed down by the incoming Howard Coalition Government in 1996, (Chapter 4), waiting

times quickly doubled to 21 months. Apart from a brief dip after the Victorian government contributed additional funding, waiting times increased to 29 months by 2003–04.

By 2014–15 waiting times had decreased to 12 months when first the Victorian government, and then the Australian government, provided additional funding (Chapter 9). From that time, waiting times started to climb as neither government continued to fund expansion of public dental care. In Victoria, when the Andrews Labor Government committed significant additional funding from 2019–20, the COVID-19 pandemic restricted the provision of dental care (Chapter 11). By June 2022, waiting times for general dental care stood at 27 months.

An injection of $27m by the Victorian Government in December 2021 (Foley, 2021) led to a reduction in waiting times to 17 months by December 2022. As the history of one-off provision of funds has shown, this recent reduction in waiting times is likely to be short lived. Recurrent funding is needed for sustained waiting time reductions.

Since state-wide data collection commenced in 1996, waiting lists have consistently exceeded 100,000 people. In December 2002 more than 185,000 people were awaiting general care, and more than 25,000 were on the waiting list for dentures (A-GV, 2002). In June 2020 waiting times had improved, but still close to 136,000 people were waiting for general care (DHSV, 2021). In 2021–22, 90,000 people on the waiting list were offered care.

While there are few data on interstate waiting times for general dental care, in 2018 the Productivity Commission reported that the wait in Victoria was the third longest in Australia at 18 months (AGPC, 2019; Duckett et. al., 2019). Only Tasmania (20 months) and the Northern Territory (26 months) had longer waiting times, while New South Wales did not provide data to the inquiry.

Attendances

Not surprisingly, the number of people treated in the public dental system has fluctuated over time in line with changes in government funding and, most recently, due to the impact of COVID-19. As numbers of attendances (or visits) to public dental services have been more commonly reported than numbers of people treated, we can go back further in time to learn about visits (Figure 5.2).

Figure 5.2 Annual visits to public dental services, Victoria, 1970–2020

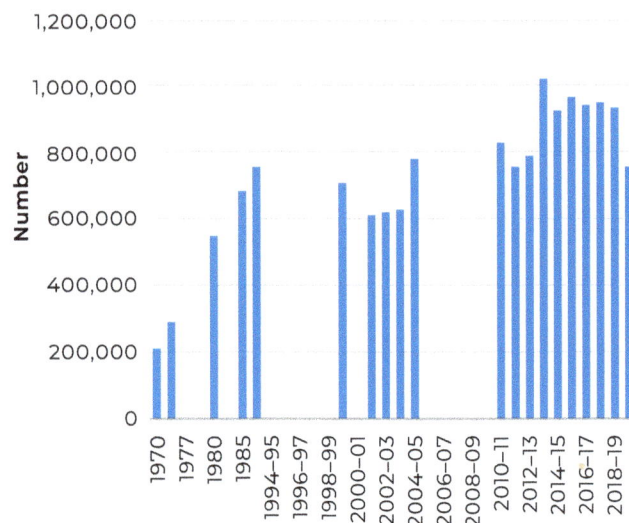

Note: Annual figures have not always been publicly reported.
Sources: 1985 and 1994 data were compiled from DHV, 1986 DH&CS and H&CS, 1995.
Other data are from DHSV annual reports.

When our history starts in 1970, just over 200,000 visits to public dental services were made by about 100,000 people (Appendix 5.1). By 1980 the number of visits had increased to more than half a million (549,500), due both to increases in the number of pre-schoolers accessing local government clinics, and school children being seen by the SDS (Section 5.2). An increase in the number of dental clinics in rural base hospitals also led to an increase in visits over this time, from fewer than 10,000 in 1975 to over 100,000 in 1980 (Appendix 5.1).

Visits increased in the 1980s with the introduction of the Victorian Denture Scheme in 1984 and community dental clinics in 1988. The 1990s saw visits rise then fall with the commencement of the CDHP in 1994 and its cessation in 1996. The 2004–05 Victorian Budget initiative (Treasury & Finance, 2004) supported an increase in visits, as did the introduction of the National Partnership Agreement (NPA) in 2012. Visits to public dental clinics peaked at more than a million (1,024,337) in 2014. In 2020, due to COVID-19 infection control restrictions which limited treatment mainly to emergency care, this figure plummeted by a quarter (26%) to 755,402.

People treated

Figure 5.3 shows the total number of people treated in public oral health services since 1999–2000, the first year in which these data were publicly released. Including those seen by private practitioners under public–private referral programs, around 300,000 people were treated in that initial year. After that, numbers increased gradually until an injection of funds from the Australian Government via the NPA allowed more than 411,000 people to be treated in 2013–14. With less NPA funding in the following years, around 400,000 people were seen each year. In 2020–21 COVID-19 curtailed treatment numbers by a quarter. In 2021–22 fewer than 300,000 people were treated.

Figure 5.3 Total persons treated in public oral health services, Victoria, 1999 to 2020, with adults and children from 2005 to 2020

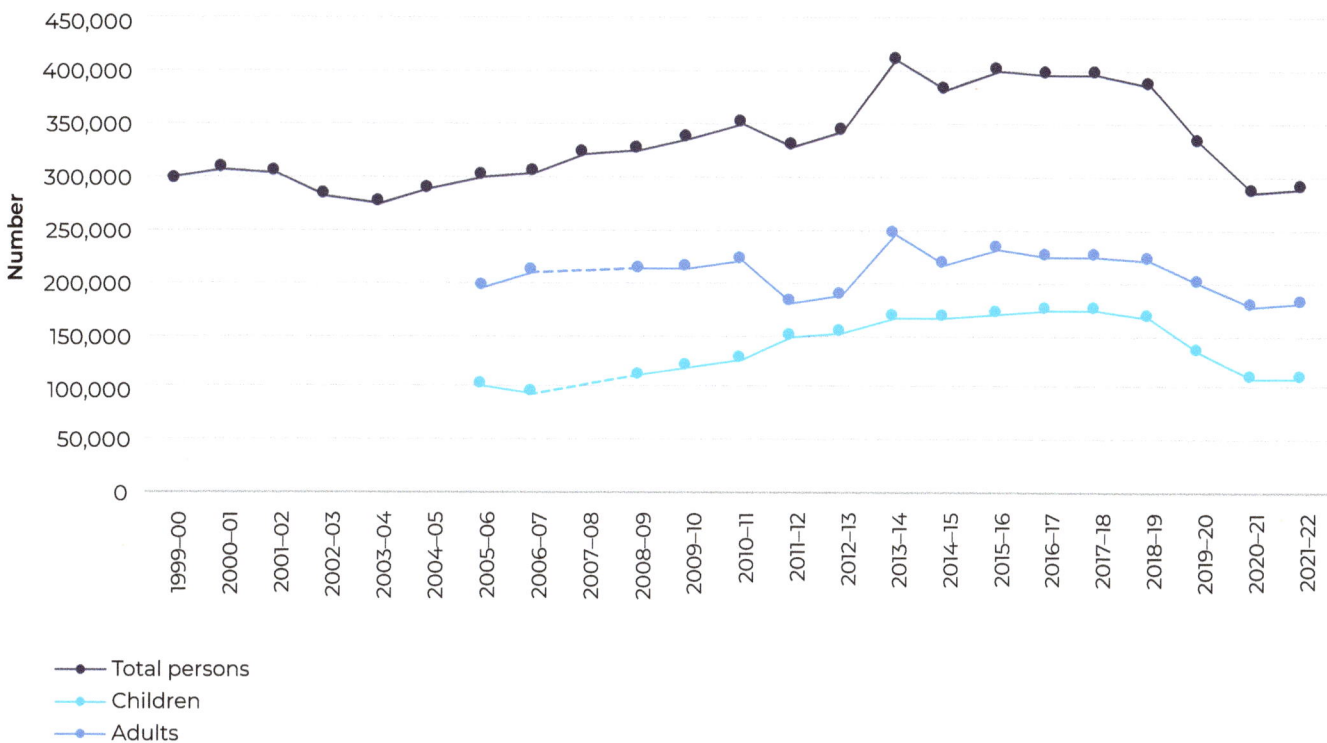

Note: The breakdown of adults and children has been reported since 2005–06.

Sources: 1985 and 1994 data were compiled from DHV, 1986 and DH&CS, 1995. Other data are from DHSV annual reports.

Since 2006, when data for adults and children treated became available, the relative proportion of children treated has increased from a third (33%) to two-fifths (40%) of all people treated in 2019–20.

Level of access – Proportion of eligible people treated

Prevention and timely treatment of oral health problems are fundamental to improving oral health. Timely treatment of decayed teeth and other oral conditions prevents tooth loss and precludes the need for expensive, complicated oral health care. However, there has been debate within the dental profession over how frequently people should visit for dental care. The message that everyone should visit every six months has been challenged for some time (Sheiham, 1977). The most recent research indicates that people should visit in accordance with their particular dental health needs (Fee et al., 2020) – for example, a visit every two years may be adequate for people with good oral health. Conservative public dental guidance holds that, on average, all adults should receive at least one course of general dental care at least every three years (AHMC, 2004).

With such variation in recommended visit frequency, it is difficult to report the proportion of people eligible for public dental care who have had timely dental visits. A proxy performance indicator for the public dental system is the proportion of the eligible group who access public dental care over a one- or a two-year period. The most recent Victorian Auditor-General's report on dental services found that, in the two years 2014 and 2016, 25% (611,288) of the 2.45 million eligible people were treated (A-GV, 2016). Before the COVID-19 pandemic in 2019 about 390,000 people received public dental care, representing less than 20% of more than two million eligible Victorians.

Earlier reports have also determined that fewer than 20% of eligible Victorians have accessed public dental services in any given year. In 1991 an estimated 15–20% of eligible people received public dental care; less than in the better-funded states of Queensland and South Australia, where the corresponding figures were 20–25% in each case (Dooland, 1992). In 1994 fewer than 15% of eligible Victorians accessed care (DH&CS, 1995), and in each year between 1997–2002, the proportion fell to 11–13% (A-GV, 2002).

Impact of funding on system performance

Since 1994 three major funding initiatives have led to considerable short-term improvements in both the number of eligible Victorians treated and waiting times for care in public dental services (Figure 5.4). It is clear that the extent of government funding is the most important factor contributing to public dental performance.

Figure 5.4 Impact of three funding initiatives on eligible Victorians treated and waiting times, 1994 to 2014

Initiative	Impact
Commonwealth Dental Health Program (CDHP) 1994–96	Waiting times for general care were reduced from up to 60 months to 10 months. There was a shift from emergency to general care with fewer extractions and more fillings.
Victorian 2004–05 Budget	Decrease in waiting time from 26 months in 2002–03 to 18 months in 2007–08. Numbers waiting decreased from 240,106 to 100,000.
National Partnership Agreement (NPA) 2013–14	Decrease in general care waiting time from 18 to 12 months compared to 2012-13. The number of people waiting decreased from 109,500 to 76,600 and an additional 70,000 people were treated.

Sources: Brennan et al, 1997; DHSV, 1997; DHSV, 2003; DHSV, 2008; DHSV, 2013; DHSV, 2014.

Mixed results in achieving oral health goals in Victorian plans and audits

In Chapter 4 we highlight uneven progress in the implementation of the recommendations of the 32 significant dental public health reviews, reports and plans released since 1970. Among the 32 reports, two were national oral health plans, and half related to Victorian initiatives. In this section we evaluate the performance of Victoria's public oral health sector by considering the impact of the five national and Victorian government oral health plans and three oral health audits conducted by the Victorian Auditor-General since 1970. We also review the achievements in meeting oral health goals reported in four major Victorian oral health documents.

Victorian governments have released oral health plans every decade from the 1980s. Their major goals, recommendations and outcomes are summarised in Appendix 5.2.

The *Dental health strategy 1988* (Chapter 4) was a response to the Cain Labor Government's 1986 *Ministerial review of dental services* (MRODS) (DHV, 1986). The review led to the decentralisation of public dental services, with dental clinics being placed in community health centres and selected hospitals. Among other outcomes, responsibility for training dental therapists moved from the Department of Health to the University of Melbourne, and extending community water fluoridation to rural Victoria assumed greater priority.

Restructure of public dental services was a key plank in the *Future directions for dental health in Victoria plan* (DH&CS, 1995) released by the Kennett Coalition Government in 1995. This was achieved through the creation of Dental Health Services Victoria (DHSV) as the peak dental health body (Chapter 4). To implement "Vision 2010", the plan promised a trifecta of initiatives; namely, funding for extension of public dental services, a review of dental legislation, and development of an oral health promotion strategy. Each of these promises was fulfilled. The partial success in achieving the oral health status goals for 2010 that ensued is discussed below.

Further system change was outlined in *Improving Victoria's oral health* released by the Bracks Labor Government in 2007 (DHS, 2007). The most significant change was the integration of the state-wide SDS managed by DHSV into the Community Dental Program (CDP) managed by independent community dental agencies. Integration was completed by 2009 and is discussed in the following section: 5.2 Victorian School Dental Service. Prevention interventions, also recommended in the plan, were partially implemented.

Action plans to prevent oral disease were released by the Napthine Coalition Government in 2013 (DHV, 2013) and the Andrews Labor Government in 2020 (DHHS, 2020). Their recommendations have been partially implemented, as discussed in Chapter 6.

The three audits undertaken by the Victorian Auditor-General are summarised in Appendix 5.3 in terms of the audit goal, key findings, major recommendations, and status of matters raised in follow-up reports. Together, the audits reviewed the effectiveness of the SDS (A-GV, 1993; A-GV, 1995); the economy, efficiency and effectiveness of community dental services (A-GV, 2002; A-GV, 2005), and timely access to public dental health services (A-GV, 2016; A-GV, 2019).

The 1993 SDS audit found that the dental health of Victorian children was generally on a par with that of children participating in similar programs in other states. However, the audit reported that Victoria's participation rate was the second lowest in Australia, and children with high dental needs were not being identified and treated. Action was taken on both issues and improvements were recognised in the follow-up report in 1995.

Service system stressors were identified in the 2002 audit, in particular, long waiting times for general treatment and a focus on emergency, rather than preventive care. A key recommendation of the audit was that Government either change public dental goals or increase funding. The latter occurred via the 2004–05 Victorian Budget (see the case study in Chapter 4 for details). Even so, long waiting times for general care have continued to dog the system, as identified earlier in this chapter.

The 2016 Auditor-General's report again identified a need to address public dental waiting times and introduce a more patient-centred, preventive approach (A-GV, 2016). The 2019 follow-up audit concluded that, in the absence of a cost–benefit analysis, it was difficult to assess whether the proposed value-based model of care would deliver the expected benefits (A-GV, 2019).

Achievements against the oral health goals included in four major Victorian oral health documents have been mixed (Box 5.1).

Box 5.1 Mixed results in achieving oral health goals in Victoria

The *Ministerial review of dental services* (MRODS) included five oral health goals to be achieved by 2000 against a 1985 baseline (DHV, 1986). Goals covered the extent of decay in children's teeth and the proportion of adults who had kept their natural teeth. These goals were met, except in relation to the proportion of 5–6-year-olds who were decay free (without dental cavities). As discussed in Chapter 10, the improvement in children's oral health has been less marked in the primary teeth than in the secondary teeth.

Future directions for dental health in Victoria also included five goals for 2010 against a 1995 baseline (DH&CS, 1995). They were similar in scope to the 1985 MRODS goals and all were met.

The *Improving Victoria's oral health* plan of 2007 did not set oral health goals but, rather, outlined minimum standards for access to dental care (DHS, 2007). One of these minimum standards required that adults should receive at least one course of general care every three years. There has been no routine audit of this standard, but it is unlikely that it has been met in Victoria. In 2016, for example, one in four Victorian adults had not had a dental visit in more than two years (DHHS, 2018).

Four oral health goals were included in the *Victorian action plan to prevent oral disease 2020–30* to be achieved by 2030 (DHHS, 2020). These are broader in scope than the goals in the earlier plans. In addition to addressing the proportion of children without dental cavities, the plan sets goals relating to gum disease prevalence, community water fluoridation coverage, and oral cancer survival rates. The Victorian Government has committed to monitoring and reviewing implementation of the action plan (DHHS, 2020).

Progress on the goals set by the national oral health plans is addressed in Chapter 4.

Government accountability requirements for public dental services have evolved over time. There have been advances in the compilation and reporting of data since consolidation of the system in the 1990s (facilitated by developments in statistical computing). However, the focus is still primarily on outputs (such as waiting times and numbers treated), rather than on oral health status. In future, it is hoped that developments in people-centred and value-based care will lead to further use of patient-reported outcome measures (PROMS) and patient-reported experience measures (PREMS), as outlined in Chapter 6.

Summary

Victorian government oral health plans have been released every decade since the 1980s, and there have been three Victorian Auditor-General reports since the 1990s. These have contributed to oral health planning through their analyses of the performance of the public dental system and recommendations for improvement. They have elevated dental public health on the crowded policy agenda (Chapter 4). The process of developing the plans has served to raise the profile of oral health problems and proposals within both the public service and government. The audit reports have kept both the Parliament and the public apprised of the performance of the Victorian public dental sector.

Implementation has been patchy, however. Public dental sector performance has fluctuated considerably over the past five decades, largely reflecting the ebb and flow of budget allocations, most markedly in Australian government funding (Chapter 9).

While there have been improvements in providing emergency care to concession card holders, waiting times for general dental care have consistently stretched to years, rather than weeks or months. In mid-2022, waiting times exceeded two years. While they decreased to 17 months in December 2022 through a one-off injection of $27 million, as history has shown, waiting times will increase if funding is not continued.

The COVID-19 pandemic has affected the provision of dental care. During 2020 and 2021 dental treatment was limited mainly to emergency care and the number of public dental clients treated declined by almost a third (30%) compared to pre-pandemic levels.

But even prior to the pandemic, less than a fifth (20%) of eligible Victorians (about 400,000) were able to access public dental care each year. Funding has simply not kept pace with increases in the eligible population (Chapter 9) and the oral health needs of disadvantaged groups continue to be unmet (Chapter 10). In summary, adequate and sustained government funding is fundamental to an effective public dental system.

5.2 The Victorian School Dental Service – Rise, decline and resurrection, 1970 to 2022

Introduction

From its commencement in 1921, the Victorian School Dental Service (SDS) has experienced highs and lows. The SDS was established within the School Medical Service following interest from dentists and mothers' committees, and in the light of examples from New South Wales and New Zealand (Robertson, 1989). Dentists provided services to children from a small number of primary schools in lower socioeconomic suburbs. The service grew from nine staff in 1921 to 77 in 1975, the first year in which dental therapists were employed (HCV, 1982).

The more recent history of school dental services in Victoria can be divided into five stages: (i) Australian School Dental Scheme (ASDS) 1973–1981; (ii) reviews and productivity increase 1982–1996; (iii) transfer of responsibility to Dental Health Services Victoria (DHSV) 1996–2009; (iv) integration with the Community Dental Program (CDP) by 2009; and (v) resurrection as the Smile Squad in 2019. The five stages, and the corresponding numbers of children seen, are shown in Figure 5.5.

Children treated

About 20,000 children were seen by the SDS in 1977, the earliest date for which data are available. Numbers increased six-fold to a peak of almost 155,000 in 1996. During the integration of the SDS with the Community Dental Program (CDP) in 2008, more children were being seen under the CDP and the number of children seen by the SDS decreased by 75% to 80,000.

The total number of children treated in Victorian public oral health services from 2002 to 2022 is shown in Figure 5.3. The Smile Squad commenced in August 2019 and examined more than 3,300 children by June 2020 (DHSV, 2020). In 2021–22, 20,777 children received care (DHSV, 2022). Figure 5.5 shows Victorian children treated in the SDS between 1977 and 2022.

Figure 5.5 Victorian children treated in the School Dental Service, selected years, 1977 to 2022

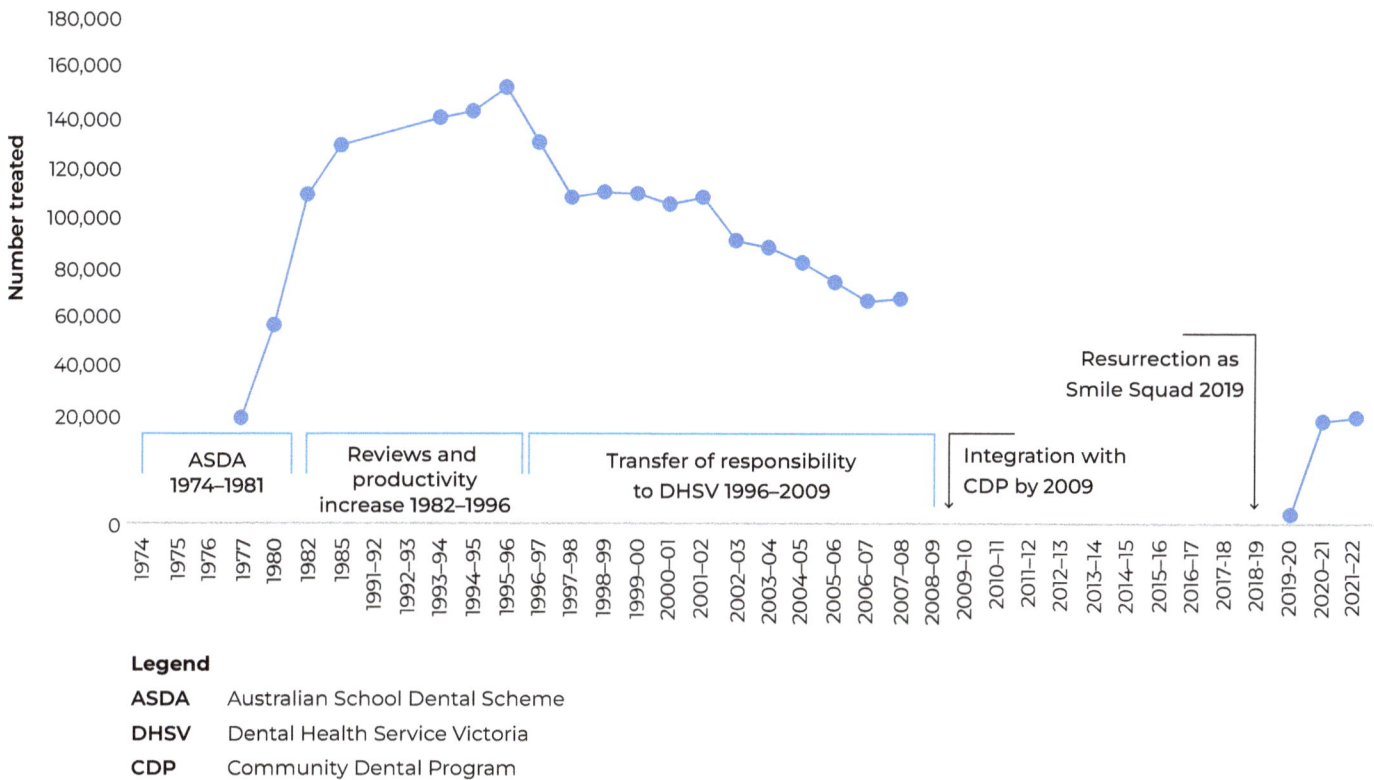

Legend

ASDA   Australian School Dental Scheme
DHSV   Dental Health Service Victoria
CDP   Community Dental Program

Note: Data were not found before 1977. There were no data between 2009-10 and 2018-19 because the School Dental Service (SDS) was integrated into the Community Dental Program (CDP).
Sources: HCV, 1982; DHV, 1986; DH&CS, 1995; DHSV Annual Reports.

Stages of the Victorian School Dental Services

1 Australian School Dental Scheme 1974–1981

The first major national government involvement in funding dental services of the 1970s was the Whitlam Labor Government's Australian School Dental Program (ASDS) established in 1973 (Biggs, 2008). The scheme offered grants to be matched by the states to build dental clinics and to employ and train dental therapists. Services were to be provided mainly by dental therapists under the supervision, direction and control of dentists. Eligibility was to be gradually extended from pre- and primary school children to secondary students under 15 years of age (HCV, 1982). The national government initially provided 100% of capital funding and 75% of operating costs, both of which decreased to 50% by 1979 under the Fraser Coalition Government.

Like New South Wales, Victoria lagged behind other states and territories in taking up the joint funding offer, mainly because the school dental programs in these larger states were less developed than in other jurisdictions. Dental therapy training commenced in Victoria in 1976 with 60 students, 10 years after Tasmania (1966) and South Australia (1967). Standards were similar to those in nursing: for example, the 1976 student handbook for dental therapy noted that white uniforms were supplied and regularly inspected for neatness and length (Satur, 2010).

In 1977 only 4% of all Victorian primary school children received care in the SDS; less than a quarter of the national rate of 18%. By 1980 the number of children seen had trebled – from around 20,000 in 1977 to 60,000 by 1980. Nevertheless, this still represented only 12% of primary school children, compared to 24% in New South Wales and 38% nationally (HCV, 1982).

In June 1981, when specific-purpose funding to states and territories for the ASDS was absorbed within general revenue grants (Duckett, 2019), Victoria was receiving less than $5 per primary school child, compared with funding of more than $20 per child flowing to South Australia, Western Australia, and Tasmania (Government bureaucrat, personal communication, 2006). These three states received the entitlements that Victorian and New South Wales had not taken up and were able to achieve participation rates above 80% in 1980 (HCV, 1982).

2 Reviews and productivity increases 1981–1996

The 1980s ushered in three reviews of the Victorian SDS and saw an increase in both the service budget and children seen. A Health Commission of Victoria review recommended a service restructure and improvements in management to address morale and low productivity (HCV, 1982). By 1982 the SDS employed 167 dental therapists (HCV, 1982). In response to Victoria's Ministerial Review of Dental Services (DHV, 1986), the 1988 Dental health strategy (Chapter 4) included additional funding to increase the number of dental therapists. The MRODS report also recognised the positive aspects of the SDS such as its universality and local and preventive focus (DHV, 1986).

In 1989 an internal review of the SDS sharpened its focus on improving oral health and increasing productivity (DHS, 1989). As a result, by 1993 the Victorian Auditor-General was able to report that the dental health of Victorian children seen by the SDS was generally consistent with that of children participating in similar programs in other states (A-GV, 1993).

Within the SDS the average number of children seen per dental therapist increased progressively over time; from 376 in 1979, to 740 in 1985 (DHV, 1986), and 1,085 in 1995-96 (DHSV, 1997). By 1992 the cost of care per child had decreased in constant dollars from $102 in 1980 to $63 in 1992 (HCV, 1982; Hollis, 1993). Productivity gains were achieved through improvements in children's oral health due to the extension of community water fluoridation, as well as through service changes. Key changes included establishing targets for area teams with regular feedback to managers, and implementation of a 12/24-month cycle in which children at lower risk of dental problems were offered care every 24 months, and those at higher risk every 12 months or less (Hollis, 1993).

The numbers of children treated each year increased until 1995-96, when 154,874 children were seen (DHSV, 1997). Almost a quarter of a million children were under care in 1993-94; with a high ratio of 2,331 children per dental therapist (DHS, 1996). The participation rate peaked at 67% of primary school children in 1993 (A-GV, 1993), with almost 90% of the dependants of health care card holders from non-English backgrounds seen (DH&CS, 1995). About a third of the children attending the service also used private dentists. The balance of children – almost 20% – used private dentists only (DH&CS, 1995).

In Victoria, while most children were examined at school, fewer than half received dental treatment at their schools (DHS, 1996) (Box 5.2).

As Victoria's School Dental Service (SDS) expanded between the mid-1970s to mid-90s, most children (91% in the 1995–96 two-year cycle) were examined at their schools; either in dental vans, fixed clinics in schools, or using portable equipment (DHS, 1996). Under half (42%) received dental treatment at their schools. The remainder were treated at another school or at a public dental clinic (DHS, 1996).

Participation rates varied by location of service delivery. In 1996, the participation rates were 75% for children who were examined and treated at their schools; 66% for those examined at their schools and treated elsewhere; and 27% for those examined and treated at another school or at a public dental clinic (DHS, 1996).

Access to the service increased markedly between 1976 and the mid-1990s. By 1981 there were 53 clinics in schools and 42 mobile vans (HCV, 1996), increasing to 83 vans in 1986 (DHV, 1986). Vans started to be phased out in the mid-1990s for various reasons, so that by 2002 only 37 were still operating (A-GV, 2005).

In the early 1990s portable equipment was used in schools to enhance access. Some dental staff disliked using this equipment because of quality concerns due to inadequate lighting, and because it was heavy, bulky, and difficult to move, even with a trolley (Hollis, 1993).

By the mid-1990s, SDS policy makers were considering getting parents more involved in accessing dental care for their children. While the mobile service ensured good access, it usually precluded parental involvement as children were normally treated without their parents present (DHSV, 1997). There were also concerns about the ageing van fleet and associated occupational health and safety issues. Older vans did not provide a good clinical environment as there was limited space and temperature control was a problem. As reported by one dental therapist, "The vans could be an ice-box in winter and a sauna in summer" (Anonymous, personal communication, January 16, 2022). Infection control could also be problematic (A-GV, 2005).

"Demobilisation" was seen to confer several benefits. Reducing the number of SDS dental vans and moving to fixed off-school clinics promised greater efficiency due to reduced staff downtime; better quality of care in an improved working environment for staff; and a higher service profile (DHSV, 1997).

Echoing this view, the 2005 Victorian Auditor-General report noted that fixed clinics provided better facilities (reception, waiting rooms, and toilets); integration with other public dental and community services; certainty of location; and an enhanced clinical environment (peer support, infection control and clinical amenity) (A-GV, 2005).

Dental Health Services Victoria's (DHSV) 1997 annual report noted that dental vans would continue to visit schools which had a high proportion of children from lower socioeconomic areas and those that were geographically isolated (DHSV, 1997). Vans and portable equipment also continued to be used to provide dental care for people with a disability.

From 2019 Victoria's Smile Squad school dental program commenced, re-establishing a mobile school dental service for all Victorian government school students (Premier of Victoria, 2019). The scheme provides dental examination and treatment services using a mix of portable equipment and treatment vans. One of the program's advantages highlighted by government is the convenience for parents who will not have to take time off work to attend dental appointments with their children. The portable equipment is also more ergonomic than that used in the 1990s and the vans have high-quality lighting. By June 2022, 52 examination and 40 treatment vans were in operation across the state (DHSV, 2022).

Other states and territories that had moved away from dental vans to fixed clinics in the 2000s have also reintroduced more school visits, using a mix of treatment vans and portable equipment.

3 Transfer of SDS to Dental Health Services Victoria 1996–2009

In August 1996 responsibility for the SDS was transferred from the Victorian Department of Health and Community Services (DH&CS) to DHSV. Following a competitive process, dental therapy training had already been transferred from the department to the University of Melbourne in January 1996.

Children's participation in the SDS declined from 1997 due to two main factors – the change in access through "demobilisation" of the van fleet (Box 5.2), and the introduction of co-payments for families who did not hold a concession card (DHSV, 1997). The latter measure was a response to the Howard Coalition Government's abolition of the Commonwealth Dental Health Program (CDHP), as the demise of the CDHP significantly reduced the Victorian public dental budget.

With further problems, including difficulty in employing dental therapists (DHSV, 1998), participation in the SDS decreased. In the 13 years to 2009, the number of children treated by the SDS almost halved – from 154,874 in 1996 to 79,983 in 2009 (DHSV, 1997; DHSV, 2009).

4 Integration into the Community Dental Program by 2009

Between 2007 and 2009 the state-wide SDS service managed by DHSV was progressively integrated into the 60 existing community dental agencies. As part of SDS "demobilisation" (Box 5.2), co-location with community dental agencies increased. The rationale for co-location, and, subsequently, complete integration, included the provision of family-oriented care; professional peer support and peer review opportunities; staffing flexibility; and greater efficiencies through economies of scale (DHSV, 1997).

There are no published studies evaluating the integration of the SDS into the CDP. Anecdotally, community agencies were supportive of the new service model, whereas DHSV staff had reservations about the loss of its "jewel in the crown" (Anonymous, personal communication, 2022). The number of children receiving public dental care almost doubled between 2007 and 2018; from 95,294 to 173,451. However, former SDS staff have remarked that the integration process could have been better managed to retain some of the strengths of the service such as the good links with schools (Anonymous, personal communication, 2022). This view was possibly vindicated by the Victorian Labor Government's introduction of a new school dental program (the Smile Squad) in 2019 (Premier of Victoria, 2019).

5 Resurrection of school dental services as the Smile Squad in 2019

Shortly before the state election in November 2018, the ALP announced its intention to restart a program orientated to preventive dental health for school children, if re-elected. It was, and the Victorian Government introduced the school dental program, the Smile Squad, in 2019, with initial funding of $321.9 million (Premier of Victoria, 2019). Impetus for the reintroduction of a school-based preventive program is discussed as a case study in Chapter 4.

The program provides free dental care for all children at government primary and secondary schools. Through embedding healthy eating and drinking policies and practices, it also aims to support schools to be health promoting environments.

The return to a more mobile service increases the focus on service accessibility. Examinations and basic treatment are being provided at schools, while community dental clinics deliver more complex care. It is predicted that the program will save families an estimated $400 a year per child in dental costs and reduce the inconvenience of parents taking time off work for appointments (Premier of Victoria, 2019).

Smile Squad operated for barely six months before all non-emergency work ceased due to the series of COVID-19 state lockdowns. More than 3,300 children had been examined by June 2020 (DHSV, 2020) and over the next two financial years 40,000 children were offered care (DHSV 2021; DHSV 2022) (Figure 5.5). As mentioned in Box 5.2, by mid 2022, 52 examination and 40 treatment vans were in operation across the state (DHSV, 2022). By March 2023 a total of more than 82,000 students had received care and 350,000 oral health packs distributed (Thomas, 2023).

When Smile Squad could fully reopen in 2022, some of the former dental assistants and oral health therapists had left the service. This was true across all staff in the public dental sector, and indeed the loss of health care workers was a worldwide phenomenon. To rebuild staffing numbers, DHSV has been offering a Dental Assisting Trainee Program through Jobs Victoria. Employment opportunities are being provided to people who are experiencing long-term unemployment, culturally diverse, women aged over 45, Aboriginal and Torres Strait Islander people and newly arrived migrants. Trainees have found positions at health services across metropolitan Melbourne and regional Victoria (Thomas, 2023). Clinical placements for new oral health therapist graduates have also been supported to rebuild pre-pandemic staffing levels.

The Smile Squad program is up and running again although there are still challenges in translating observed treatment needs into actual treatment in vans or community dental clinics. It will be important to monitor uptake and oral health outcomes under this service model. Student participation rates in Victoria's SDS have historically been lower than those of other state and territory programs, except for New South Wales.

Many questions remain to be answered; for example, what proportion of parents will want to be present when their children are being treated? Will the high proportion of school children who already attend private dentists access the SDS as well, and what are the implications for continuity of care for them? Will the potential equity advantages of the model be realised? Is this the most cost-effective use of resources compared with, say, further targeting to disadvantaged preschool children and their families?

Summary

The SDS has experienced highs and lows since 1970. The period has been book-ended by two significant initiatives – the Whitlam Government's national school dental program in 1973, and the Andrews Government's Smile Squad from 2019. In the early 1980s the Victorian Department of Health questioned whether the school dental program should continue. It did continue but by 2009 it was absorbed into the community dental program. Revitalisation has now come about by way of the Smile Squad.

How successful have the various iterations of the SDS been? There has been no published overall examination of the impact of school dental services in Victoria. Children in Australian states and territories with more developed school dental programs have better oral health than Victorian children. However, other socioeconomic and cultural variations between jurisdictions also influence the extent of tooth decay (Chapter 10).

Despite the lack of a definitive evaluation, Victoria's SDS has clearly delivered a range of benefits through the decades. It has focussed mainly on preventive care, encompassing screening and early intervention, and targeting of children at higher risk of poor oral health has improved over time. The service also triggered the introduction of dental therapists, and they have proved able to provide cost-effective quality care. As a result, millions of Victoria children have benefited from a preventive approach to dental care provided by an innovative workforce.

It can seem disappointing, and possibly self-serving, when researchers conclude that further research is required to resolve remaining questions or form a broad consensus. The well-funded Smile Squad potentially allows Victoria to develop school dental services that match or surpass other jurisdictions. Even so, the school dental service has not been well studied and important questions about its role, performance and potential remain unanswered.

Appendices

Appendix 5.1 Annual visits to public dental services, Victoria, 1970 to 1994

Year	RDHM	Base hospitals	Pre-school clinics	SDS visits	Other	Total
1970	167,551		22,686	18,400		**208,700**
1975	237,297	8,143	24,139	23,000		**292,600**
1980	296,421	94,252	36,418	122,400		**549,500**
1985	264,277	114,196	46,766	262,800		**688,000**
1994	183,000	103,800	23,000	348,745	98,200	**756,700**

Notes and sources:
- RDHM, base hospitals and pre-school clinics data from 1970 to 1985 from DHV, 1985 and RDHM Annual Reports.
- 1985 data from DHV, 1985 and RDHM Annual Report, 1986
- SDS data from HCV, 1982 and DHV, 1985.
- 1994 data from DH&CS, 1995. 'Other' visits comprised of 43,800 visits to community health centres, 4,400 visits to aged care centres, and 50,000 visits to private dental practices.

Appendix 5.2 Major goals, recommendations and outcomes of Victorian government oral health plans, 1986 to 2030

Plan (*Government*)	Major goals	Major recommendations	Outcomes
Ministerial review of dental services, 1986 (MRODS) (DHV, 1996) (*Cain Labor*)	Increase access to dental services for those most in need. Prevent dental disease.	• Integrate and decentralise public dental services at a regional level. • Relocate dental therapist training to the Royal Dental Hospital of Melbourne (RDHM). • Extend community water fluoridation. • Focus on priority groups in settings such as community health centres and schools.	1988 Dental Health Strategy – 29 new community dental clinics established (Chapter 4). Therapist training moved to the University of Melbourne in 1994. Extension of fluoridation to 95% of Victorian population occurred by 2007.
Future directions for dental health in Victoria, 1995 (DH&CS, 1995) (*Kennett Liberal National Coalition*)	Provide a significant improvement in the dental health of Victorians. Restructure and improve the planning, integration, coordination and management of public dental services.	• Prevent dental disease and promote dental health. • Target public dental services to groups at high risk. • Conduct population-wide dental surveys. • Set and promote oral health goals. • Establish a lead dental agency, Dental Health Services Victoria (DHSV), by amalgamating the School Dental Service and the RDHM. • Update dental legislation.	*Promoting oral health 2000–2004 action plan* released.[1] 2004–06 adult oral health survey conducted. DHSV formed in 1996. *Dental Practice Act 1999.*

Plan (Government)	Major goals	Major recommendations	Outcomes
Improving Victoria's oral health, 2007 (DHS, 2007) *(Bracks Labor)*	All Victorians to enjoy good oral health and have access to health care when they require it.	• New oral health service planning framework. • Integrate public adult and children's services. • Workforce strategy. • Oral health promotion. • Respond to high-needs groups. • Oral health funding, accountability and evaluation.	Partly implemented. Integration completed in 2009.[2] Partly implemented. Partly implemented.[3] Partly implemented. Partly implemented.[4]
Action plan for oral health promotion 2013–2017 (DHV, 2013) *(Napthine Liberal National Coalition)*	Improve the oral health of all Victorians including population groups at higher risk.	• Build partnerships and environments. • Improve oral health literacy. • Strengthen prevention programs. • Improve workforce oral health promotion skills. • Improve oral health data and research.	Stronger links made with the settings-based Achievement Program (Chapter 6). Prevention programs implemented (Chapter 6). Partially implemented.
Victorian action plan to prevent oral disease 2020–30 (DHCS, 2020) *(Andrews Labor)*	Achieve oral health for all Victorians by 2030 and reduce the gap in oral health.	• Improve the oral health of children. • Promote healthy environments. • Improve oral health literacy. • Improve oral health promotion, screening, early detection and prevention services. • Four targets set for 2030.	*Smile Squad* program implemented in schools but constrained by COVID-19 in 2019 and 2020. Prevention programs implemented (see Chapter 6).

Notes and sources:

1. *Promoting oral health 2000–2004: Strategic directions and framework for action* (DHS, 1999).
2. Involved the integration of the School Dental Service into the Community Dental Program.
3. Oral health promotion was to become, "a vital component in the integrated health promotion approach ... led by Primary Care Partnerships" (DHS, 2007).
4. Included finding ways, "to support service integration, workforce strategies, demand management and oral health promotion" (DHS, 2007).

Appendix 5.3 Victorian Auditor-General oral health audits: Conclusions, recommendations, and outcomes, 1993 to 2019

Audit goal	Key findings	Major recommendations	Status of matters raised in follow-up reports
Review of the Schools Dental Health Service (SDHS), 1993, with follow-up in 1995			
Assess the effectiveness of the Schools Dental Health Service	The dental health of children was generally consistent with that of children participating in similar programs in other states. Only 67% of eligible school children participated in the service; the lowest rate in Australia, except for New South Wales. Failure to fully identify and treat children with high dental needs contributed to potentially poorer dental health outcomes. Taxpayers could not be assured that school dental services were provided in the most cost-effective manner.	Improve participation rates, particularly for children with high dental needs. Determine the potential for cost savings from the establishment of alternative program delivery arrangements.	Relatively low participation: – Survey undertaken by Department showed that 99% of Victorian primary school children had received dental care in the public or private system in the previous 3 years. Not fully identifying and treating children with highest dental needs: – Increase in children treated had occurred. Failure to examine outsourcing: – Department was considering becoming a purchaser of dental services, rather than a provider, so that services would be purchased on an output basis at the lowest cost consistent with service and quality standards.

Examine the economy, efficiency and effectiveness of community dental services	A system under stress facing increasing demand pressure, leading to a mismatch between the Government's stated priority for oral health promotion and the mix of services being delivered.[1] Issues in 4 main areas: • Inadequate access for the eligible population. • Efficiency, health and safety performance, and conditions in clinics vary widely. • Workforce shortages, database shortfall, scope to expand role of allied dental professionals. • Strategic direction requires revisiting, role confusion between DHS & DHSV, inadequate data on costs of service provision, need to focus more on outcomes.	15 recommendations regarding the 4 areas: • Service access. • Efficiency of service delivery. • Workforce issues. • Program management. Change goals or increase funding, "that the government address the increasingly low levels of effective access to public dental services. This will require either reduction in the eligibility, for and/or nature of service offerings or increased resources, or both" (A-GV, 2005, p. 52).	Some progress made but slow progress in: • improving waiting list management practices. • developing agency level information on costs and agency level benchmarks. A further 9 recommendations made in the 4 areas.

Assess the extent of timely access to the public dental system	Current treatment model is less cost effective than a preventive approach. Need to shift focus from treatment to a more patient-centred model aimed at prevention, early intervention and improving health outcomes.	Eleven recommendations in 3 areas: • A new approach to delivering public dental services. • Access to care during the transition. • Measuring and reporting performance.	Oral health promotion recommendation completed. Ten recommendations in progress. With no cost-benefit analysis, it is difficult to assess whether the value-based health model of care that has been piloted will deliver the expected benefits.

References

Australian Dental Association Victorian Branch. (ADAVB). (2022, February 23). *Drop in waiting times for public dental care, but concerns remain over long-term access.* [Media release]. <https://adavb.org/news-media/media-releases/drop-in-waiting-times-for-public-dental-care--but-concerns-remain-over-long-term-access>

Australian Health Ministers' Conference. (AHMC). National Advisory Committee on Oral Health. & South Australia. Department of Health. (2004). *Healthy mouths, healthy lives: Australia's national oral health plan 2004–2013.* Adelaide: South Australian Department of Health. <https://catalogue.nla.gov.au/Record/3298219>

Auditor-General of Victoria. (A-GV). (1993). *Report on ministerial portfolios, May 1993.* <https://www.audit.vic.gov.au/sites/default/files/19930501-Ministerial-Portfolios-May-1993.pdf>

Auditor-General of Victoria. (A-GV). (1995). *Report on ministerial portfolios, May 1995.* <https://www.audit.vic.gov.au/sites/default/files/19950501-Report-on-Ministerial-Portfolios.pdf>

Auditor-General Victoria. (A-GV). (2002). *Community dental services.* <https://www.audit.vic.gov.au/report/community-dental-services?section=.>

Auditor-General Victoria. (A-GV). (2005). *Results of special reviews and other investigations.* May 2005. <https://www.audit.vic.gov.au/sites/default/files/20050504-Special-Reviews-and-other-Investigation-May2005.pdf>

Auditor-General Victoria. (A-GV). (2016). *Access to public dental services in Victoria.* <https://www.audit.vic.gov.au/report/access-public-dental-services-victoria?section=32003--4-addressing-barriers-to-access#page-anchor.>

Auditor-General Victoria. (A-GV). (2019). Follow up of *Access to public dental services in Victoria.* <https://www.audit.vic.gov.au/report/follow-access-public-dental-services-victoria>

Australian Government Productivity Commission (AGPC). (2019). *Report on Government Services 2019.* Chapter 10, Primary and community health. <https://www.pc.gov.au/ongoing/report-on-government-services/2019/health/primary-and-community-health>

Biggs, A. (2008). *Overview of Commonwealth involvement in funding dental care.* <https://parlinfo.aph.gov.au/parlInfo/search/display/display.w3p;adv=yes;orderBy=customrank;page=0;query=Content%3ABiggs%20Content%3A%22Overview%20of%20Commonwealth%20involvement%20in%20funding%20dental%20care%22%20Date%3A01%2F01%2F2008%20%3E%3E%2031%2F12%2F2008%20Dataset%3Aprspub,jrnart,jrnart88;rec=1;resCount=Default>

Brennan, D.S., Carter, K.D., Stewart, J.F., & Spencer, A.J. (1997). *Commonwealth dental health program evaluation report 1994–1996.* Adelaide: University of Adelaide.

Dental Health Services Victoria (DHSV). *Annual reports* 1997 to 2022. Melbourne: DHSV.

Department of Health. Victoria. (DHV). (1986). *Ministerial review of dental services: Final report.* Melbourne: Department of Health.

Department of Health. Victoria. (DHV). (2013). *Action plan for oral health promotion 2013–2017.* <https://content.health.vic.gov.au/sites/default/files/migrated/files/collections/research-and-reports/1/1303009_htv_oral_health_web---pdf.pdf>

Department of Health and Community Services (DH&CS). Victoria. (1995). *Future directions for dental health in Victoria.* Melbourne: VGPS.

Department of Health and Human Services. (DHHS). (2020). *Victorian action plan to prevent oral disease 2020–30.* <https://www.health.vic.gov.au/sites/default/files/migrated/files/collections/research-and-reports/o/victorian-action-plan-to-prevent-oral-disease-2020.pdf>

Department of Human Services. (DHS) (1989). *On site analysis for change of dental health services.* Unpublished manuscript. Melbourne. Victoria.

Department of Human Services (DHS). (1996). *Victorian School Dental Service Core Data.* Dental Health Branch, November 1996. Unpublished manuscript. Melbourne. Victoria.

Department of Human Services. Victoria. (DHS). (2007). *Improving Victoria's oral health.* <https://vgls.sdp.sirsidynix.net.au/client/search/asset/1291900>

Dooland, M. (1992). *Improving dental health in Australia.* Background Paper No. 9. Melbourne: National Health Strategy.

Duckett, S., Cowgill, M., & Swerrisen, H. (2019). *Filling the gap: A universal dental care scheme for Australia.* <https://grattan.edu.au/wp-content/uploads/2019/03/915-Filling-the-gap-A-universal-dental-scheme-for-Australia.pdf.>

Fee, P., Riley P., Worthington H.V., Clarkson J.E., Boyers D., & Beirne P.V. (2020). *Recall intervals for oral health in primary care patients.* Cochrane Database of Systematic Reviews 2020, Issue 10. Art. No.: CD004346. <https://www.cochranelibrary.com/cdsr/doi/10.1002/14651858.CD004346.pub5/full>

Foley, M. (2021, December 22). *Boost for dental catch-up care.* [Media release]. <https://www.premier.vic.gov.au/sites/default/files/2021-12/211222%20-%20Boost%20For%20Dental%20Catch-Up%20Care.pdf?utm_source=miragenews&utm_medium=miragenews&utm_campaign=news>

Health Commission Victoria (HCV). (1982). *Report of internal committee reviewing the Victorian School Dental Service.* Unpublished.

Hollis, M. (1993). *Review of the dental program for school children.* Unpublished manuscript. Melbourne. Victoria.

Premier of Victoria. (2019, May 26). *The Smile Squad – Free dental vans to hit schools soon.* [Media release]. <https://www.premier.vic.gov.au/smile-squad-free-dental-vans-hit-schools-soon>

Robertson, J. (1989). *Dentistry for the masses?* Master of Arts Thesis, History Department. University of Melbourne. Victoria.

Satur, J. (2010). The establishment of dental therapy and hygiene in Victoria. In A. Tsang. (Ed.), *Oral health therapy programs in Australia and New Zealand.* Knowledge Books and Software. Queensland, Australia.

Sheiham A. (1977). Is there a scientific basis for six-monthly dental examinations? *The Lancet. 310*(8035), 442–44.

Storen, R., & Corrigan, N. (2020). *COVID-19: a chronology of state and territory government announcements (up until 30 June 2020).* <https://www.aph.gov.au/About_Parliament/Parliamentary_Departments/Parliamentary_Library/pubs/rp/rp2021/Chronologies/COVID-19StateTerritoryGovernmentAnnouncements>

Thomas, M-A. (2023, March 20). *Bringing more smiles to Victorian students.* [Media Release]. Victorian State Government.

Treasury and Finance, Victoria. (2004). *Service delivery 2004–05. Budget paper No. 3.* <https://www.dtf.vic.gov.au/previous-budgets/2004-05-state-budget>

Chapter 6
Prevention interventions – Better than cure?

John Rogers

Introduction

Prevention of oral disease, promoting oral health, and reducing longstanding inequities in health requires action by all sectors in civil society. How has this challenge been managed in Victoria? What are the lessons that could help shape future prevention interventions?

In this chapter, we discuss prevention initiatives that have been implemented in Victoria over the past 50 years. Particular attention is paid to evidence-based interventions that have improved the oral health of Victorians or at least achieved intermediate health promotion or health outcomes.

While scope to address the social, economic, political and environmental determinants of poor oral health – "the causes of the causes", such as income, education and housing – lies largely outside the health system, these determinants can be influenced by health policy and practice. Health policy, for example, can help promote healthy environments, influence early childhood development, and provide access to affordable health services of decent quality, all of which are social determinants of health (PAHO & WHO, 2023).

Key prevention and health promotion concepts that have shaped the Victorian prevention story are shown in Box 6.1.

Prevention interventions encompass primary prevention (stopping the occurrence of a disease), secondary prevention (reducing progression of a disease), and tertiary prevention (minimising the impact of a disease). Quaternary prevention (protecting people from medical interventions that are likely to cause more harm than good) has been identified more recently.

Health promotion is the process of enabling people to increase control over, and improve their health (WHO, n.d.). It moves beyond a focus on individual behaviour to encompass a wide range of social and environmental interventions (PAHO & WHO, 2023).

The Ottawa Charter for Health Promotion is recognised as a useful framework for categorising health promotion and prevention interventions (WHO, 1986a). There are five action areas: Build healthy public policy; create supportive environments; develop personal skills; strengthen community action; and reorient health services. A series of WHO international conferences have further developed health promotion policy and practice in areas such as bridging the equity gap and addressing the social determinants of health (Watt, 2005).

Development of a prevention and promotion focus in Victoria

While national interest in oral health promotion developed slowly – it took until 2004 for the first national oral health plan to be released (AHMC, 2004), a greater focus on prevention and promotion began to emerge in oral health in Victoria in the 1980s. The 1970s saw expansion of the School Dental Service (SDS) and the introduction of community water fluoridation, but there was a need for a broader focus on prevention policy and practice.

Victorian community development initiatives to improve oral health and reduce oral health inequality emerged in the 1980s. Internationally these approaches were articulated in the Declaration of Alma Ata (WHO, 1978) and the Ottawa Charter (WHO, 1986a) as part of the New Public Health (Lewis, 2003). District Health Councils were established in Victoria to support community involvement in health promotion and health planning, strengthen health system accountability, and educate people about factors which influence their health (Legge & Sylvan, 1990).

Brunswick and Kensington Community Health Centres in Melbourne, with District Health Council support, undertook community development activities to advocate for greater access to public dental services (Chapter 8). An outcome of such advocacy, echoed in the recommendations in the Ministerial Review of Dental Services (MRODS) (DHV, 1986), was the establishment of the Community Dental Program (CDP) in 1998 (Chapter 4). Twenty-nine new public dental clinics were created to provide preventively focused public dental care, managed by community health centres or hospitals.

Comprehensive planning of oral health promotion occurred in 1995. The Public Health Division of the Department of Health and Human Services released a discussion paper (DHS, 1997) and the Faculty of Dentistry at the University of Melbourne was commissioned to undertake a literature review of prevention best practice (DHS, Wright, Satur & Morgan, 2000). A broad consultation process was established to develop a prevention plan titled *Promoting oral health 2000–2004: Strategic directions and framework for action* (DHS, 1999). Coordination was facilitated by the establishment of Dental Health Services Victoria (DHSV) which brought together the SDS, the Royal Dental Hospital of Melbourne (RDHM), and the coordination of community dental agencies (Chapter 4).

When the Promoting Oral Health plan was released, a funding round for oral health promotion projects was announced and a broadly representative committee was established to oversee the implementation of the plan and associated projects. The planning process and plan were recognised internationally as best practice in public health (Watt, 2005).

Extension of community water fluoridation to rural areas and expansion of pre-school dental services occurred with funds from the 2004–05 State Budget. The best practice review has been updated several times since 2010 (Satur et al., 2010; Rogers & DHS, 2011; Hegde & de Silva, 2013; Rana et al., 2022); two oral health prevention plans have been released (DHV, 2013; DHHS, 2020) facilitated by Dental Health Services Victoria (DHSV) as part of their state wide oral health promotion role; and new programs have been introduced for preventing oral disease in preschool children, for smoking cessation, and for oral cancer screening. The SDS has also been resurrected as the Smile Squad with significant funding (Chapter 5).

A timeline of prevention and health promotion interventions introduced in Victoria over the past 50 years and a list of key policy and planning documents, are presented in Appendix 6.1. These are described in more detail in Chapter 4 as many encompass broader oral health policy and planning activities.

Victorian interventions and the Ottawa Charter for Health Promotion

In broad terms, the intention of prevention and health promotion activities in oral health is to make the healthy choices the easy choices and, ideally, to reduce inequality in oral health. The Charter embodies the concept that "health promotion is not just the responsibility of the health sector but goes beyond healthy lifestyles to wellbeing" so as to "to address the political, economic, social, cultural, environmental, behavioural and biological factors that can favour health or be harmful to it" (WHO, 1986a, p. 1).

In this section, key Victorian oral health interventions of the past 50 years are examined within the framework of the Ottawa Charter for Health Promotion. Interventions are discussed in terms of their rationale, the Victorian experience and achievements, and remaining challenges. Interventions were identified through a systematic literature review as outlined in Appendix 6.2.

The success of an intervention is considered within a hierarchy, where improvement in oral health status is the ultimate measure, but progress on intermediate health promotion or health outcomes is also acknowledged. Promising interventions are included with the caveat that further evaluation is required before broader implementation can be considered.

1 Build healthy public policy

Building healthy public policy is the overarching action area of the Ottawa Charter. Interventions can occur through legislation, regulation, guidelines or fiscal measures.

1.1 Progressive implementation of community water fluoridation, 1962 – ongoing

Rationale

Fluoridation is the controlled adjustment of the underlying fluoride concentration in drinking water to the level that prevents tooth decay. It is a safe and cost-effective way to prevent tooth decay in children and adults, regardless of socioeconomic status or access to dental care (NHMRC, 2017; IADR, 2022). Community water fluoridation has been identified as one of the ten great public health achievements of the 20th century (CDC, 1999).

The Victorian experience

While Victoria was the site of one of the first community water fluoridation initiatives (in Bacchus Marsh in 1962) and passed the *Health (Fluoridation) Act* in 1973, fluoridation of Melbourne's water supply did not occur until 1977, which was later than in most Australian capital cities. Extension of community water fluoridation in rural Victoria occurred only after a 2004–05 State Budget allocation of $3.1m for this purpose which was part of a four-year $97.2m dental health package (Treasury & Finance, 2004).

Achievements and remaining challenges

By 2017, more than 90% of Victorians had access to fluoridated drinking water (NHMRC, 2017). It has been estimated that fluoridation has saved the Victorian community about $1 billion over a 25-year period through avoided costs of dental treatment and days absent from work or school (Jaguar Consulting, 2016). In addition, fluoridation is significantly associated with a reduction in dental hospitalisations of young Victorian children for removal of badly decayed teeth under general anaesthetic (Rogers et al., 2018).

While Melbourne and large regional centres have community water fluoridation, people living in regional and rural Victoria have less access to fluoridated drinking water. The *Victorian action plan to prevent oral disease 2020–30* includes a target to "increase the proportion of rural and regional Victorians accessing fluoridated drinking water to 95%" by 2030, from the baseline of 87% (DHHS, 2020, p. 6). While fluoridation of Cohuna's water supply in 2021 increased this coverage to 88% (see Section 4.1), further extension of fluoridation is required to meet the 2030 target.

1.2 Expanding the role of non-dental professionals, 2019 – ongoing

Rationale

Applying fluoride varnish to preschoolers at high risk of tooth decay is preventive (WHO, 2019) and the application of fluoride varnish by non-oral health clinicians can be cost effective (Quinonez et al., 2006).

The Victorian experience – Workforce legislation and regulation changes

Amendments to the Victorian Drugs Poisons and Controlled Substances Regulations 2017 authorised dental assistants (in 2019) and Registered Aboriginal Health Practitioners (in 2022) to obtain, possess and administer fluoride varnish in certain community settings. It is expected that these changes will facilitate timely, cost-effective application of fluoride varnish to children. In the case of dental assistants, this will take place in pre-school settings and, for Aboriginal children, in an environment that is culturally appropriate, inclusive of, and easily accessible to their families.

Achievements and remaining challenges

As these are recent initiatives, there has not yet been an economic evaluation to determine the cost effectiveness of using non-oral health clinicians to apply fluoride varnish in Victoria. Such economic evaluations should be supported. There is scope to trial application of varnish by other health professionals, for example, pharmacists, maternal and child health nurses, and paediatricians.

There is also further scope for non-dental professionals to become oral health promoters. Collaboration in Victoria with midwives, maternal and child health nurses, early childhood professionals and community mental health professionals is supported under Ottawa Charter action area 2. A challenge for many professionals is that they have limited knowledge and understanding of oral health issues, as was identified for paediatricians (Dickson-Swift et al., 2020) and pharmacists (Calache et al., 2017; Chuanon, 2019; McMillan, 2021). Oral health advice is available for 13 different professional groups on the DHSV website.[19]

---

19 See <https://www.dhsv.org.au/oral-health-advice/Professionals>

1.3 Oral health prevention policies and plans, 1970 – ongoing

Rationale

The introduction of significant prevention interventions requires an authorising environment and effective policies and plans that clearly outline the issues and put forward proposals to address these.

The Victorian experience, achievements and remaining challenges

There have been ten Victorian and Australian government policies and plans for the prevention of oral disease and the promotion of oral health since 1970: three in the first 30 years, and seven since 2000 (Appendix 6.1). Some have proved more influential than others. The national plans released in 2004 (AHMC et al., 2004), and 2015 (COAG, 2015), have outlined oral health issues and possible solutions, but there is no allocation of responsibility for funding and implementation. The latest Victorian plan released in 2020 includes oral health targets for 2030 (DHHS, 2020). Chapter 5 includes an analysis of the extent to which plans have been implemented.

1.4 Oral health in all health policy, 2011 – ongoing

Rationale

Recognition and integration of oral health in relevant policies and public health programs is a key strategy for improving oral health and reducing inequities. In Victoria, the *Public Health and Wellbeing Act 2008* gives state and local governments specific responsibilities to plan for and contribute to the protection and improvement of health and wellbeing. The Act requires both state and municipal public health and wellbeing plans to be prepared sequentially every four years. Victorian public health and wellbeing (VPHW) plans provide an opportunity to raise the profile of oral health and incorporate oral health prevention and promotion activities.

The Victorian experience – Victorian Public Health and Wellbeing Plans

The 2011–15 *Victorian public health and wellbeing plan* included oral health as one of nine priority areas (DHV, 2011). However, while the 2015–19 and 2019–23 VPHW plans used a common risk factor approach that included promotion of healthy food and smoking cessation, oral health was not included as a priority (SGV, 2015; SGV, 2019).

Achievements and remaining challenges

Inclusion of oral health in local government VPHW plans has fluctuated. An unpublished review found that two thirds (41%) of the 79 local governments included oral health as a priority in their 2014 plans. In the 2017 plans there was a reduction with only four of 48 rural municipal plans including oral health-specific actions or strategies (Dickson-Swift & Crocombe, 2021). However, a third (34%) of the 79 plans in 2021 included oral health as a priority, and all but three of the plans included initiatives that would prevent dental disease, such as tobacco control and reduction of sugar (DHSV, 2022a). Actions that local government can take to improve oral health are outlined in the *Improving oral health – Local government action guide* (DHSV & DHHS, 2020).

A further opportunity to promote oral health in all health policy is to integrate oral health promotion into the implementation of the *National preventive health strategy 2021–2030* (DH-A, 2021) (Appendix 12). While oral health is not specifically included as one of the seven strategic focus areas, five of the areas are common risk factors for oral disease.

2 Create supportive environments

2.1 Healthy families, healthy smiles, 2012 – ongoing

Rationale

The period of early childhood is crucial for establishing lifelong oral health (Trinh et al., 2022). There is promising evidence that health and early childhood professionals can be effective in promoting oral health (Rogers & DHS, 2011; Trinh et al., 2022).

The Victorian experience

The *Healthy families, healthy smiles* preventive program commenced in 2012 and aims to improve the oral health of young children and pregnant women (DHSV, 2022b). Managed by DHSV with funding from the Department of Health, the focus is on building the knowledge, skills and confidence of health and early education professionals to promote oral health when they interact with children and families. The professions involved include midwives, maternal and child health nurses, Aboriginal health workers, physicians, dieticians, pharmacists, and professionals who work in early childhood settings and supported play groups. The approach has been to support these professionals to incorporate oral health promotion into their routine activities. Training has included "lifting the lip" to identify tooth decay in the upper anterior teeth; encouraging screening and early intervention, including referral for dental care; and encouraging toothbrushing.

Achievements and remaining challenges

Over the ten-year history of the program, more than 6,300 professionals and students have received occupationally specific training in oral health promotion (DHSV, 2022c). A range of resources (position statements, practice guides, flipcharts, tooth packs, videos, flyers, mouth models and tip cards) have been developed and distributed. Partnerships have been established with professional associations, such as in pharmacy and nutrition, to facilitate training and develop oral health promotion policies (DHSV, 2015a; DHSV & DA, 2021). Systems-level changes have included incorporation of oral health prompts in general health screening, introduction of clinical guidelines, and the development of referral pathways.

Three key initiatives of *Healthy families, healthy smiles* have involved midwives, maternal and child health nurses, and supported playgroups. Each of these interventions has shown health promotion impacts, but they require further economic evaluation, also of their impacts on children's behaviour and, ideally, on their oral health.

Monitoring and evaluation of the program has been extensive (DHSV, 2015b; George et al., 2016; DHSV, 2020a; DHSV, 2020b; Heilbrunn-Lang et al., 2020). Positive health promotion actions have occurred and intermediate health outcomes achieved. However, there has been no published economic evaluation or evaluation of the program's impact on the oral health of participating children. The latter can be methodologically challenging as *Healthy families, healthy smiles* works primarily with health professionals (to enable them to promote oral health), rather than directly with families.

2.1.1 Role of midwives

Rationale

Oral health is an integral part of antenatal care with a dental check-up recommended early in pregnancy. An online *Midwifery initiated oral health education program* (MIOH) course for midwives has been shown in New South Wales to be both cost effective (Tannous et al., 2021) and to improve the oral health outcomes of the pregnant women under these midwives' care (George et al., 2018).

The Victorian experience

The MIOH course has been revised to make it relevant to the Victorian context and training places have been made available. By 2022, more than 390 midwives working in Victoria had completed the program (DHSV, 2022d).

Achievements and remaining challenges

Course participants have reported significant increases in oral health knowledge and higher confidence levels in performing mouth checks, communicating oral health and nutritional information, and supporting pregnant women with their dental referral (Heilbrunn-Lang et al., 2015; George et al., 2016; DHSV, 2022d). Oral health questions have been added to the Birthing Outcome System, a clinical information management system used in around 75% of Victorian hospitals.

Further evaluation is required with Victorian midwives who have completed the MIOH course to determine whether their strong intention to change their professional practice has translated into the actual care delivered, whether there has been an increase in pregnant women attending for dental care, and what impact there has been on the oral health of children.

2.1.2 Role of maternal and child health nurses

Rationale

Integrating oral health promotion into nursing practice is a promising initiative for preventing oral disease and reducing oral health inequities (Abou El Fadl et al., 2016).

Victorian experience

The Victorian Maternal and Child Health (MCH) Service is a free universal primary health service available for all Victorian families with children from birth to school age. The Healthy families, healthy smiles initiatives have built on earlier oral health promotion interventions in Victoria such as the Country Kids program (Neumann et al., 2011). Anticipatory guidance, health promotion and prevention all aim to give children, mothers and families the best likelihood of optimal health, wellbeing, safety, learning and development outcomes. There are ten key age and stage assessments. "Lift the lip" mouth checks occur at the 8-month, 18-month, and 3–5-year visits. Tooth tips fact sheets are provided at the 8-, 12- and 18-month visits, and a toothbrushing demonstration at the 18-month visit (DHV, 2022). Referral to dental clinics is facilitated when oral health problems are found.

Achievements and remaining challenges

The MCH nurses in disadvantaged communities have been provided with toothbrushes and toothpaste for low-income families. Provision of these "tooth packs", along with mouth checks and referrals for dental care, has been found to significantly increase the likelihood of children attending a dental clinic (by 28 times); self-reported parent assisted toothbrushing twice daily (by 1.8 times); and toothpaste use once a day (by 2.8 times) (Heilbrunn-Lang et al., 2020). Further evaluation is required to determine the viability and cost effectiveness of expanding this approach to all disadvantaged children in Victoria.

2.1.3 Supported playgroups
– Brush Book Bed, 2018 – ongoing

Rationale

Young children are at higher risk of tooth decay if they go to bed with dirty teeth. Government-supported playgroups are a key setting for oral health promotion as they target vulnerable population groups who are likely to have poorer oral health (Chapter 10).

The Victorian experience

Brush book bed was developed as a pilot project in supported playgroups to trial an innovative approach to engage and encourage parent-child toothbrushing (DHSV, 2020c). Facilitators were trained to provide toothbrushing demonstrations using a puppet alligator. Parents received family packs with information, a book, and family toothbrushes and paste.

Achievements and remaining challenges

Over the two years to June 2020, 200 supported playgroup facilitators attended workshops, and 3,000 families were reached. More than 90% of facilitators reported that they felt confident and planned to deliver a toothbrushing demonstration (DHSV, 2020d). Follow-up research to determine if the demonstrations had occurred, and their impact on the frequency of parent-child toothbrushing, was not possible because of the COVID-19 pandemic. Such research is necessary to determine the impact of the program.

2.2 *Smiles4Miles,* 2004 – ongoing

Rationale

By instituting healthy food policy and practices and promoting oral hygiene (Anopa et al., 2015) and dental visits, early childhood services can be oral health promoting environments for young children. The same is true for health promoting schools (Moysés et al., 2003).

The Victorian experience

Dental Health Services Victoria works in partnership to implement *Smiles 4 Miles,* an oral health promotion award program for early childhood services in disadvantaged areas. Services can become accredited when they meet criteria as an oral health promoting setting.

Achievements and remaining challenges

Partners include 34 local community health organisations, the Statewide Achievement Program,[20] Healthy Eating Advisory Service,[21] Cancer Council Victoria, Nutrition Australia, Victorian Aboriginal Community Controlled Health Organisation (VACCHO), and the early childhood care and education sectors. The Smiles4Miles program began in 2004 in 16 early childhood centres with 776 children. In 2021–22, the program reached more than 56,000 children and their families in 750 early childhood services (DHSV, 2022e). Further research is required to determine the impact of the program on oral health.

---

20 An initiative of the Victorian State Government and Cancer Council Victoria – see <https://www.achievementprogram.health.vic.gov.au>
21 See <https://heas.health.vic.gov.au>

2.3 Disability Support Services, 2008 – ongoing

Rationale

The oral health of people with intellectual and developmental disability is poorer than that of the general community (Kisely et al., 2015; Wilson et al., 2022). Group homes can potentially become oral health promoting settings and community mental health professionals can become oral health champions.

The Victorian experience

Three oral health projects have forged partnerships with disability services providers. In the early 2000s, Plenty Valley Community Health Service and DHSV worked with staff from the disability accommodation services of the Department of Human Services to strengthen oral health practices in group homes (DHSV, 2008b). Subsequently, the non-government disability provider, genU, worked with DHSV from 2014 to develop a staff-led oral health champions program in group homes (DHSV, 2018). Thirdly, the Melbourne Dental School at the University of Melbourne have been in partnership with Neami National, an Australian community mental health service, to deliver the Smile for Health program (Ho et al., 2017; Meldrum et al., 2018; McGrath et al., 2021).

Achievements and remaining challenges

These projects established oral health policy and practice guidelines and built the capacity of staff to support oral health. The two initiatives in group homes established an oral health champion in each home and individual oral health care plans were developed or planned (DHSV, 2008b; DHSV 2018). *Smile for Health* provided training to develop the capacity of Neami staff to promote the oral health of people living with severe mental health problems in the community. Training was provided initially in Victoria and then nationally. Participation in oral health training led to higher knowledge, confidence and more positive attitudes to oral health promotion (McGrath et al., 2021). Similar results were found after information sessions with genU staff (DHSV, 2018). A website has been developed by DHSV with information, resources, tips and strategies to build the knowledge, confidence and skills of the disability support workforce to promote healthy environments.[22]

The creation of the National Disability Insurance Scheme (NDIS) has enhanced greater client choice of service providers and affected the sustainability of some previous providers. Further partnership models need to be tested.

---

22 See <https://www.dhsv.org.au/oral-health-programs/disability>

3 Develop personal skills

Behavioural choices are influenced by information, resources and social support, as well as by personal skills. The relatively low levels of oral health literacy among Victorians is discussed in Chapter 10, particularly concerning gum disease and parents' understanding of diet.

Programs such as *Healthy families, healthy smiles* and *Smiles4Miles* provide information and resources, and help develop personal skills. A degree of social support is also provided to families in the settings in which these programs operate. Other Victorian programs that develop personal skills include the following.

3.1 Smokefree Smiles, 2014 – ongoing

Rationale

Smoking significantly increases the risk of oral cancer and periodontal (gum) disease. Oral health professionals can play an important role in helping clients to quit smoking (Holliday et al., 2021).

The Victorian experience

The Smokefree Smiles project trains and supports oral health staff to deliver brief interventions to help their patients quit smoking, as well as initiate referrals to Quitline (DHSV, 2022f).

Achievements and remaining challenges

Smoking cessation support strategies for the oral health setting have been incorporated within an online training resource (DHSV, 2017, p. 17). There is the opportunity for a brief discussion with a patient about smoking cessation when an oral health professional is undertaking an oral cancer screening exam. The latter is being promoted by the Victorian Oral Cancer Screening and Prevention Program.[23] Further evaluation of both programs is required.

3.2 Mouthguards

The use of mouthguards in contact sports to prevent trauma is well accepted and Victorian programs to increase their use have been shown to be effective (Jolly, 1996).

4 Strengthen community action

4.1 Advocacy for community water fluoridation, 1962 – ongoing

Rationale

Water fluoridation is a safe and effective way of reducing tooth decay across the population (NHMRC, 2017), as presented in Section 1.1.

The Victorian experience

Public advocacy has been crucial for the extension of community water fluoridation in Victoria. Support has come from various alliances of health workers, professional associations and universities, and from community-based initiatives. A local dentist was the driving force behind fluoridating the Bacchus Marsh water supply in 1962 (Head, 1978). Dentists and dental academics worked with Australian Dental Association Victorian Branch (ADAVB) to advocate for the fluoridation of Melbourne

---

23 See <https://www.dhsv.org.au/oral-health-programs/oral-cancer-screening-and-prevention>

in the 1970s (Chapter 8). The Department of Health established a Water Fluoridation Advisory Committee in the late 1990s with a broad membership of academics, clinicians and policy makers to support local activity, speak at forums, and undertake media activity.

Achievements and remaining challenges

The most recent fluoridation initiative, in the Victorian rural town of Cohuna, came about through a process of community engagement, planning and implementation. The Rural ECOH (Engaging Communities in Oral Health) project obtained a partnership grant from the National Health and Medical Research Council (DHSV, 2019). The partners for this grant included La Trobe Rural Health School, James Cook University, the Royal Flying Doctors, DHSV and Murray Primary Health Network (formerly Loddon Murray-Mallee Medicare Local). The aim was to attain dental/oral health improvement in rural Australia through community participation in population health planning (Dickson-Swift, 2019).

Academics worked with the local community to identify oral health problems, plan strategies to address these (such as water fluoridation) and advocate for them to be implemented (Dickson-Swift, 2019). The first community meeting was held in 2014 and, despite challenges in achieving meaningful community engagement (Wilson et al., 2017; Taylor et al., 2018; DHSV, 2019), Cohuna's water supply was fluoridated in 2021 (Gannawarra Shire Council, 2021; Dickson-Swift & Crocombe, 2021).

As mentioned in Section 1.1, further extension of fluoridation is required to meet the 2030 target outlined in the *Victorian action plan to prevent oral disease 2020–30* (i.e., access to fluoridated drinking water for 95% of rural and regional Victorians) (DHHS, 2020).

4.2 Teeth Tales, multicultural community-based oral health promotion program, 2010–2014

Rationale

Culturally and linguistically diverse (CALD) communities often have higher prevalence of oral disease and face more barriers to obtaining oral health care than the general population (Chapter 10). Community development approaches can increase community interest and networks to support oral health (DHS & Wright et al., 2000).

The Victorian experience

Teeth Tales was a community-based participatory research project that brought together the University of Melbourne, Merri Community Health Service and organisations working with CALD communities. The aim was to establish a model for feasible, replicable and affordable child oral health promotion for culturally diverse local governments in Australia.

There were three phases in a co-designed "bottom-up" approach. Interviews were conducted in their own languages with mothers from Iraqi, Lebanese and Pakistani communities to gain an understanding of existing knowledge, beliefs and practices about dental development and oral health. The second phase was a pilot study of possible interventions, and the third was a series of "peer support" focus groups, in which non-dental personnel recruited for the project provided oral health education and promotion (Gibbs et al., 2014).

Achievements and remaining challenges

The outcome of the project was a significant change in the knowledge, attitudes and practices surrounding the dietary intakes and behaviours of the participating families, as manifested by drinks purchased and children's tooth-brushing routines and plaque indices (Riggs et al., 2014; Gibbs et al., 2015). Other beneficial outcomes were the establishment of mutual support networks among the families, a lower likelihood of feeling isolated, improved self-esteem for many mothers, and increased knowledge of how and where to access dental and health care (Riggs et al., 2014; Gibbs et al., 2015).

While *Teeth Tales* was a successful pilot program, funds were not available to continue the program. Further resources are required to continue and expand programs such as *Teeth Tales.*

4.3 Community-based oral health promotion programs for elderly migrants, 2004–2015

Rationale

Culturally and linguistically diverse communities often have higher prevalence of oral disease and face more barriers to obtaining oral health care than the general population (Chapter 10).

The Victorian experience

A community-based health promotion model for older Greek and Italian migrants attending community clubs in Melbourne was developed based on the extent and impact on quality of life of oral conditions and access to dental care: *Oral Health Information Seminars/ Sheets* (ORHIS) (Marino et al., 2004; Marino et al., 2005). Subsequently, peer educators were used to provide further seminars and brushing sessions at the clubs (Marino, 2013). A further

development was multimedia-based health education (eORHIS) for older adults using social media web technologies (Marino et al., 2016).

Research has been conducted with a range of cultural groups to determine the barriers and enablers to improve oral health as a starting point for community-based oral health promotion initiatives. Programs have been conducted with Chinese (Marino et al., 2012) and Sri Lankan older migrants (Abuzar et al., 2009).

Achievements and remaining challenges

ORHIS led to improved oral health knowledge, attitudes, quality of life and dental care attendance compared to the control group (Marino et al., 2004; Marino et al., 2005; Marino et al., 2013). The peer education sessions led to significant improvements in denture hygiene and self-reported oral health compared to the control group (Marino et al., 2013). An analysis of costs determined that community-based oral health interventions can be cost-effective compared to chair-side oral health promotion in a dental clinic (Marino et al., 2014). The eORIS program was found to improve oral health knowledge, attitudes and self-efficacy (Marino et al., 2016).

Further research is required to determine the long-term impact and broader cost-effectiveness before these programs can be expanded.

5 Reorient health services

5.1 School-based programs – ongoing

Rationale

School-based oral health programs provide preventive-focused and accessible oral health care that can provide children with a good oral health foundation for life.

The Victorian experience

There have been a range of preventive initiatives based in Victorian schools. These include support for the integration of oral health promotion into subjects such as maths, science and biology. A *Dental health education kit – A curriculum approach, prep to year six* was developed by the SDS and the Directorate of School Education. The resource was released in 1993 and over 1,000 copies were sold to schools (DHS, 1993). No evaluation of the impact of the resource has been identified.

Economic evaluation determined that a school-based fissure sealant and fluoride mouth rinsing program was effective in non-fluoridated regional Victoria (Morgan et al., 1998). Also, school-based dental check-up programs targeted to children from low-income families have shown some success in increasing dental visits (Nguyen et al., 2020).

In 2019, the Smile Squad[24] was established as a preventive school dental program which aims to provide free dental care for all children at government primary and secondary schools in Victoria. The program also aims to embed oral health promotion policies into practice in schools, including healthy eating and drinking. At the announcement of the program in 2019, it was anticipated that this initiative funded at the level of $321m over four years would save families around $400 a year per child in dental costs (Premier of Victoria, 2019).

Achievements and remaining challenges

The COVID-19 pandemic has restricted implementation of the Smile Squad (Chapter 5). A comprehensive evaluation is being planned which needs to include oral health impacts.

5.2 Preventive and value-based dental care

Rationale

Screening and early and minimal intervention approaches prevent oral disease and the hospitalisation of young children (Arrow & Klobas, 2015) and can be cost-effective Tonmukayakul & Arrow, 2017). Value-based health care is a person-centred approach that has the potential to deliver improved health outcomes that matter most to people at a lower cost (Porter, 2010).

The Victorian experience

Community dental agencies have varied in their focus on prevention and oral health promotion. Some do so through partnership in programs such as *Smiles4Miles* or have developed their own outreach programs in aged care facilities, childcare settings and schools. The 2016 Victorian Auditor-General's report noted that the ability of community dental agencies to carry out oral health promotion activities depended on available resources (A-GV, 2016, p.15). The report goes on to say that DHSV will need to collaborate with agencies to identify ways to deliver health promotion effectively and efficiently, and, importantly, allocate the necessary resources (A-GV, 2016, p.16).

---

24 See <https://www.smilesquad.vic.gov.au>

Agencies have collaborated in a wide range of research projects with DHSV, universities and research institutes. North Richmond Community Health Service has implemented a "health promoting minimally invasive oral disease management model of care" (Hall & Christian, 2017). Barwon Health has undertaken relevant practice-based research. The health service participated in the Romp & Chomp program, which was shown to reduce childhood obesity and improve young children's diets through a community-wide focus on healthy eating and active play (de Silva et al., 2010). Barwon Health has also prevented tooth decay through the application of fluoride varnish to children in childcare settings (Mason et al., 2015; Rogers et al., 2016), and successfully managed decayed molar teeth by using Hall crown techniques (Barwon Health, 2022). A trial run by DHSV with two community dental agencies found that using silver diamine fluoride to manage tooth decay significantly prevented the dental hospitalisation of children (Yawary & Hegde, 2022).

Value-based oral health care has been trialled at the RDHM with high levels of client satisfaction (Mckee et al., 2019). However, the Victorian Auditor-General's 2019 report on access to public dental services in Victoria noted that without a cost–benefit analysis it was difficult to assess whether the value-based model piloted will deliver the expected benefits (AG-V, 2019, p. 7). New models of care have been introduced in the RDHM's general and primary care clinics and within the Smile Squad (DHSV, 2021). State-wide roll-out to community dental agencies is planned.

A key aspect of a value-based care model that can provide a more preventive approach in the delivery of public dental services is having a funding model that rewards optimal client outcomes rather than treatment outputs (AG-V, 2016, p. 29). Blended funding models with a risk-adjusted capitation base and outcome-based components have been proposed as a means to re-orient funding from volume to value (Hegde & Haddock, 2019). The Department of Health and DHSV are reviewing funding models (AG-V, 2019, p.7).

Being able to measure client satisfaction has been enhanced through a best-practice initiative instigated by DHSV. A standard set of oral health outcome measures has been developed with the International Consortium for Health Outcome Measures. These comprise patient-reported outcome measures (PROMS) and patient reported experience measures (PREMS) (Riordain et al., 2021). These measures are being used to analyse the effectiveness of services and prioritise high-value care (that is, care that contributes to patient oral health outcomes, and is cost effective), while eliminating low-value care (care that does not improve health outcomes and is less cost effective) (Hegde & Haddock, 2019).

Achievements and remaining challenges

The challenge is to scale up value-based care with a prevention focus across the public oral health system. This will require close collaboration between DHSV and community dental agencies. Strong monitoring and evaluation elements are necessary. If the high demand on the sector continues, it is likely that a shift to a more preventive focus in the public sector will require considerable additional funding, at least in the short term (Chapter 4).

The Ottawa Charter in action in Victoria

This brief historical overview of prevention and oral health promotion initiatives in Victoria emphasises the importance of action in each of the five action areas of the Ottawa Charter. It recognises the key determinants of health and the shared responsibility of individuals, communities and governments. It highlights the need for effective partnerships in health promotion, through which the work of relevant sectors and stakeholders combines to achieve better oral health outcomes.

System infrastructure

System infrastructure to provide continuity, coordination and dissemination of best practice for prevention and promotion has improved since 1970. On its release in 2004, the first national oral health plan – *Healthy mouths healthy lives: Australia's national oral health plan 2004–2013* (AHMC, 2004) – identified the priority need for strategic leadership to assist states and territories to build oral health promotion research and practice capacity.

In 2006 the National Oral Health Promotion Steering Group (NOHPSG) was established with a broad membership of public oral health managers from each state and territory, professional associations and researchers. The NOHPSG's primary objective was to provide national leadership in the delivery of the health promotion components of the first national oral health plan and the subsequent plan, *Healthy mouths healthy lives: Australia's national oral health plan 2015–2024* (COAG, 2015). However, a formal mechanism for NOHPSG to perform such a role, via reporting to the National Dental Directors Group, was not achieved until a review of the terms of reference in 2016.

In the meantime, NOHPSG, with a membership primarily of state and territory oral health promotion managers, continued to meet and served as a useful conduit to coordinate interstate resource sharing and communicate best practice in oral health promotion. The group also provided detailed input into the development of the second national oral health plan.

Within Victoria, the DHSV Population Health Committee has played an important role in developing the Victorian *Action plan for oral health promotion 2013–2017* (DHV, 2013) and the subsequent *Victorian action plan to prevent oral disease 2020–30* (DHHS, 2020). Committee membership has included representatives from community dental agencies, the Victorian Aboriginal Community Controlled Health Organisation (VACCHO), and professional associations such as the Australian Dental Association Victorian Branch (ADAVB). These organisations have been directly involved in prevention programs as well as advocacy to increase access to dental care (Chapter 8).

The ADAVB through its Oral health Committee has contributed to prevention initiatives through management and advisory roles for programs such as the Oral Cancer and Screening program, Smokefree Smiles and *Healthy families, healthy smiles*. It runs Dental Health Week and participates in World Oral Health Day which have become important annual avenues for enhancing community oral health literacy.

In the future, there are two opportunities to integrate oral health promotion within broader health promotion using a common risk factor approach. The first is to include oral health promotion in the implementation of the *National preventive health strategy 2021–2030* (DH-A, 2021) as mentioned in Section 1.4 of this chapter. Secondly, oral health could be included in the remit of the Australian Centre for Disease Control being established by the Commonwealth health department.

Summary

What has been learnt from the Victorian experience that can applied in future oral health policy and interventions?

Improving oral health and reducing longstanding inequities between populations calls for action across all five Ottawa Charter action areas by all sectors of the society. It requires tackling the broader determinants of health in addition to the more proximal factors that cause oral disease. The rationale for this approach is further strengthened by the fact that these broader determinants – such as poor diet, smoking and excessive alcohol consumption – are common risk factors for a range of other health issues including obesity, heart disease, and cancers (Watt & Sheiham, 2012).

In addition to the common risk factors, the prevention of oral disease also requires a "FOD approach" – the use of **f**luoride, **o**ral hygiene, and preventive **d**ental visits. These interventions are specific to oral health and need to be included in broader health promotion programs.

It is apparent that while there have been successful prevention programs in Victoria over the past 50 years, they have often been on a relatively small scale. Community water fluoridation has been a standout example; however, further opportunities for prevention of oral disease and reduction of inequity have not been realised. Indeed, inequality has increased (Chapter 10). Budgets for prevention have been small and successful pilot programs have often not been funded to proceed. Indeed, from a macro perspective, funding for oral health care is considerably misaligned in favour of post-disease treatment, rather than prevention.

To achieve substantial improvements in oral health, population-wide programs and programs targeted to those at highest risk are required. The following interventions could be extended or introduced:

1. Expand community water fluoridation to meet or exceed the current target that 95% of rural and regional Victorians have access to fluoridated drinking water by 2030 (DHHS, 2020).

2. Scale up Victorian prevention programs that have been evaluated to be cost effective, for example:

   - Collaborate with health, education and welfare professionals who interact with young children and their families (Section 2.1)
   - Create oral health promoting environments in pre-school, school, and aged care settings (Section 2.2)
   - Extend preventive value-based dental care by employing minimal intervention approaches such as fissure sealants, Hall crowns, silver diamine fluoride and community-based fluoride varnish programs (Section 5.2)
   - Trial the involvement of other health professionals in applying fluoride varnish (Section 1.2)
   - Support peer-led oral health promotion programs (Section 4.2)
   - Introduce oral health assessment on entry into residential care such as aged care and disability facilities, and develop oral health care plans and provide support to residents in these settings

3. Enhance access to preventive and value-based dental care (Section 5.2) through secure, ongoing Australian government funding (WHO Strategic Objective 4, Chapter 12).

4. Advocate for inclusion of oral health in all health plans, including in local government Public Health and Wellbeing plans and in the implementation of the *National preventive health strategy 2020–2030* (Section 1.4).

5. Consider introducing new evidence-based initiatives:

   - Further restrict advertising of sugar-rich foods to children through regulation
   - Introduce a (national) sugar levy (WHO, 2022). (It has been estimated that a 20% tax on sugar-sweetened beverages in Australia would prevent 3.9 million decayed-missing-filled teeth and save $666m over 10 years [Sowa et al., 2019])
   - Implement a national oral health literacy campaign
   - Include oral health prompts in routine health checks

6. Support the training of dental practitioners to achieve the health promotion competencies required by the Australian Dental Council for newly qualified dental practitioners[25] (WHO Strategic Objective 3, Chapter 12).

7. Include the prevention of oral disease and oral health promotion in the remit of the Australian Centre for Disease Control that is currently being established[26] (WHO Strategic Objective 1, Chapter 12).

8. Include a focus on prevention in broader oral health information systems that need to be developed (as outlined in WHO Strategic Objective 5, Chapter 12).

9. Undertake prevention research, monitoring and evaluation (WHO Strategic Objective 6, Chapter 12) focussing on addressing oral health inequalities (Tsakos et al., 2023), economic evaluation, community-based participatory research, and interdisciplinary research.

---

25 <https://adc.org.au/files/accreditation/competencies/ADC_Professional_Competencies_of_the_Newly_Qualified_Practitioner.pdf>
26 <https://www.health.gov.au/our-work/Australian-CDC>

Appendices

Appendix 6.1 Timeline of oral health prevention and promotion initiatives in Victoria, 1970 to 2021

1970   Dental services for Australians. Fabian Society, Pamphlet No. 21 (Lane, 1970).

Recommended the introduction of community water fluoridation, dental therapists to provide preventive measures, and dental health education to the community (Chapter 2).

1972   *Dentists Act 1972* (Vic) allows dental therapists to operate in Victoria.

1973   *Health (Fluoridation) Act 1973* (Vic).

1977   Fluoridation of Melbourne's drinking water commenced.

First Victorian-trained dental therapists graduate.

1978   Review of the water fluoridation of Melbourne commenced prior to a by-election in Ballarat.

1980   Report of the Committee of Inquiry into the Fluoridation of Victorian Water Supplies for 1979–80 (Myers et al., 1980). Fluoridation had been suspended from March 1979 until September 1980.

1986   Ministerial Review of Dental Services (MRODS) final report released (DHV, 1986).

Recommended the extension of community water fluoridation, and the provision of health promotion and education through institutions and organisations which are part of people's day to day living, for example, infant welfare centres and schools.

1989   Fissure sealants introduced into the School Dental Service (SDS).

Hygienists allowed to operate in Victoria.

1992   Monash Preschool Dental Program commenced – which informed development of *Smiles4Miles*.

1993   *Dental health education [kit] – A curriculum approach, prep to year six* (DHS, 1993) released.

The resource was developed for schools by the SDS and the Directorate of School Education. Over 1,000 copies were sold to schools. The authors were Catherine Thompson and Robin Gillmore.

1996   The *Victorian school dental service child dental health promotion strategy 1995–2000* (DHS, 1996) released by the Child and Adolescent Health Promotion Unit, Primary Health Division, Department of Health and Community Services.

| 1997–2000 | Health Development Public Health Division, Department of Human Services commenced a process to develop an oral disease prevention strategy. The stages were: |

- *Towards better oral health: Background and issues for Victoria's oral disease prevention and health promotion strategy.* Discussion paper released in 1997 (DHS, 1997).
- *Promoting oral health 2000–2004: Strategic directions and framework for action,* released in 2000 (DHS, 1999).
- *Evidence-based health promotion: Resources for planning. No. 1 Oral health,* released in 2000 (DHS, Wright, Satur & Morgan, 2000).
- 16 oral health promotion projects sponsored.
- The Victorian Oral Health Promotion Partnership Group (VOHPPG) established to coordinate oral health promotion and oversee the implementation of the 2000 strategic directions.

2004
Healthy mouths healthy lives: Australia's national oral health plan 2004–2013 (AHMC, 2004) released.

Smiles4Miles commenced – an oral health promotion award program for kindergartens and early childhood centres.

Defenders of the Tooth created – cartoon characters Munch Girl, Water Boy and Brush Boy.

2005–2011
Extension of community water fluoridation in rural Victoria.

2007
Improving Victoria's oral health plan (DHS, 2007) released.

2008
DHSV Statewide oral health promotion strategic plan 2008–2012 released (DHSV, 2008a)

2010
Australian Population Health Improvement Research Strategy for Oral Health (APHIRST-OH) established. A DHSV collaboration with The Jack Brockhoff Child Health and Wellbeing Program (University of Melbourne) (TJBH, n.d.) to support oral health promotion monitoring, evaluation and research..

2011
Oral health messages for the Australian public released (National Oral Health Promotion Clearing House, 2011).

Evidence-based oral health promotion resource (Rogers & DHS, 2011) released.

2011–2014
Teeth Tales, community-based participatory research project (Gibbs et al., 2014) implemented.

2012
Healthy families, healthy smiles program commenced (DHSV, 2022b).

2013   Victorian *Action plan for oral health promotion 2013–2017* (DHV, 2013) released.

Update of the oral health promotion evidence base for the National Oral Health Promotion Committee (Hegde & de Silva, 2013) released.

National oral health promotion plan (Wright, 2013) completed but not released.

2014   *Smokefree Smiles* commenced – a program to train oral health professionals to support their clients to quit smoking through brief interventions (DHSV, 2022c).

2015   *Healthy mouths healthy lives: Australia's national oral health plan 2015–2024* (COAG, 2015) released.

2018   Victorian Oral cancer screening and prevention program commenced (DHSV, n.d.).

2019   The Smile Squad commenced – a school dental program which provides free dental care for all children at government primary and secondary schools (Premier of Victoria, 2019).

2020   *Victorian action plan to prevent oral disease 2020–30* (DHHS, 2020) released.

2021   *National preventive health strategy 2021–2030* (DH-A, 2021) released.

2022   Amendment to the Victorian Drugs Poisons and Controlled Substances Regulations 2017 to authorise Registered Aboriginal Health Practitioners to obtain, possess and administer fluoride varnish to Aboriginal children.

Update of the oral health promotion evidence base (Rana et al., 2022).

Appendix 6.2 Review of the literature

A systematic database search carried out in September 2022 included MEDLINE, ERIC and CINAHL via the EBSCOhost platform; PubMed, EMBASE, DARE, NHSEED, HTA, Cost-Effectiveness Analysis Registry, PEDE and Cochrane reviews via EMBASE Classic and Evidence-Based Medicine Reviews; Scopus; Science Direct; and Google Scholar.

Search terms included 'oral health' or 'dental health' or 'dentistry' or 'dental care' and 'promotion' and 'Victoria Australia'. Inclusion criteria were English-language peer reviewed studies examining oral health promotion/ prevention interventions and showing oral health impacts.

Grey literature including government and relevant health organisation plans, papers and reports were sourced through content experts in oral health promotion and website searches. Reference lists of documents were also searched.

The time period for documents that related to interventions in Victoria was between 1970 and September 2022.

References

Abou El Fadl, R., Blair, M., & Hassounah, S. (2016). Integrating maternal and children's oral health promotion into nursing and midwifery practice-a systematic review. *PloS one, 11*(11), e0166760.

Abuzar M, Mariño R, Perera I, & Morgan M. (2009). Oral Health Awareness of Sri Lankan Older Adults Living in Melbourne, Australia. *2nd Meeting of IADR Pan Asian Pacific Federation, Wuhan China, September 2009*. <https://iadr.abstractarchives.com/abstract/papf09-126039/oral-health-awareness-of-sri-lankan-seniors-living-in-australia>

Australian Health Ministers' Conference. (AHMC). (2004). National Advisory Committee on Oral Health. & South Australia. Department of Health. *Healthy mouths, healthy lives: Australia's national oral health plan 2004–2013*. Adelaide: South Australian Department of Health. <https://catalogue.nla.gov.au/Record/3298219>

Anopa, Y., McMahon, A. D., Conway, D. I., Ball, G. E., McIntosh, E., & Macpherson, L. M. (2015). Improving child oral health: cost analysis of a national nursery toothbrushing programme. *Plos one, 10*(8), e0136211.

Arrow, P., & Klobas, E. (2015). Minimum intervention dentistry approach to managing early childhood caries: a randomized control trial. *Community Dentistry and Oral Epidemiology, 43*(6), 511-520.

Auditor-General Victoria. (AG-V). (2016). *Access to public dental services in Victoria*. <https://www.audit.vic.gov.au/report/access-public-dental-services-victoria?section=32003--4-addressing-barriers-to-access#page-anchor>

Auditor-General Victoria. (AG-V). (2019). *Follow up of access to public dental services in Victoria*. <https://www.audit.vic.gov.au/sites/default/files/2019-11/20191128-Follow-up-Dental-report.pdf>

Barwon Health. (2022). *Oral health*. Barwon Health Research Areas. <https://www.barwonhealth.org.au/research/our-research/item/oral-health#pain-free-dentistry-for-children-the-hall-technique>

Calache, H., Christian, B., Ford, P., Freeman, C. R., Gussy, M., Jackson, J. K., ... & Taing, M. W. (2017). Supporting Oral Health Services in Pharmacy. June 7. *Australian Pharmacist*.

Centers for Disease Control and Prevention. (CDC). (1999, April 2). *Ten great public health achievements – United States, 1900–1999*. MMWR Weekly, 48(12), 241–243. <https://www.cdc.gov/mmwr/preview/mmwrhtml/00056796.htm>

Chuanon, J. J. (2019). *Exploring the oral health curriculum in Australian pharmacy schools*. [Master's thesis, University of Melbourne]. <https://minerva-access.unimelb.edu.au/items/3fa18b2e-fa3a-5faf-a453-336ef15e4840>

COAG Health Council. (2015). *Healthy mouths, healthy lives: Australia's national oral health plan 2015–2024*. <https://www.health.gov.au/resources/publications/healthy-mouths-healthy-lives-australias-national-oral-health-plan-2015-2024?language=en>

Dental Health Services. (DHS). (1993). *Dental health education [kit]: A curriculum approach, prep. to year six*. Melbourne: Dental Health Promotion Unit, Dental Health Services. Department of Health and Community Services. <https://www.vgls.vic.gov.au/client/en_AU/VGLS-public/search/detailnonmodal/ent:$002f$002fSD_ILS$002f0$002fSD_ILS:423545/ada?qu=School+mental+health+services.&d=ent%3A%2F%2FSD_ILS%2F0%2FSD_ILS%3A423545%7EILS%7E18&ic=true&ps=300&h=8>

Dental Health Services Victoria. (DHSV). (n.d.). *The Victorian oral cancer screening and prevention program*. Retrieved December 9, 2022 from <https://www.dhsv.org.au/oral-health-programs/oral-cancer-screening-and-prevention>

Dental Health Services Victoria. (DHSV). (2008a). *DHSV Statewide oral health promotion strategic plan 2008–2012*. <https://www.dhsv.org.au/__data/assets/pdf_file/0010/3412/dhsv-statewide-oral-health-promotion-strategic-plan-2008-2012.pdf>

Dental Health Services Victoria. (DHSV). (2008b). Disability Accommodation Services Department of Health, Dental Health Services Victoria, Plenty Valley Community Health Inc *Final project report 2008*.

Dental Health Services Victoria. (DHSV). (2015a). *Victorian joint position statement on pharmacy and oral health*. <https://www.dhsv.org.au/__data/assets/pdf_file/0018/155052/PSA_Joint-position-statement-on-oral-health_final_2015-03.pdf>

Dental Health Services Victoria. (DHSV). (2015b). *Healthy families healthy smiles. Overview of implementation and evaluation findings 2012–2015 (June)*. <https://www.dhsv.org.au/__data/assets/pdf_file/0008/155753/Report_Overview-of-Healthy-Families-Healthy-Smiles-2012-15.pdf>

Dental Health Services Victoria. (DHSV). (2017). *Annual report 2016–17*. <https://www.parliament.vic.gov.au/file_uploads/Dental_Health_Services_2016-2017__complete__1tG2xt90.pdf>

Dental Health Services Victoria. (DHSV). (2018). *Building the capability of disability support services to improve oral health of people with disabilities, 2014–2018.* Final process evaluation report. Dental Health Services Victoria.

Dental Health Services Victoria. (DHSV). (2019). *Case study: Water fluoridation in Cohuna.* Rural ECOH – Engaging Communities in Oral Health. <https://www.dhsv.org.au/__data/assets/pdf_file/0017/170441/Final-ECOH-Case-study.pdf>

Dental Health Services Victoria. (DHSV). (2020a). *Healthy families heathy smiles – Evaluation report 2015–19, July 2020.* <https://www.dhsv.org.au/__data/assets/pdf_file/0020/171812/HFHS-Report-2015-19_FINAL_2020-07-28.pdf>

Dental Health Services Victoria. (DHSV). (2020b). *Healthy families healthy smiles – Evaluation report, July 2020. Appendices.* <https://www.dhsv.org.au/__data/assets/pdf_file/0019/171811/HFHS-Report-2015-19_Appendices_20191114_FINAL.pdf>

Dental Health Services Victoria. (DHSV). (2020c). *Brush book bed. Toothbrushing in supported playgroups. Final Report July 2018–June 2019.* Health Promotion Team. Dental Health Services Victoria.

Dental Health Services Victoria. (DHSV). (2020d). *Brush book bed. Toothbrushing in supported playgroups. Report July 2019–June 2020.* Health Promotion Team. Dental Health Services Victoria.

Dental Health Services Victoria. (DHSV). (2021). *Annual report 2020–21.* <https://www.dhsv.org.au/__data/assets/pdf_file/0011/176672/2021-DHSV-Annual-Report-and-Financial-Statements-291121.pdf >

Dental Health Services Victoria. (DHSV). (2022a). *Oral health and Municipal Public Health and Wellbeing Plans* 2021–2025 Audit Report 2022.

Dental Health Services Victoria. (DHSV). (2022b, July 30). *Healthy families, healthy smiles.* <https://www.dhsv.org.au/oral-health-programs/hfhs>

Dental Health Services Victoria. (DHSV). (2022c). *Healthy families, healthy smiles* [Newsletter], *Issue 22, March 2022.* <https://www.dhsv.org.au/__data/assets/pdf_file/0006/178971/HFHS-March-Newsletter-Issue-22.pdf>

Dental Health Services Victoria. (DHSV). (2022d). *Evaluating the impact of MIOH over time.* Advancing oral health in midwifery practice, July 2022 [Newsletter]. <https://www.dhsv.org.au/__data/assets/pdf_file/0018/182520/MIOH-Newsletter-July-2022.pdf>

Dental Health Services Victoria. (DHSV). (2022e). *Annual report 2021–22.* <https://www.dhsv.org.au/__data/assets/pdf_file/0011/187337/Dental-Health-Services-Victoria-Annual-Report-2021-2022-FINAL-021222-small.pdf>

Dental Health Services Victoria. (DHSV). (2022f, December 8). *Smokefree Smiles.* <https://www.dhsv.org.au/oral-health-programs/smokefree-smiles>

Dental Health Services Victoria & Department of Health and Human Services. (DHSV & DHHS). (2020). *Improving oral health – Local government action guide.* <https://www.health.vic.gov.au/sites/default/files/migrated/files/collections/policies-and-guidelines/o/oral-health-local-government-action-guide---aug-2020---pdf.pdf>

Dental Health Services Victoria & Dieticians Australia. (DHSV & DA). (2021). *Joint position statement on interdisciplinary collaboration between accredited practising dietitians, nutrition and oral health professionals for oral health and nutrition.* <https://dietitiansaustralia.org.au/sites/default/files/2022-06/FINAL%20VERSION%20JPS%20OH_Nutrition%20Collab_20062022.pdf>

Department of Health. Australia. (DH-A). (2021). *National preventive health strategy 2021–2030.* <https://www.health.gov.au/resources/publications/national-preventive-health-strategy-2021-2030#:~:text=National%20Preventive%20Health%20Strategy%202021–2030%20–%20Glossary&text=Description%3A,over%20a%2010%2Dyear%20period>

Department of Health. Victoria. (DHV). (1986). *Ministerial review of dental services: Final report.* Melbourne: Health Department of Victoria.

Department of Health. Victoria. (DHV). (2011). *Victorian public health and wellbeing plan 2011–2015.* Government of Victoria, Department of Health, Melbourne. <https://www.health.vic.gov.au/publications/victorian-public-health-and-wellbeing-plan-2011-2015>

Department of Health. Victoria. (DHV). (2013). *Action plan for oral health promotion 2013–2017.* Government of Victoria, Department of Health, Melbourne.

Department of Health. Victoria. (DHV). (2022, July 18). *Maternal and child health service practice guidelines 2019.* <https://www.health.vic.gov.au/publications/maternal-and-child-health-service-practice-guidelines>

Department of Health and Human Services. (DHHS). (2020). *Victorian action plan to prevent oral disease 2020–30*. <https://www.health.vic.gov.au/sites/default/files/migrated/files/collections/research-and-reports/o/victorian-action-plan-to-prevent-oral-disease-2020.pdf>

Department of Human Services. (DHS). (1996). *The Victorian school dental service child dental health promotion strategy 1995–2000*. Melbourne: DHS.

Department of Human Services. (DHS). (1997). *Towards better oral health: Background and issues for Victoria's oral disease prevention and health promotion strategy*. Discussion paper. Melbourne: DHS.

Department of Human Services. (DHS). (1999). *Promoting oral health 2000–2004: Strategic directions and framework for action*. <https://www.vgls.vic.gov.au/client/en_AU/search/asset/1159746>

Department of Human Services. (DHS), Wright, F. A. C., Satur, J., & Morgan, M. V. (2000). *Evidence-based health promotion: resources for planning, No. 1 Oral health*. <https://www.vgls.vic.gov.au/client/en_AU/search/asset/1160073/0>

Department of Human Services. Victoria. (DHS). (2007). *Improving Victoria's oral health*. Melbourne: DHS. <https://vgls.sdp.sirsidynix.net.au/client/search/asset/1291900>

Department of Human Services. (DHS). (2019, May 26). *The Smile Squad – free dental vans to hit schools soon* [Media release]. State Government of Victoria. <https://hnb.dhs.vic.gov.au/web/pubaff/medrel.nsf/3cf90a23430db5a9852562840073ae37/15705120dbf022e3ca258407000ab3b3?OpenDocument>

De Silva-Sanigorski, A.M., Bell, A.C., Kremer, P., Nichols, M., Crellin, M., Smith, M., Sharp, S., de Groot, F., Carpenter, L., Boak, R., Roberson, N., & Swinburn, B.A. (2010). Reducing obesity in early childhood: results from Romp & Chomp an Australian community-wide intervention program. *The American Journal of Clinical Nutrition 91*, 831–840.

Dickson-Swift, V. (2019). Gannawarra Shire Council. (2021). *Case study: Water fluoridation in Cohuna*. <https://www.dhsv.org.au/__data/assets/pdf_file/0017/170441/Final-ECOH-Case-study.pdf>

Dickson-Swift, V., & Crocombe, L. (2021). Missed opportunities for improving oral health in rural Victoria: The role of municipal public health planning in improving oral health. *Health promotion journal of Australia, 33*(2), 509–518.

Dickson-Swift, V., Kenny, A., Gussy, M., McCarthy, C., & Bracksley-O'Grady, S. (2020). The knowledge and practice of pediatricians in children's oral health: A scoping review. *BMC oral health, 0*(1), 1–10.

Gannawarra Shire Council. (2021, May 3). *Cohuna town water supply fluoridation achieved*. [Press release]. <https://www.gannawarra.vic.gov.au/News-Media/Cohuna-town-water-supply-fluoridation-achieved>

George, A., Dahlen, H. G., Blinkhorn, A., Ajwani, S., Bhole, S., Ellis, S., Yeo, A., Elcombe, E. & Johnson, M. (2018). Evaluation of a midwifery initiated oral health-dental service program to improve oral health and birth outcomes for pregnant women: A multi-centre randomised controlled trial. *International journal of nursing studies, 82*, 49–57. Epub 2018 Mar 12. PMID: 29605753.

George, A., Lang, G., Johnson, M., Ridge, A., de Silva, A. M., Ajwani, S., Bhole, S., Blinkhorn, A., Dahlen, H. G., Ellis, S., Yeo, A., Langdon, R., Carpenter, L., & Heilbrunn-Lang, A. (2016). The evaluation of an oral health education program for midwives in Australia. *Women and birth, 29*(3), 208–213.

Gibbs, L., Waters, E., De Silva, A., Riggs, E., Moore, L., Armit, C., Johnson, B., Morris, M., Calache, H., Gussy, M., Young, D., Tadic, M., Christian, B., Gondal, I., Watt, R., Pradel, V., Truong, M. & Gold, L. (2014). An exploratory trial implementing a community-based child oral health promotion intervention for Australian families from refugee and migrant backgrounds: a protocol paper for Teeth Tales. *BMJ open, 4*(3), e004260.

Gibbs, L., Waters, E., Christian, B., Gold, L., Young, D., de Silva, A., Calache, H., Gussy, M., Watt, R., Riggs, E, Tadic, M., M Hall, Gondal, I., Pradel, V., & Moore, L. (2015). Teeth Tales: a community-based child oral health promotion trial with migrant families in Australia. *BMJ open, 5*(6), e007321.

Hall, M., & Christian, B. (2017). A health-promoting community dental service in Melbourne, Victoria, Australia: protocol for the North Richmond model of oral health care. *Australian Journal of Primary Health, 23*(5), 407-414.

Head, B. W. (1978). The fluoridation controversy in Victoria: Public policy and group politics. *Australian Journal of Public Administration, 37*(3), 257–273.

Hegde, S., & de Silva, A. (2013). *Update of the oral health promotion evidence base for the National Oral Health Promotion Committee*. Dental Health Services Victoria. <https://www.dhsv.org.au/__data/assets/pdf_file/0016/32227/Update-of-the-evidence_final_12032013.pdf>

Hegde, S., & Haddock, R. (2019). *Re-orienting funding from volume to value in public dental services. Issues brief 32*. Deeble Institute for Health Policy Research. <https://ahha.asn.au/system/files/docs/publications/deeble_issues_brief_no_32_reorienting_funding_from_volume_to_value__0.pdf>

Heilbrunn-Lang, A. Y., Carpenter, L. M., de Silva, A. M., Meyenn, L. K., Lang, G., Ridge, A., Perry, A., Cole, D. & Hegde, S. (2020). Family-centred oral health promotion through Victorian child-health services: a pilot. *Health promotion international, 35*(2), 279–289.

Heilbrunn-Lang, A. Y., De Silva, A. M., Lang, G., George, A., Ridge, A., Johnson, M., Bhole S., & Gilmour, C. (2015). Midwives' perspectives of their ability to promote the oral health of pregnant women in Victoria, Australia. *BMC pregnancy and childbirth, 15*(1), 1–11.

Ho, H. D., Satur, J., & Meldrum, R. (2018). Perceptions of oral health by those living with mental illnesses in the Victorian community – The consumer's perspective. *International journal of dental hygiene, 16*(2), e10-e16.

Holliday, R., Hong, B., McColl, E., Livingstone-Banks, J., & Preshaw, P. M. (2021). Interventions for tobacco cessation delivered by dental professionals. *Cochrane Database of Systematic Reviews, 2*(2).

International Association for Dental Research. (IADR). (2022, June 20). *Position statement on community water fluoridation.* <https://www.iadr.org/science-policy/position-statement-community-water-fluoridation>

Jaguar Consulting. (2016). *Impact analysis: Expanding water fluoridation in Victoria*. 2016. [Unpublished data]. Melbourne: Department of Health and Human Services Victoria.

Jolly, K. A., Messer, L. B., & Manton, D. (1996). Promotion of mouthguards among amateur football players in Victoria. *Australian and New Zealand journal of public health, 20*(6), 630–639.

Kisely, S., Baghaie, H., Lalloo, R., Siskind, D., & Johnson, N. W. (2015). A systematic review and meta-analysis of the association between poor oral health and severe mental illness. *Psychosomatic medicine, 77*(1), 83–92.

Lane, J. (1970). *Dental services for Australians. [Pamphlet 21]*. Melbourne: Victorian Fabian Society.

Legge, D., & Sylvan, L. (1990). Consumer participation in health: the Consumers' Health Forum and the Victorian District Health Council Program. In Evers, A., Farrant, W., & Trojan, A. (Eds.), *Healthy public policy at the local level*. Boulder: Westview Press. 176-198.

Lewis, M. (2003). *The people's health: Public health in Australia, 1950 to the Present*. Praeger Publishers, Westport, CT, USA.

McMillan, S. S., Hu, J., El-Den, S., O'Reilly, C. L., & Wheeler, A. J. (2021). Pharmacy participation in dental and oral health care: a scoping review protocol. *JBI Evidence Synthesis, 19*(7), 1651-1658.

Mariño, R., Calache, H., & Morgan, M. (2013). A community-based culturally competent oral health promotion for migrant older adults living in Melbourne, Australia. *Journal of the American Geriatrics Society, 61*(2), 270-275.

Mariño, R., Calache, H., Wright, C., Schofield, M., & Minichiello, V. (2004). Oral health promotion programme for older migrant adults. *Gerodontology, 21*(4), 216–225.

Mariño, R. J., Fajardo, J., Calache, H., & Morgan, M. (2014). Cost-minimization analysis of a tailored oral health intervention designed for immigrant older adults. *Geriatrics & Gerontology International, 14*(2), 336–340.

Mariño, R. J., Marwaha, P., & Barrow, S. Y. (2016). Web-based oral health promotion program for older adults: Development and preliminary evaluation. *International journal of medical informatics, 91*, e9-e15.

Mariño, R., Morgan, M., Kiyak, A., Schwarz, E., & Naqvi, S. (2012). Oral health in a convenience sample of Chinese older adults living in Melbourne, Australia. *International Journal of Public Health, 57*, 383-390.

Mariño, R., Wright, C., Minichiello, V., Schofield, M., & Calache, H. (2005). A qualitative process evaluation of an oral health promotion program for older migrant adults. *Health Promotion Journal of Australia, 16*(3), 225–228.

Mason, A., Mayze, L., Pawlak, J., Henry, M. J., Sharp, S., & Smith, M. C. (2015). A preventative approach to oral health for children in a regional/rural community in South-West Victoria, Australia. *Dentistry, 5*(7), 1.

McGrath, R., Marino, R., & Satur, J. (2021). Oral health promotion practices of Australian community mental health professionals: A cross sectional web-based survey. *BMC Oral Health, 21*(1), 1–9.

Meldrum, R., Ho, H., & Satur, J. (2018). The role of community mental health services in supporting oral health outcomes among consumers. *Australian Journal of Primary Health, 24*(3), 216–220.

Mckee, S., McGrath, R., & Hedge, S. (2020). Oral health for better health – A value based oral health care model in Australia. *International Journal of Integrated Care, 20*(S1), 98.

Morgan, M. V., Crowley, S. J., & Wright, C. (1998). Economic evaluation of a pit and fissure dental sealant and fluoride mouthrinsing program in two nonfluoridated regions of Victoria, Australia. *Journal of public health dentistry, 58*(1), 19–27.

Moysés, S. T., Moysés, S. J., Watt, R. G., & Sheiham, A. (2003). Associations between health promoting schools' policies and indicators of oral health in Brazil. *Health promotion international, 18*(3), 209–218.

Myers, D. M. & Committee of Inquiry into the Fluoridation of Victorian Water Supplies, & Victoria. Parliament. Legislative Assembly. (1980). *Report of the committee of inquiry into the fluoridation of Victorian water supplies for 1979–80*. <https://www.parliament.vic.gov.au/papers/govpub/VPARL1980-81No14.pdf>

National Advisory Committee on Oral Health. (NACOH). (2004). *Healthy mouths healthy lives: Australia's national oral health plan 2004–2013*. Adelaide: South Australia. Department of Health. <https://catalogue.nla.gov.au/Record/3298219>

National Health and Medical Research Council. (NHMRC). (2017). *NHMRC public statement 2017. Water fluoridation and human health in Australia.* <https://www.nhmrc.gov.au/sites/default/files/documents/reports/fluoridation-public-statement.pdf>

National Oral Health Promotion Clearing House. (2011). Oral health messages for the Australian public. Findings of a national consensus workshop. *Australian dental journal, 56*(3), 331–335.

Neumann, A. S., Lee, K. J., Gussy, M. G., Waters, E. B., Carlin, J. B., Riggs, E., & Kilpatrick, N. M. (2011). Impact of an oral health intervention on pre-school children < 3 years of age in a rural setting in Australia. *Journal of paediatrics and child health, 47*(6), 367–372.

Nguyen, T. M., Christian, B., Koshy, S., & Morgan, M. V. (2020). A validation and cost-analysis study of a targeted school-based dental check-up intervention: Children's Dental Program. *Children, 7*(12), 257.

Porter, M. E. (2010). What is value in health care. *N Engl J Med, 363*(26), 2477–2481.

Pan American Health Organization. (PAHO) & World Health Organization. (WHO). (2023). *Social determinants of health*. <https://www.paho.org/en/topics/social-determinants-health>

Premier of Victoria. (2019). *The Smile Squad – Free Dental Vans To Hit Schools Soon*. [Media release]. <https://www.premier.vic.gov.au/smile-squad-free-dental-vans-hit-schools-soon>

Quinonez, R. B., Stearns, S. C., Talekar, B. S., Rozier, R. G., & Downs, S. M. (2006). Simulating cost-effectiveness of fluoride varnish during well-child visits for Medicaid-enrolled children. *Archives of pediatrics & adolescent medicine, 160*(2), 164–170.

Rana, K., Ekanayake, K., Chimoriya, R., Palu, E., Do, L., Silva, M., Tadakamadla, S., Bhole, S., Leshargie, CT., Wen, LM., Ha, D., & Arora, A. (2022). *Effectiveness of oral health promotion interventions: an Evidence Check rapid review*. Sax Institute 2022. <https://www.health.vic.gov.au/preventive-health/oral-health-planning>

Riggs, E., Gussy, M., Gibbs, L., van Gemert, C., Waters, E., & Kilpatrick, N. (2014). Hard to reach communities or hard to access services? Migrant mothers' experiences of dental services? *Australian dental journal, 59*(2), 201–207.

Riordain, R. N., Glick, M., Al Mashhadani, S. S. A., Aravamudhan, K., Barrow, J., Cole, D., … & Williams, D. M. (2021). Developing a standard set of patient-centred outcomes for adult oral health–an international, cross-disciplinary consensus. *International dental journal, 71*(1), 40–52.

Rogers, J. G. (2011) & Department of Human Services (DHS). *Evidence-based oral health promotion resource*. Melbourne: Prevention and Population Health Branch, Department of Health, Victoria. <https://www.health.vic.gov.au/sites/default/files/migrated/files/collections/policies-and-guidelines/f/final-oral-health-resource-may-2011-web-version---pdf.pdf>

Rogers, M. J., Pawlak, J. A., Mason, A., Mayze, L., Sharp, S., & Smith, M. (2016). The prevalence of caries free deciduous teeth upon visual examination in kindergarten settings: a preventative approach to oral health for children in a regional/rural community in South-West Victoria. *Journal of Preventive Medicine,1*(1), 2.

Rogers, J. G., Adams, G. G., Wright, F. A. C., Roberts-Thomson, K., & Morgan, M. V. (2018). Reducing potentially preventable dental hospitalizations of young children: A community-level analysis. *JDR clin trans res, 3*(3), 272–278.

Satur, J. G., Gussy, M. G., Morgan, M. V., Calache, H., & Wright, C. (2010). Review of the evidence for oral health promotion effectiveness. *Health Education Journal, 69*(3), 257–266.

Sowa, P. M., Keller, E., Stormon, N., Lalloo, R., & Ford, P. J. (2019). The impact of a sugar-sweetened beverages tax on oral health and costs of dental care in Australia. *European journal of public health, 29*(1), 173–177.

State Government of Victoria. (SGV). (2015). *Victorian public health and wellbeing plan 2015–2019.* <https://www.health.vic.gov.au/publications/victorian-public-health-and-wellbeing-plan-2015-2019>

State Government of Victoria. (SGV). (2019). *Victorian public health and wellbeing plan 2019–2023.* <https://www.health.vic.gov.au/publications/victorian-public-health-and-wellbeing-plan-2019-2023>

Tannous, K. W., George, A., Ahmed, M. U., Blinkhorn, A., Dahlen, H. G., Skinner, J., Ajwani, S., Bhole, S., Yaacoub, A., Srinivas, R., & Johnson, M. (2021). Economic evaluation of the midwifery initiated oral health-dental service programme in Australia. *BMJ open, 11*(8), e047072.

Taylor, J., Carlisle, K., Farmer, J., Larkins, S., Dickson-Swift, V., & Kenny, A. (2018). Implementation of oral health initiatives by Australian rural communities: factors for success. *Health & social care in the community, 26*(1), e102-e110.

The Jack Brockhoff Foundation (TJBG). (n.d.). *The Jack Brockhoff Foundation child health & wellbeing program. Five year review.* Melbourne School of Population & Global Health. The University of Melbourne. <https://mspgh.unimelb.edu.au/__data/assets/pdf_file/0008/2172284/JBCHWBP_5_Year_Review-circulated.pdf>

Tonmukayakul, U., & Arrow, P. (2017). Cost-effectiveness analysis of the atraumatic restorative treatment-based approach to managing early childhood caries. *Community dentistry and oral epidemiology, 45*(1), 92–100.

Treasury & Finance, Victoria. (2004). *Service delivery 2004–05. Budget paper No. 3.* <https://www.dtf.vic.gov.au/previous-budgets/2004-05-state-budget>

Trinh, M. V., Rhodes, A. L., Measey, M. A., & Silva, M. (2022). Dental visits in early life: patterns and barriers among Australian children. *Australian and New Zealand Journal of Public Health, 46*(3), 281-285.

Tsakos, G., Watt, R. G., & Guarnizo-Herreño, C. C. (2023). Reflections on oral health inequalities: Theories, pathways and next steps for research priorities. *Community Dentistry and Oral Epidemiology, 51*(I), 17–27.

Watt, R. G. (2005). Strategies and approaches in oral disease prevention and health promotion. *Bulletin of the World Health Organization, 83*, 711–718.

Watt, R. G., & Sheiham, A. (2012). Integrating the common risk factor approach into a social determinants framework. *Community dentistry and oral epidemiology, 40*(4), 289–296.

Wilson, E., Kenny, A., & Dickson-Swift, V. (2017). Rural health services and the task of community participation at the local community level: a case study. *Australian health review, 42*(1), 111–116.

Wilson, N. J., Lin, Z., Pithouse, M., Morrison, B., Sumar, B., & George, A. (2022). Qualitative insights from a novel staff-led oral health champions program within a residential service for people with intellectual and developmental disability. *Journal of intellectual disabilities*, 17446295221095654.

World Health Organization. (1978). *Declaration of alma-ata* (No. WHO/EURO: 1978-3938-43697-61471). World Health Organization. Regional Office for Europe. <https://apps.who.int/iris/handle/10665/347879>

World Health Organization. (WHO). (1986a). *Ottawa charter for health promotion.* <https://www.who.int/publications/i/item/ottawa-charter-for-health-promotion>

World Health Organization. (WHO). (2019). *Ending childhood dental caries: WHO implementation manual.* <https://apps.who.int/iris/bitstream/handle/10665/330643/9789240000056-eng.pdf>

World Health Organization. (WHO). (2022). *WHO manual on sugar-sweetened beverage taxation policies to promote health diets.* <https://www.who.int/publications/i/item/9789240056299>

World Health Organization. (WHO, n.d.). *Health promotion.* <https://www.who.int/health-topics/health-promotion#tab=tab_1>

Wright, F.A.C. (Ed). (2013). *National Oral Health Promotion Plan.* Unpublished manuscript Commissioned by Australian Government. Canberra.

Yawary, R., & Hegde, S. (2022). Silver diamine fluoride protocol for reducing preventable dental hospitalisations in Victorian children. *International Dental Journal, 72*(3), 322–330.

Chapter 7
The Evolution of Dental Services – Extract and replace becomes restore and enhance

Jamie Robertson

Introduction

This chapter traces the continuity of change in what dentists and other dental practitioners do in their daily practice. By 1970, the smell of vulcanite denture base had been banished from dental surgeries due to the introduction of methyl methacrylate after the World War II. The smell of eugenol (oil of cloves), however, was still redolent of most practices. Now, even that has faded in favour of alternatives that entail very little hand-mixing of materials. In 1970 amalgam was the restorative material of choice for posterior teeth but its use now is very limited. The introduction and rapid uptake of computers since the 1980s have facilitated and forced better record keeping and the abandonment of scribbled notes that were scarcely legible even to the writer. Higher legal standards of record-keeping have also been imposed. Accompanying these changes have been great developments in bioengineering and materials to permit standards of aesthetics, form and function unknown to practitioners 50 years ago.

Social context

Depending on one's point of view, in 1949 Australia either avoided or missed out on a nationalised dental health service when the Chifley-led national ALP Government lost an election to a Menzies-led Coalition. Plans for a scheme had been well advanced but from this point in time, as before, the subsequent series of Coalition governments opted to play a very minor role in the provision of dental services beyond dispensing tax funds to state governments. By 1970 nothing had changed regarding funding although much had changed in terms of Australia's population, dental technology and the decline in the number of dentists per 100,000 of the population from 37 to 32 (Chapter 3, Table 3.3).

In 1970, the air turbine handpiece had been in widespread use for barely ten years. Cutting tooth structure had become much faster and easier, perhaps too easy sometimes, and so procedures for tooth restoration had become more comfortable and acceptable for patient and dentist alike. Long sessions of slow drilling were no longer a disincentive to preferring a restoration of a tooth to its extraction. Nevertheless, folk memories were long and only changed slowly. The saving in tooth cutting time greatly increased output for dentists, particularly if they adopted "four-hand" restorative techniques with chairside assistants, and revealed the truth of Ben Franklin's aphorism that "time is money". Incomes for private practitioners were rising but the small number of public sector dentists on fixed salaries were being left behind.

The growing disparity in incomes between the private and public sectors made it difficult to recruit dentists to the relatively small public sector and, as stated (Chapter 3), most of the dentists at the Royal Dental Hospital of Melbourne (RDHM) in the 1970s were either older dentists easing back or young novices starting out. Public clinics for routine dental care were few and far between apart from the RDHM, hence there were long waiting lists for treatment. There was time for sound teeth to become decayed and even minimal problems could become unrestorable. It was akin to having to book a maternity bed six months before conception.

The introduction of professional dental therapists and advanced dental technicians slightly relieved the pressure for care at both ends of the age spectrum. By the end of the 1970s, people needing full dentures could receive them at lower cost from prosthetists than from most dentists. However, when advanced dental technicians (ADT) began opening their denture clinics from 1975 onwards, they found that the cost savings in making dentures directly for patients fell short of their expectations because the costs of compliance for a legitimate business, including infection control, occupational health and safety, and income tax were much higher than in the more "informal" pre-regulated era when nothing was declared. The new ADTs were like former poachers who became game keepers to protect their patch.

Families with children at government primary schools began to benefit from a better funded School Dental Service (SDS). It was staffed by a new workforce of dental therapists who provided a free dental service for children's teeth, which, in the 1980s, were slowly becoming more resistant to decay thanks to the fluoridation of town water and toothpaste. The small numbers of these new service providers merely scratched the surface of need, however, and it was only when the firestorm of dental caries began to be quenched by fluoridated water and toothpaste fluoridation became the norm, and when higher numbers of dentists were added to the workforce annually, that the sense of being overwhelmed by disease lessened.

The great success of water fluoridation in preventing disease occurred in conjunction with other successful preventive health measures in Victoria. In the 1970s, compulsory wearing of car seat belts and the introduction of random breath testing of drivers began to dramatically reduce road trauma. In 1981 the Cancer Council of Victoria started the *Slip, Slop, Slap* campaign which reduced the incidence of basal and squamous cell carcinomas, and in 1987 the National government produced the Grim Reaper campaign to educate the public about a deadly new disease called AIDS. All of these measures have been highly effective in lessening death and disease rates and have raised the profile of preventive public health in practice and in status.

At much the same time as these preventive health measures were being introduced, the clinical approaches to the treatment of human illnesses were being re-evaluated. Initially set in train by a few individuals, this reassessment gained momentum as their ideas got more exposure. It is important to note that the dissemination and uptake of new ideas and concepts has generally been slower in a profession of mainly cottage-industry practitioners like dentistry compared with the medical profession. While there are isolated (or solo) practitioners of medicine, unlike dentistry, the medical profession also has many large concentrations of practitioners in hospitals and in teaching and research institutions.

For populations anywhere, dental services have been broadly divided into two categories: namely, activities designed to prevent the onset of disease or disorder, and activities designed to respond to disease or disorders once established. Some preventive activities can take place outside a clinical setting – for example, the fluoridation of water supplies – while others occur within the clinical setting, such as the sealing of fissures of intact molar teeth. During the period of this study, a more nuanced view of the onset of dental decay has developed, thanks in part to pioneering research by Professor Eric Reynolds and his team at the Melbourne Dental School. It has been established that there is a liminal stage at which damage to enamel may be reversed or proceed to irreversibility, depending on actions taken by a practitioner or the owner of the teeth. The decision to pick up a handpiece to tackle oral health problems has become, or ought to have become, more considered and complex. We now have more tools than a hammer.

Leaving aside the number of clinicians practising, the quantity of clinical treatment provided each year in Victoria is determined by a personal capacity to pay for it in the private sector and the level of government funding in the public sector. Currently in the private sector, about 58% of costs are borne directly by the consumer (Duckett et al., 2019) and almost 15% by the National government through a combination of health insurance tax rebate and targeted dental health programs. The public sector relies on annual budgetary allocations from the State government and, since 1997, a small patient co-payment which is capped and has several categories of exemption (A-GV, 2002). Over a two-year period the public sector can still only afford to supply care to about 23–26% of those eligible for its services (A-GV, 2016, p. 19).

This is in spite of staffing levels and efficiency having increased since the 1980s, partly in response to political pressure from all parties and partly to reach the primary health goals *of the Ottawa Charter for Health Promotion* of 1986 by decentralising treatment centres.

Historically, fee schedules have shown a bias towards rewarding operative interventions rather than interventions involving counselling, giving advice and applying protective measures. This bias is reflected in the clinicians' preferred treatments and the patients' perceptions of value: "He didn't DO anything; just talked and still charged me!" This has been true in both the private and public sectors, even when dentists in the latter have been paid salaries unrelated to the number of procedures performed. The evolution of the dental profession has seen much of the work of disease prevention delegated to dental hygienists, therapists and, more recently, to dental assistants while dentists, in the main, have continued to perform the responsive procedures of restoration, removal or replacement of damaged teeth. This is seen by dental governance and management as an efficient use of scope of practice training, but it has done little to alter the perception that prevention is less important than repair. Alternatively, it could be viewed as an acceptance that changing human behaviour, in this case dietary and oral hygiene choices, is the most difficult and frustrating endeavour and therefore the least satisfying to the ego.

Prevention

As described in Chapters 2, 4, 6 and 8, the fluoridation of Melbourne's water supplies began in 1977 although this was 20 years after it had been adopted as a policy position by the Australian Dental Association Victorian Branch (ADAVB). Adjusting the levels of fluoride to reticulated water supplies has been accepted as one of the ten greatest achievements in public health during the 20th century (CDCP, 2011). Its great advantages lie in its universal reach in reticulated supplies, its social equity, low cost and high effectiveness and the fact that it does not rely on actions of the population other than drinking and using the water. However, even in 2022 some small rural areas of Victoria have still to receive the benefit of fluoridated water supplies so that the project is unfinished (Chapter 6).

Apart from fluoride in water, most toothpastes now have fluoride salts added to them in varying levels to act as topical agents on erupted teeth. These days it is harder to avoid fluoridated toothpaste than it is to find it, and, coupled with higher rates of tooth brushing now (Chapter 10), aided by repeated commercial campaigns for dental hygiene products, more people are protecting more teeth today than in the past.

Much oral disease including dental caries and oral cancer is preventable. A major factor in the prevention of disease and trauma is making people aware of cause and effect, or, of actions and their probable consequences. Giving people oral health education in terms which they understand, and information on what to do about any problems, in an encouraging environment can be an effective tool in promoting healthier diets and behaviours. This is known as raising oral health literacy but individuals still have a free choice in their actions or, rather, still have to confront the social circumstances in which they find themselves.

The association between dental caries and diets high in fermentable carbohydrates has been hypothesised since Aristotle's time (National Research Council, 1989). In the early 20th century the Dental Board of Victoria (DBV), in the first flush of funds following annual, as opposed to life-long registration, began to produce information about dental health and diet. Leaflets for the public were produced in the 1930s and a booklet for dentists was written in 1940 (DBV, 1993). After 1945 there were no more DBV funds for disease prevention.

Before the introduction of dental hygienists to Victoria in 1989, only a minority of dentists spent much time with their patients on oral health education for the reasons given above. Since that time, studies have revealed in greater detail associations of dental diseases with other chronic systemic disorders such as diabetes mellitus, cardiovascular disease and obesity. This has increased the need for oral health education to be provided to patients, the general public and medical practitioners and the impetus to involve the whole dental team in the task. In 2014 Dental Health Services Victoria (DHSV) started to run courses for midwives and maternal and child health nurses (Chapter 6) to broaden the outreach of oral health literacy, and in the public sector diabetes educators and clinicians have interacted more closely in the past ten years. Private sector dental assistants can now be formally trained to provide oral health education in clinical and non-clinical settings (DHSV, 2015).

These initiatives reflect a greater awareness of the intimate relationship between oral health and general health and psychological wellbeing. The depth and breadth of new programs emphasising the links have accelerated in the past 20 years and have encouraged the medical and dental professions to recognise the importance of each other in achieving better health outcomes.

The phrase "putting the mouth back in the body" has been used by medical and dental agencies since at least 2009 (Flieger & Doonan, 2009) and, like many concepts which appear to be self-evident but only in retrospect, it has spread quickly around the world through seminars, articles and books. It has been easier to introduce this in the public sector since the co-location of dental clinics into community health centres in Victoria and better computerised record keeping, although a major impediment to fuller integration is the incompatibility of all dental software with the national medical software because the latter is centred on Medicare, from which dentistry is excluded.

Clinical treatment

During the past 50 years there have been enormous changes in technology, materials and attitudes affecting the delivery of clinical care in dentistry. These range from the apparently banal change from reusable to disposable single use needles for local anaesthetic – which has saved an unquantifiable amount of pain, let alone infection, and even death from viral hepatitis – to the success of osseointegrated titanium implants, which have gone from exotic marvel in the 1980s to commonplace by 2020. In addition, older discarded practices have been reinvented with success: for example, nitrous oxide sedation was reintroduced to Australia by Dr Harry Langa as Relative Analgesia in the early 1970s and, in the early years of the 21st century, the topical use on teeth of a silver salt – this time fluoride – solution to arrest the process of tooth decay mainly in primary teeth. Nevertheless, the rush to capitalise on unproven inventions and materials has left in its wake storerooms full of discarded equipment. The injunction not

to be the first nor the last to adopt a technology has been sound advice for many a practitioner. The philosophy of evidence-based dentistry has always had to compete with short-term entrepreneurism.

In general, technological progress is neither predestined nor linear. It comes in fits and starts with an element of serendipity about it and the potential for causing what Thomas Kuhn called a "paradigm shift" in his work titled *The Structure of Scientific Revolutions* (1962). Innovation has to happen in the right place at the right time, which means that there are many cultural determinants, if it is to take hold and change the way things are done. In dentistry two examples have shown the extremes of change and acceptance.

In 1957 Borden's air turbine contra-angle drill improved on the earlier invention of Melbourne-trained John Walsh, and it became a runaway success with ramifications for reclining chairs, better operating lights, high volume water evacuation and four-handed dentistry. It greatly reduced operating time and patient discomfort with no loss of precision. In contrast to the air turbine's success, an alternative, non-drill removal of damaged tooth structure using air abrasion, a form of sand blasting, came on to the market in the 1990s when composite resins had largely replaced amalgam for restoring posterior teeth. Its selling points were its silent operation, even less discomfort to the patient, and the prospect of not requiring injections of local anaesthetic. Alas, its drawbacks included lack of precision, pain in deeper cavities without local anaesthesia and the inability to deal with large amounts of gritty sand residue. It was another case of "too good to be true", although it has found a niche for some minimally invasive dentistry.

Box 7.1 A Melbourne dentist's reminiscences from 1970

- In my time through the dental course there were about 20 females in the whole of the course[27] out of a little over 250 students.[28] There were very few Asian students, perhaps six in our year, and they returned to their country of origin after graduating. Almost all of these were on the Colombo Plan. The course was basically Caucasian males.[29]

- When I graduated the dentist down the road was my colleague, but by the time I retired, he/she was my competitor. This loss of collegiality saddened me.

- I stood to work. The patient sat upright with their head under my armpit while I balanced on one leg and controlled the speed of the drill with the other foot. No wonder dentists had bad backs and other posture-related problems.

- In the 1960s, over 80% of the population over the age of 30 had full dentures. It was often difficult to persuade some adult patients to keep their teeth. Parents in my area wanted their children to keep their teeth. Decay was rampant and we had an anaesthetist who, for many years, came to the surgery on the first Monday of every month and I would spend the day filling and removing teeth for young children. Fluoridation thankfully changed this and eventually we rarely required his service.

- When I graduated, we certainly used the same needle (to inject local anaesthetic) for a number of patients. From memory I had four syringes, two with short needles for infiltrations and two with long needles for lower blocks,[30] all with a covering metal sheath.

- Infection control: In the 1960s the instruments were washed under running cold water in a sink and then placed in a boiling water bath for at least 15 minutes. The headrest of the chair and the bracket table were wiped with alcohol. The handpieces, which were rarely changed between patients, were also wiped with alcohol and the burrs removed and cleaned with a small brass-wire brush and placed in a container in the boiler for re-use. Gloves were almost never used, even when extracting teeth. The 1970s saw the introduction of the autoclave. The 1990s saw everything "bagged"[31] before entering an automatic autoclave with a printer attached and the requirement to keep the print-out records.

- After the arrival of AIDS in the mid-1980s – the first death in Australia was 1984 – the new disease altered infection control enormously. Almost overnight, and before legislation, dentists started wearing gloves, masks and protective eyewear.

- Whilst we all practised aesthetic dentistry, the rise of "cosmetic dentistry" to pre-eminence is both disappointing and staggering. The idea of bleached, vivid white front teeth as being a requirement of good dentistry and the mark of a "good" dentist beggars belief. It is a sad state of affairs to see the amount of media advertising related to bleaching.

- The involvement of third parties in practice ownership and treatment planning was unheard of in the early days. By law a dental practice could only be owned by a dentist who had to practise in his/her own name. In the 1960s, 70s and 80s single person practices were common, then group practices became more common. Now anyone can own a dental practice. The non-dental owner can set fees, dictate treatment plans and has control of the practice.

- Computers were unknown in dental practices before the 1980s, while now all records, including radiographs, are stored in a computer. A dentist has to be computer-competent just to keep up with the legislative requirements. Everything is done online. I certainly could not cope and am very thankful I retired when I did.

27 Five years.
28 Now (2021) about 360 students in the four-year course.
29 In 2020 majority was Asian background and about 52% of the total were female.
30 Injections to anaesthetise one side of the lower jaw.
31 In plastic and/or paper.

After a false start in the 1980s, the use of lasers in dentistry has found a more limited but effective role for soft tissue manipulation and their use is likely to expand. Digital x-ray imaging with ever improving definition has largely superseded hard copy, chemically processed x-ray film. Images can now be seen almost instantaneously, stored with computerised records and sent anywhere by email or on disk. In Orthodontics and Prosthodontics the need for mouth impressions is giving way to the scanning of arches and emailing results to laboratories where virtual images may be stored and hard copy models can be made with no loss of precision or dimensional change. Clear benefits are patient comfort and the obviation of storage space for an ever-expanding collection of models of mouths held for the required legal period of time. These are only a few examples of innovations which have made life easier for both patient and dentist while keeping costs down despite initial capital outlays. Innovations will, however, keep developing at irregular intervals – probably using Artificial Intelligence, virtual reality and holograms – regardless of perceived need.

Not all technological advances need to have large capital investment, nor must they disrupt existing systems and procedures. Examples include the evolution of matrix bands used when placing restorations, and the disposable needle. Somewhat more complex change has occurred in endodontics with the introduction of rotary instrumentation in the 1990s. Improved nickel–titanium alloy for instruments has permitted faster, more thorough and less taxing biomechanical preparation of root canals, leading to more successful outcomes across a wider spectrum of practices. One can say with considerable certainty that the evolution of materials and procedures will continue regularly.

A revolution in technology that has wider ramifications for the practice of dentistry and prevention of disease will occur infrequently but will have more impact.

In addition to the evolution of clinical technology since 1970, there has been a revolution in the administration of dentistry from pen to keyboard. It went from pre-Gutenberg scribbles to post-Gutenberg clarity but in a much-collapsed time frame. In 1970 there were no computers in dentistry; in 2020 it is a rare and fading practice without one. In the private sector software packages initially handled the financial affairs of a practice but soon spread to appointment books, procedures performed, patient record keeping and the storing of digitised radiographs. A time traveller from 1970 would scarcely believe the amount of data gathered and recorded about each patient and the entire operations of a practice, the mandatory nature of this, and safeguards for the privacy of patients' records.

A problem when introducing IT changes and an impediment to change arises when the entire remuneration system for dentists has been based on an existing system. An example has been the slow introduction of minimal intervention dentistry (Dawson & Makinson, 1992) or minimally invasive dentistry (MID). (In fact, minimal invasion is only one component of minimum intervention; prevention, remineralisation and reduction of the rate of restoration replacement are the others) (Dawson & Makinson, 1992). Even though the concept has been given wider exposure through the textbook by Mount and Hume (1998) in which they devised a new classification of caries damage, it has been hard to dislodge the old model of treatment items based on the American dentist, G. V. Black's cavity classification which dates from 1896.

The legal requirements for record keeping, which represent a recognition of patients' rights, have risen markedly over the period of study. Gone are the days of illegible scrawls, ink blots and caustic comments, or even no records at all. Deficient or non-existent records mean no defence against random audits or patient challenges. Beyond the legal requirements, in this virtual mountain of data lies the possibility of retrospective research – whether at a single practice level or aggregated to a "big data" level – for more understanding of actual evidence-based practice.

Such practice-based research has already started through the ADAVB-sponsored eviDent Foundation, which was established in 2011. Despite there being a wide range of practice management software systems in the private sector, there is a universally accepted code for treatment items which was formulated by the Australian Dental Association (ADA) to facilitate record keeping and standardise procedures. The public sector uses one software system, Titanium, but it too uses the same item codes for procedures as the Australian government does for the purposes of insurance and its Defence Force clinics. In theory, information relating to treatment items could be extracted from all sources provided de-identification could be guaranteed.

Mention is made in Chapter 10 of the public's gradual change in attitude towards its own dental wellbeing in terms of function and appearance. By 1970 the era of a perfect white smile being achieved by full dentures was still common but in decline. The functional limitations of dentures were obvious and the process of restoring teeth had become faster and relatively cheaper with the spread of the air turbine drill. As preventive measures lessened the level of tooth decay, restorative and reparative procedures became less like valiant but doomed transitions to full dentures, and more like pathways to good health.

Clearly, this was generally truer for those born after 1970 because their dentitions developed in the more favourable environment of protection, easier treatment and higher expectations. With ever-improving technology and greater understanding being revealed about biological processes through research, itself assisted by technology, dentists' expectations of themselves also rose.

In the twenty-first century, in the wake of the human genome project, it became possible to conceive of treatments for some disorders to be tailored to the level of an individual. With this the era of personalised medicine was born which has morphed into precision dentistry and value-based dentistry, although it is less easy to conceive how gene splicing or substitution will greatly change the incidence of dental caries most of which is already preventable through existing measures. Beyond that, affordability will continue to shape ultimate treatment decisions as it has in the past.

Dental specialists

In 1970, although several dentists limited their areas of practice and had acquired further training, there was no formal recognition of specialisation within the dental profession. That changed with the Dentists Act of 1972 which enabled formal processes for naming specialist areas and methods of qualifying for specialist status. Initially, five disciplines were chosen for the first specialist register in 1978 and that had grown to 13 by the year 2020.[32] The five original groups were ones which were economically viable for their practitioners who had hitherto been de facto specialists. These disciplines also had the strongest representation in the dental curriculum. Other disciplines such as oral medicine and oral pathology had academic status and prestige but no independent practitioners. However, the very creation of a specialist register brought these two as well as paediatric, or children's dentistry, into contention for addition to the list as areas of expertise.

Forensic dentistry, which became forensic odontology later, began in Victoria as a side interest of a general dentist, Gerald Dalitz, who assisted Victoria Police. While its relevance and importance grew slowly, the Ash Wednesday bushfires of 1983 gave it a dramatic and sudden importance through disaster victim identification.[33] Its establishment as a speciality was formalised by the arrival of John Clement from England as Professor of Forensic Odontology at the Melbourne Dental School in 1989. He established a postgraduate diploma for dentists and

a close link with the Victorian Institute of Forensic Medicine. However, by 2020 only Monash University offered an academic course which is a Master of Forensic Medicine (Forensic Odontology).

The growing focus on access to care indirectly led to the creation of two other specialties: Special Needs Dentistry and Public or Community Dentistry. The former predominantly deals with people with congenital or acquired illnesses or injuries but also others with psychosocial difficulties, while the latter focuses on the study of society's oral health, its contributing factors, policy, planning and its administration.

Oral and Maxillofacial Surgery (OMS), the training for which incorporates medical qualification, has largely replaced Oral Surgery which may eventually become redundant as current practitioners retire. The scope of OMS has become broader and more adventurous even though the removal of wisdom teeth still helps to pay bills. The newest speciality, Dental and Maxillofacial Radiology has only one specialist in Victoria so far but, unlike Oral Surgery, its numbers will grow.

Among the original group of five dental specialties,[34] orthodontists were the most numerous and that is still true today. Numbering 150, they represent nearly one third of all specialists. The second and third highest groups are way behind with periodontists at 63 and oral and maxillofacial surgeons at 60. Orthodontics is a good example of the conflicted motives for treatment, professionally observed need, and aspiration for patient-imagined perfection.

---

32 The *Dentists Act 1972* nominated Endodontics, Oral Surgery, Orthodontics, Periodontics and Prosthodontics. By 2020 the field had become Dento-maxillofacial Radiology, Endodontics, Forensic Odontology, Oral and Maxillofacial Surgery, Oral Medicine, Oral Pathology, Oral Surgery, Orthodontics, Paediatric Dentistry, Periodontics, Prosthodontics, Public Health (Community) Dentistry, Special Needs Dentistry as per The Dental Board of Australia, Registrant Data, March 2020.

33 Among these early Disaster Victim Identification dentists were Ross Bastiaan, Ian Hewson and Lloyd O'Brien.

34 Dental Board of Australia, Registrant Data, p. 8, March 2020.

Children and teenagers growing up without having lost any teeth to decay have been presenting in ever growing numbers with problems of crowded and irregular teeth. The cost of improving function and appearance by specialist orthodontists has been beyond the reach of many families. Further, the rate at which specialists can be trained has never been sufficient to meet the growing demand.

Over time general dentists have sought to fill the void in orthodontic care by training themselves. Through short courses and, in more recent years, by surrendering diagnostic and treatment planning control to offshore computerised programs, they are becoming providers of sequential plastic splints, or aligners, with no clear end of treatment. Paradoxically, this last form of treatment can be more expensive than that provided by specialists in many instances.

Further training and its implications

The private courses in Orthodontics mentioned above have been replicated across a broad spectrum of dental activities. This is understandable given that innovation in technology, materials and knowledge occurs continuously. Since the nascent profession organised itself as the Odontostomatological Society of Victoria (OSV) in 1884 there have been meetings, seminars and conferences for practitioners to upgrade their knowledge and skills. These grew in frequency and diversity as special interest groups formed in the second half of the 20th century. However, attendance was not compulsory and many dentists rarely informed themselves of new ideas. That said, lectures on practice management and financial planning have always been popular.

In 2005 Victoria was the first state in Australia to make further self-education, called continuing professional development (CPD), a mandatory requirement for annual registration, and since 2010 this has become a nationwide requirement. In a three-year cycle the required hours vary from 40 for a dental therapist to 60 for a dentist. A main factor in the decision was to protect the public from complacent and out-of-touch practitioners. Since CPD was mandated, it has become a major industry with dental schools, dental companies and public sector agencies joining in to compete in the market for the bums and eyeballs of all types of fee-paying practitioners. While proof of attendance for the number of hours must be logged by each practitioner to comply with Dental Board of Australia regulations, there is no standard set for the course or lecture provider; lectures may provide cutting-edge knowledge or infotainment.

Beyond these minimum requirements for continuing education, it has always been possible for a dentist, and now an oral health therapist, hygienist and prosthetist to undertake postgraduate training to further their knowledge and skills in a field of dentistry. Dentists can go on to become specialists with a higher degree but they may also remain general dentists and study for membership or fellowship of the Royal Australasian College of Dental Surgeons (RACDS). The College itself was established in 1965 to provide high quality post-graduate education to dentists and it has succeeded over time to stem the flow of bright young dentists going overseas to study for and collect Fellowships from Colleges in England, Scotland and Ireland. Many specialists pursue both university and College qualifications.

Another avenue for gaining knowledge about research methods or pursuing interest in a topic has opened up in recent years. The program, known as eviDent, is a research-focussed alliance between ADAVB and dental academia. It was launched in 2010 as a collaboration between ADAVB and the Collaborative Research Centre for Oral Health (CRCOH) at the University of Melbourne. One aim was to harness the enthusiasm and resource power of many disparate clinicians in their own practices and for them to involve themselves in research which could have outcomes to inform oral health policy. The program could also speed up the translation of research results into clinical practice. Participating in an eviDent project does not confer a formal qualification but can spark the desire to embark on a higher degree.

Although other dental practice-based research networks based in the USA and UK predated eviDent, it is the foremost such network in Australia. It has continued to grow and develop beyond Victoria into South Australia and New South Wales. At the start of 2022 it has involved 76 dental practitioners on 32 projects which all have academic chief investigators (M. Quinn, CEO, eviDent, personal communication, May 13, 2022). It might be expected that most research topics would be clinical, given that most participants are in general practice, but the 32 projects to date have covered a wide range of subjects. One quarter of the projects have focussed on disease prevention and only one third have been directly clinical. Results have mostly suggested incremental changes in attitude, procedure and refinement of techniques. Nevertheless, each result adds to the corpus of knowledge and participants gain greater insight into both the routine of their daily work and the need to question the blizzard of new information that confronts all practitioners.

Practice accreditation

In addition to an individual practitioner's pursuit of excellence through mandatory and voluntary courses of education, practice owners can submit their practices to continuing development, or accreditation, in order to promote the safety of patients and consumers and the provision of high-quality health care services.

Separate to the Australian Health Practitioner Regulation Agency (Ahpra) is the Australian Commission on Safety and Quality in Health Care (ACSQHC) (Chapter 3). It has created a set of standards, the National Safety and Quality of Health Service (NSQHS) Standards, which must be attained by submitting to an external audit. A practice which achieves the standards gains accreditation by the Commission. Accreditation is mandatory for all public sector health agencies and voluntary for private dental clinics. The Commission was formed in 2011 and the first set of quality-assurance tests was published in 2013. Public hospitals and clinics, including dental, are subject to external auditing. Private dental clinics which choose to take part undertake internal audits, although in each state the ADA provides advice, education and encouragement.

The Commission has set up eight NSQHS standards but only six are relevant to the practice of dentistry. The six standards cover clinical governance; partnering with consumers; preventing and controlling healthcare-associated infections; medication safety; comprehensive care; and communicating for safety (ACSQHC, 2021). The ADA encourages and assists practices to go through the accreditation process, the aim of which is to promote continuous quality improvement in all its functions, to minimise clinical and business risk and, in so doing, to improve each patient's experience and confidence (ADA, 2022).

Once a practice has invested time and money in the process to be accredited it cannot rest on its laurels; the status of accreditation has to be renewed every three or four years. This means that staff, new and old, maintain their levels of administrative, patient management and clinical skills. The staff engagement required raises competence and self-confidence because the staff know that they are following best-practice guidelines.

By 2016, 633 private practices across Australia had been accredited and this had jumped to 1,745 by the end of 2018 (AIHW, 2020). Only 256 Victorian practices were included in the 2018 total. However, this had risen to 570 by the end of 2021[35] and it is possible that early adopters of the accreditation process have been using it as a marketing exercise as a point of differentiation. Nevertheless, as with RACDS membership and fellowship, if the end result has been the raising of standards of service, then the aims of the Commission will be achieved across the sector over time.

While the voluntary nature of practice accreditation means that the process and its achievement could be used as a marketing advantage, that should not detract from the ensuing benefits to staff and patients alike. The relationship between accreditation and dental public health may be difficult to quantify but raising standards in the delivery of care across public and private clinics should be beneficial. Over time, it may be possible to discern a reduction in notifications to Ahpra concerning dentists in accredited practices as opposed to those in non-accredited ones.

Corporates

In 1970 private sector dentistry was still being run in much the same way as it had in the days of apprenticeship. It was mainly a cottage industry full of solo practitioners, each at one location. Group practices and part-time branch practices existed but they were a small minority. Dentists rarely went beyond the confines of their walls unless perhaps to give pro bono oral health talks to schools and kindergartens. With the exception of the RDHM, even the few public sector clinics had only one or two chairs. Dental chairs and units had been upgraded to accommodate the changes brought about by the adoption of air turbine drills and seated dentistry in the late 1950s, but they were still expected to last nearly a lifetime of practice. The rate of change in just about every aspect of dentistry and dental health has accelerated since then; particularly with regard to the size of practices, the gender mix of their workforces, the higher cost and turnover of capital equipment, and the legal structures around oral health provision.

The first iteration of dental corporatisation occurred in the late 1980s and served simply as a vehicle for permitting an increase in annual superannuation contributions for individual owners of private dental practices. It did not change the practice of dentistry itself, nor were practice owners (themselves all dentists) given any enhanced legal protection. The impulse to seek incorporation was due to dentists seeing that self-employed doctors and tradesmen and -women had already achieved that status and could put large tax-deductible sums into their superannuation funds, whereas dentists were severely limited in this. The Dental Board of Victoria eventually convinced the Australian

---

35 In comparison, by the end of 2021 there 937 NSW, 753 Queensland and 330 WA practices accredited.

Tax Office that it was illogical for medical practitioners to be allowed to incorporate while dentists could not (D. Hurley, personal communication, August, 2022). By 1987, the DBV had won its fight and changes to regulations of the Act were made.

The second iteration has emerged in the 21st century, since non-dentists have been allowed to own dental practices and since the popularisation of private health insurance "extras" including dentistry.

In the private dental sector, the practice owner, who may or may not be a dental practitioner, creates a corporate body which separates all aspects of administration from the staff who deliver clinical services. Practitioners are thus free to treat more patients and are relieved of the time and the stress involved in management. Management itself can be centralised and standardised across many clinical outlets regardless of size. In theory, it is a win–win situation for clinicians; for patients, who save through reduced overhead costs; and for owners who are rewarded for their entrepreneurial and management skills.

Corporatised practices are expanding through the purchase and corporatisation of traditional ones and the establishment of corporate practices in dormitory suburbs. The latter have the attraction of being open at weekends and most public holidays. In 2012 Genna Levitch gave a good insider's account of the rationale and description of five of the main dental corporates in Australia up to that time. He was also wise enough to say that "the viability of corporate practices can only be gauged over time once the original owner stops working" and the sense of embedded goodwill and ethics of a sole practice has gone (Levitch, 2012,).

In the time since Levitch's article, the number of corporate players and practices has grown. For example, in 2001, Pacific Smiles had 35 practices in Australia, and, at the start of 2022, it owned nearly 120. In 2001, Dental Corp had 182 practices in Australia and New Zealand and in 2022 it has 220. Along the way, group ownerships have changed and private health insurance companies have entered the field.

Dental Corp is now part of British United Provident Association (BUPA) and Pacific Smiles is allied to NIB (originally Newcastle Industries Benefits). There are likely to be more start-ups and takeovers, which is what one would expect in a free-market economy. One can see parallels between the rise of corporates out of what has been called the "cottage-industry" stage of dentistry and the replacement of 18th century hand-loom weavers by 19th century cotton and woollen factories. The new model is arising out of the old one.

However, is there a natural ceiling for corporate clinics? Can the two approaches co-exist like K-Mart and bespoke tailoring? There may be a price differential but other factors come into play apart from out-of-pocket expenses. Another unknown factor is the longevity of private health insurance. It has been said that private health insurance is in a "death spiral" (Davey, 2021) and although people can have "extras" policies without the high premiums of full cover, they often drop the dental extras when a course of care is completed, feeling that they have had their money's worth. If enough people do that, this could result in corporate practices, reliant on their association with health insurance companies, becoming victims of a virtual pyramid scheme.

Alexander Holden and colleagues have studied Australian corporate practices through the lens of George Ritzer's theory of the "McDonaldisation" of health services and its four key tenets of efficiency, predictability, calculability and control (Holden et al., 2021). Through interviews, they found that the clinicians can have different values and attitudes to administrative staff, causing an inherent tension or even conflict of interests. They also found that patients can start to form loyalty to the corporate brand rather than to any particular clinician, a development no doubt caused or heightened by a high turnover of clinical staff.

At the same time patients can and do differentiate between minor dental problems needing immediate resolution at an ever-ready corporate clinic, and more serious, strategic issues, which they prefer to have managed by an experienced independent practitioner likely to be available for a number of years.

A different perspective was provided by Paul Batchelor in a British Dental Journal editorial when he noted that, by 2020, 25% of dental practices in Britain were corporate owned (Batchelor, 2020). Batchelor identified three risks in this development; namely, standardisation, commodification and oligarchic structures. The first two of these are congruent with Ritzer's ideas (Holden et al., 2021) while the third risk – oligarchic structures – is inherent to the nature of capitalism. In the corporate world, patients can be made to fit the treatment even though the professional ethic should place patient wellbeing at the centre of decision making. In reference to somnambulism, Batchelor argued that governing bodies (in his case, the General Dental Council and General Medical Council) have not paid sufficient attention to problems which may arise when a corporate body collapses and patients and front-line staff are abandoned as a consequence.

Ahpra says that each practitioner has a duty of care, but how is that to be exercised in such a situation? There does not seem to be a clear pathway of redress within the current Australian system.

There is another issue which the existence of corporates has brought into sharp relief rather than created, and that is the possibility of overservicing patients. All health practices in the private sector are run as businesses to provide a living for the owner and staff. An ethical boundary is crossed when treatment is provided solely for the benefit of the provider and not the recipient. The Ahpra code of conduct states that health practitioners should "provide treatment options that are based on the best available information and are not influenced by financial gain or incentives" (Ahpra, 2022) In many instances dentists employed by corporate entities are given monthly financial targets or targets for high-value treatment items. A conflict of interest can, and often does, arise when targets cannot be met except by overservicing. It is the dental practitioner and not the corporate entity, who is in jeopardy for unethical conduct, although proof for prosecution would be hard to come by. The more that corporate practices become the domain of private equity companies that exist solely for profit, the more this dilemma will be encountered.

Summary

The main points covered in this chapter have been as follows: People's attitudes towards dental care have been shaped by their own experiences and the hearsay of that of others. It took time for new restorative technology to improve the dental experiences of patients and for that to percolate through society.

Following the fluoridation of public water supplies, the gradual reduction in rates of tooth decay helped to change attitudes towards treatment choices.

There has been a concurrent rise in disease prevention measures at the clinical level. These have often been performed by non-dentist providers.

Further preventive measures for some people have been led by known associations between certain systemic disorders and their oral health status.

Developments in dental technology and materials have permitted better treatment options and their prognoses. However, progress has been punctuated by occasional mis-steps and failures.

The rapid spread of computerisation and information technology has completely changed administration, strategic planning and the pooling of data for research.

The itemisation of procedures for the purpose of funding or payment needs constant updating and redefinitions of the items.

Although some dental fields of interest predated the period under study, their formal recognition as specialties, allied to improved attitudes in society towards the benefits of good oral health, have led to the proliferation of specialties and specialists.

Ever rising base levels of acceptable standards in health care settings have spread to dental clinics of all kinds. These cover premises, procedures and personnel. These are mandated in all publicly funded clinics but are still voluntary in the private sector though with increasing peer pressure to comply.

The commodification of nearly everything and the spread of franchising in the "free market" have encouraged the corporatisation of many health practices. In theory, the added layers of administration are more than offset by increased efficiency and lead to reductions in costs to patients. In practice, this has not always been so. This process is still unfolding and there will always be evolution in health delivery models.

Notwithstanding many discoveries and innovations over time, much medical and dental treatment as practiced during the 20th century was based on remembered precepts and unsystematic clinical experience. Sometimes retrospectively called "eminence-based medicine", this gave way to "evidence-based medicine" in the mid-1990s,[36] although Archie Cochrane had stated its principles as some two decades earlier in his book, *Effectiveness and Efficiency* (1972).

The take-up of paradigm shifts in attitudes, ideas and technology can be slow because they necessarily challenge and change the world views of established and eminent practitioners and educators in whichever field. This has been true in the provision of dental services when changing from preceptor-dictated to evidence-based practice. Two aspects are involved here: One is when new developments in technology, materials and equipment offer new possibilities of care but need to be measured against existing treatment options to assess which offers more durable and affordable benefits to patients. The other is when new biological understanding challenges the premises on which former treatment decisions were made.

One hopes that the history of the next 50 years will see G. V. Black relegated to an honourable footnote as it is hard to imagine anyone else casting such a long shadow over operating orthodoxy.

---

36 The term was coined by Gordon Guyatt in 1991 at McMaster University, Canada when introducing a new system of medical education.

References

Auditor-General Victoria. (A-GV). (2002). *Community dental services report*. <https://www.parliament.vic.gov.au/papers/govpub/VPARL1999-2002No186.pdf>

Auditor-General Victoria. (A-GV). (2016). *Access to public dental services in Victoria*. <https://www.audit.vic.gov.au/report/access-public-dental-services-victoria>

Australian Dental Association. (ADA). (2022, April 25). *Why should you seek accreditation?* <https://www.ada.org.au/Dental-Professionals/Practice-Accreditation-(1)/Introductory-Practice-Accreditaiton/Why-seek-practice-accreditation.>

Australian Commission on Safety and Quality in Health Care. (ACSQHC). (2021). *National safety and quality health service standards. Second edition – 2021.* <https://www.safetyandquality.gov.au/publications-and-resources/resource-library/national-safety-and-quality-health-service-standards-second-edition>

Australian Health Practitioner Regulation Authority. (Ahpra). (2022). *Code of conduct for health practitioners*. <https://www.dentalboard.gov.au/codes-guidelines/policies-codes-guidelines/code-of-conduct.aspx>

Australian Institute of Health and Welfare. (AIHW). (2020). *Australia's national oral health plan 2015–2024: Performance monitoring report. In brief.* <https://www.aihw.gov.au/reports/dental-oral-health/national-oral-health-plan-2015-2024-in-brief/contents/summary>

Batchelor, P. (2020). A case of somnambulism?, *British Dental Journal, 228*(8), 565–565.

Centers for Disease Control and Prevention. (CDCP). (2011). Morbidity and mortality weekly report, 60(24). <https://www.cdc.gov/mmwr/pdf/wk/mm6024.pdf>

Cochrane, A. L. (1972). *Effectiveness and efficiency. Random reflections on health services.* Oxford: The Nuffield Provincial Hospitals Trust. <https://www.nuffieldtrust.org.uk/files/2017-01/effectiveness-and-efficiency-web-final.pdf>

Davey, M. (2021, May 20). Australia's private health insurance industry in a 'death spiral', report says. *The Guardian.* <https://www.theguardian.com/australia-news/2021/may/20/australias-private-health-insurance-industry-in-a-death-spiral-report-says#:~:text=Australia's%20private%20health%20insurance%20industry%20is%20in%20a%20%E2%80%9Cdeath%20spiral,thinktank%20the%20Grattan%20Institute%20says.>

Dawson, A. S., & Makinson, O. F. (1992). Dental treatment and dental health, Part 2. An alternative philosophy and some new treatment modalities in operative dentistry. *Aust Dent J, 37*(3), 205–210. <doi: 10.1111/j.1834-7819, 1992.tb00744.x.>

Dental Board of Victoria. (DBV). (1993). *A history of its first hundred years.* Melbourne: DBV.

Dental Health Services Victoria. (DHSV). (2015). *Annual report 2014/2015.* <https://parliament.vic.gov.au/file_uploads/Dental_Health_Services_Victoria_Report_2014-15_5pKbVZwB.pdf>

Department of Health Victoria. (DHV). (October 26, 2021). Is my water fluoridated? <https://www.health.vic.gov.au/water/is-my-water-fluoridated>

Duckett, S., Cowgill, M., & Swerissen, H. (2019). *Filling the gap. A universal dental scheme for Australia.* Melbourne: Grattan Institute. <https://grattan.edu.au/wp-content/uploads/2019/03/915-Filling-the-gap-A-universal-dental-scheme-for-Australia.pdf>

Flieger, S. P., & Doonan, M. T. (2009). *Putting the mouth back in the body. Improving oral health across the Commonwealth.* Massachusetts Health Policy Forum, June 16, 2009. <https://heller.brandeis.edu/mass-health-policy-forum/categories/oral-health/pdfs/improving-oral-health-across-the-commonwealth/putting-mouth-back-body-issue-brief.pdf>

Holden, A., Adam, L., & Thompson, W.L. (2021). Rationalisation and 'McDonaldisation' in dental care: Private dentists' experiences working in corporate dentistry, *British Dental Journal* [online], June 25, 2021.

Kuhn, T. (1962). *The structure of scientific revolutions.* (Phoenix books in science). Chicago: University of Chicago Press.

Levitch, G. (2012). Corporatised dentistry 10 years on. *Australasian Dental Practice*, September/October 2012.

Mount, G. J., & Hume, W. R. (1998). *Preservation and restoration of tooth structure.* London: Mosby.

National Research Council. (NRC). (1989). *Diet and health. Implications for reducing chronic disease risk.* Washington, DC: The National Academies Press. <doi.org/10.17226/1222>

Chapter 8
Alliances and Advocacy – You gotta have friends

Jamie Robertson

Introduction

Since Plato's *Republic* and perhaps before, people who have identified and proposed their own solutions to problems in society have sought a broad support base to bring about the changes or reforms they advocate. In democracies, widespread, persistent support for change has often led to new legislation or, at least, a change in regulations. Generating and garnering that support is critical to success in the adoption of new ideas. This short chapter looks at how ideas can be spread and reinforced through alliances with like-minded people acting at opportune times in election cycles or at other serendipitous moments. It surveys advocacy activities undertaken since 1970 to argue for improvements in oral health and access to dental health care for all Victorians.

Box 8.1 Public health advocacy

Advocacy is the act of

❛ Taking a position on an issue, and initiating actions in a deliberate attempt to influence private and public policy choices. ❜

(Labonte, 1994, p. 255).

OR

❛ Advocacy is necessary to steer public attention away from disease as a personal problem to health as a social issue... Advocacy is a strategy for blending science and politics with a social justice value orientation to make the system work better, particularly for those with least resources. ❜

(Baum, 2015, p. 566).

Convergence of goals

A glance at the titles in airport bookstands and at the multiplicity of courses supposedly teaching it, shows that leadership is a much praised and analysed quality in the broad range of human endeavours. What is usually meant in discussion of leadership is a person conveying a sense of purpose, explaining how to achieve it and instilling enthusiasm in the group or team commissioned with executing the task. Different leadership styles, ranging from "the great man" to the "servant leader", have been hypothesised. Nevertheless, the personal qualities required for running an organisation are not necessarily best suited to swaying public opinion on issues of public health, especially if the issues have a low priority in the public's imagination. In such situations, good leaders reach out for allies with shared interests and goals.

Over the years some dental issues have been so acute that they have required little support from other agencies. For example, the social injustice of unaffordable private dental care, lack of access to care and long public sector waiting times have created potent electoral pressure on different Victorian governments. More often, health issues alone do not lead to changes in government, but they can be a critical force for change when combined with other perceived deficiencies when the social gradient of disease is more clearly revealed. Dental health issues rarely have the emotional impact of the life-and-death matters that arise in general health as, for example, with cancer or sudden infant death syndrome (SIDS). It has therefore made sense for proponents of dental health to highlight and jointly advocate on any links between dental and systemic health issues.

Another reason for seeking alliances on a health issue is that it can look like self-interest if only aired by the profession that deals with it, in this case, if dental practitioners were commenting on oral health. By forming alliances with respected but non-dental groups, issues on oral health can be shown to be for the public good rather than for the benefit of a few. Furthermore, alliances confer more power and legitimacy to the issue and nullify any adverse comment or even consequences that could ensue were the issue to be advocated by a specific group.

When certain behaviours such as high consumption of refined carbohydrates or smoking are common risk factors for diseases – such as tooth decay and diabetes mellitus, both of which are associated with dietary choices; or oral and lung cancer, which are both associated with smoking, it makes sense for dental and medical agencies to act jointly for their minimisation. Even where no linked association in disease predisposition is demonstrable, health professions are ultimately likely to endorse any actions directed at better overall health outcomes. Water fluoridation helps to reduce the prevalence of dental decay, especially in children, but has no other direct health benefit: however, reduced dental decay means fewer visits to medical practitioners for repeat and subsidised prescriptions of analgesics or antibiotics as palliative care.

As with measles and whooping cough, in the 21st century most young families in Victoria have little understanding of the pain and suffering caused by the high rates of dental disease before 1970. Sadly, the first two diseases are slowly returning, aided by complacency and ignorance about their possible severity.

So too, while the pain of childhood dental decay may be happening to fewer Australian children these days, it is still real and slowly increasing despite its preventable nature.

Throughout the 50 years covered in this history, formal and informal liaisons between organised dentistry and other agencies have existed to advocate for governmental policy and social behaviours to improve dental health and, by extension, general wellbeing. The earliest such initiative dates to the 1970s, when a committee, composed mainly of Australian Dental Association Victoria Branch (ADAVB) members, was established to advocate for water fluoridation. An example of one of the most recent liaisons has been a publication called the *Oral Health Tracker*, which is a periodic report card on various dental data and their progress towards target improvement levels by a future date (ADA, 2021). It is a collaboration between the federal ADA (Australian Dental Association) and the Australian Health Policy Collaboration unit at Victoria University.

When the timing was thought to be propitious, often in the lead up to elections, various groupings have formed to promote single issues, canvass support for specific policies, or simply to secure additional funding. The ADAVB has often led these campaigns – as with fluoridation of water supplies – but was not always the prime mover. For example, the ADAVB endorsed, but did not lead, *Quit*, an anti-smoking campaign which began in 1985 (Quit, 2021), and the *Rethink sugary drink* campaign launched in 2013 (CCV, 2021) to reduce the sugar content in soft drinks. In both cases there was a clear convergence of goals among a range of health and community organisations; a demonstration that oral health cannot be separated from general health.

In the mid-1980s, the same questioning of the status quo that prompted the 1986 Ministerial Review of Dental Services (MRODS) in Victoria (HDV, 1986) also encouraged fresh thinking about community input to the design and planning for dental services in the public sector. The Alma-Ata Declaration on Primary Care (WHO, 1978) had been given additional impetus by the Ottawa Charter of 1986 (WHO, 1986) to seek community involvement in designing health services. Primary Health academics and bureaucrats were aware of these drivers and the Cain Government's Minister for Health, David White had the drive to champion this fresh thinking.

Water fluoridation

In 1962 Bacchus Marsh became the first Victorian municipality to have its water supplies fluoridated. It came about following a local referendum, thanks largely to the vigorous efforts of a local dentist, and in spite of the efforts of local anti-fluoridationists. However, the campaign aroused little interest beyond Bacchus Marsh and that is probably why it succeeded. It was led by a respected local dentist with apparently nothing to gain, other than a reduction in children presenting in pain, in a tight-knit community. After that it became harder to influence the public in favour of fluoridation. The Victorian Anti-Fluoridation Society, though few in number, worked hard and the State Premier of the time, Sir Henry Bolte was an avowed opponent of the measure. Although individual medical practitioners supported the ADA's efforts, no attempt was made to seek a wider support base among other health agencies or organisations and no progress was made until Bolte retired in 1972. As seen in Chapter 2, legislation to permit water fluoridation was passed in 1973.

Even after water fluoridation commenced in Melbourne, opposition to it did not disappear, especially in rural Victoria. Indeed, opposition exists to this day in 2022. In October 1978, a by-election campaign for the Legislative Council seat of Ballarat gave anti-fluoridationists an opportunity to pressure the government of Victorian Premier Dick Hamer. During the campaign Hamer announced a suspension of further fluoridation procedures and another inquiry into the effects of water fluoridation (Sun, 1978). The ADAVB hired a public relations company, International Public Relations, to advocate its case and to promote the cause and benefits of water fluoridation.

Nevertheless, as the National Rifle Association in the USA has shown, a vocal minority with political influence can successfully impede beneficial public health measures even though a majority of the population may be in favour.[37] Advocacy is a two-way street. Hamer's Liberal Government lost that Ballarat by-election battle but won the war; the ALP's David Williams was successful in the 1978 election, but the inquiry found in favour of the fluoridation of water supplies and the roll-out recommenced. Hamer was astute enough to follow the old politician's adage; never set up an inquiry without knowing the outcome in advance.

---

37 Pew Research Center, survey results, 13 September, 2021 show 53% of adults favour stricter gun control. This has fluctuated in recent years but has been a majority for past ten years.

With hindsight, one might ask, would the ADAVB have made faster progress towards water fluoridation if it had sought a broad "coalition of the willing" among other social and health agencies? Karen Block has analysed how much the pro- and anti-fluoridationists were talking past each other in the contest of collective versus individual human rights, and how challenging their respective deeply held beliefs affected their psyches (Block, 2009). Rational debate only goes so far before it hits deeper layers of self-protection, and this is replicated in current controversies on climate change and energy policies. Henry Bolte's opposition to fluoridation was implacable and progress had to wait until his retirement. *Realpolitik* demonstrated that no matter how persuasive the advocacy on an issue, opposition from an incumbent premier or prime minister can often only be challenged at the ballot-box.

Community beginnings

The Victorian Department of Human Services created the first of 16 District Health Councils in May 1986 to elicit community and consumer feedback on their health needs and priorities (HDV, 1987). To the surprise of some, Kensington Community Health Centre clients named poor access to dental care as one of their main health priorities (Tony McBride, personal communication, December 10, 2019) (Chapter 2). Meanwhile, the CEO of Brunswick Community Health Centre, Meredith Kefford contributed to a Health Issues Forum pamphlet in which she sought support for action on the MRODS recommendations, writing: "It is timely for community groups to put their weight behind this report which will put Victoria in the direction of more accessible and accountable dental services" (Kefford, 1987, pp. 6–7).

These community groups had formed an alliance to create the *Molar Energy Campaign* (a word play on a then current solar energy campaign) and it was a forerunner, but not progenitor, of the later Victorian Oral Health Alliance (VOHA). Further pressure on the state ALP government filtered through from its local branches who could see electoral advantage in the issue among their constituents. This helped to get the first dental clinic in Brunswick Community Health Centre and 20 other centres soon followed (Chapter 4). This decentralisation reduced pressure on the Royal Dental Hospital of Melbourne (RDHM) and improved geographic access to public care for eligible people.

In the run-up to the national election in 1993, the Australian Council of Social Service (ACOSS) and the Consumers' Health Forum led a push for a national dental program for people on low incomes. They produced a pamphlet, *Getting your teeth into health care*, which was endorsed by 12 other sectional interest groups (ACOSS & CHF, 1993).[38] The advocacy from this broad coalition provided more solid support to the 1992 report, *Improving dental health in Australia* (Dooland, 1992) (Chapters 2 and 4). The combined efforts, and the not incidental fact of the ALP victory in the election, resulted in the Commonwealth Dental Health Program (CDHP), which was introduced following the report of the National Health Strategy in January 1994 under the Keating-led Labor Government (Chapter 4). The intention of the program was to reduce reliance upon emergency treatment by providing more timely general care.

38 Association of District Health Councils, Australian Community Health Association, Australian Consumers' Association, Australian Council on the Ageing, Australian Pensioners' and Superannuants' Association, Australian Youth Policy and Action Coalition, Disabled Persons International, Family Planning Australia, Health Issues Centre, Mental Health Coordinating Council, National Council for Single Mothers and their Children, and Public Health Association of Australia.

Bite-Back Campaign

In 1996 Martin Dooland, CEO of the new DHSV, approached the Brotherhood of St Laurence (BSL) to run a campaign to save the CDHP which was under threat by the incoming Coalition Federal Government. The BSL took up the challenge and launched the *Bite-Back campaign* – which was a pun on the Fight Back campaign of the then Liberal leader John Hewson in the lead-up to the 1993 Federal election.

The supporters of the campaign were extremely broad – representing a wide range of interests. They included the Victorian Farmers Federation, Council on the Ageing Victoria, the Health Issues Centre, Combined Pensioners and Superannuants Association, the Uniting Church in Victoria, the Victorian Council of Social Services (VCOSS) and a number of influential individuals, including Brian Howe, who was the Minister responsible for introducing the CDHP in the first place and who had recently retired from Federal politics. The Uniting Church got involved via Bronwyn Pike who was head of its social justice unit at that time and who later became a Victorian Health Minister.

As part of its advocacy, the BSL undertook research into low-income people's access to dental services through its Changing Pressures project.

What made Bite-Back interesting was that the issue cut across the usual dividing lines of left and right; the rural disadvantage caused by a lack of public dental clinics demonstrated that. While the Bite-Back campaign was ultimately unsuccessful, it did lead to future collaboration between the BSL and DHSV when the former was invited to provide consumer input into the design of the new dental hospital being constructed in Swanston Street.

Victorian Oral Health Alliance

Although the Health Issues Centre (HIC) was conceived in 1980, it only took form later in the 1980s with Shane Solomon as its first CEO (T. McBride, personal communication, August 16, 2021). Its purposes were to analyse health policies and economics and to give health service consumers a forum, in which to voice their complaints, opinions and ideas. Tony McBride, who had been involved with oral health issues since his time at Kensington CHC, was its CEO from 2003 until 2009. Since the cessation of the Commonwealth Government's CDHP in 1997, funding for public sector dental care and the heightened need to advocate for funds in state government budgets were recurring issues. Discussions between HIC and ADAVB identified shared concerns about the lack of funding and limited access to public sector dental services. The Victorian Oral Health Alliance (VOHA) was formed in June 2004 to campaign for improvements (G. Pearson, former CEO of ADAVB, personal communication, February 12, 2020). Its founding members were the HIC, ADAVB, Australian Dental and Oral Health Therapists Association (ADOHTA), VCOSS, Victorian Aboriginal Community Controlled Health Organisation (VACCHO) and the BSL, which, itself, had produced a report on poor dental health and its causes and ramifications among its clientele.

Although VOHA was formed too late to influence the May 2004 Victorian state election, it campaigned for the October federal election of the same year and had agreed-upon National Oral Health Plan (NOHP) goals to support its efforts. Between elections the individual organisations which make up a broad advocacy alliance typically concentrate on their respective core priorities: this was true for VOHA members and there may have been misalignment of policies on other matters.

Nevertheless, as subsequent election campaigns have come round, VOHA has reliably come out of hibernation to press for public dental sector funding and more resources for the NOHP.

The early years of the 21st century were conducive to new thinking in a wide range of Australian enterprises and organisations. It was both the beginning of a new century and the centenary of Australian Federation which had united separate colonies into one nation state. A stable national Coalition Government presided over a prospering economy, an encouraging environment for federal departments to progress further ideas of nationhood. One product of these times was the Australian Research Centre for Population Oral Health (ARCPOH), established in 2001 and attached to the Dental School at Adelaide University. As its name suggests, ARCPOH's remit was to study the nation's oral health and offer suggestions for improvement. Its early work formed the basis of Australia's first NOHP which was endorsed by the Council of Australian Governments (COAG) at its meeting in Adelaide in May 2004. A national plan provided baseline data, a set of goals and a timeline for progress in achieving them.

Beyond 2004 – with moves leading to national governance of health professions rather than state-based boards, and with results of early research by ARCPOH including a report on the National Survey of Adult Oral Health 2004–06 (Slade et al., 2007) – it was logical that advocacy for better funding and resources for oral health should be directed to a national government. In the 2007 Federal election, the reinvigorated VOHA campaigned again and helped to force the issues of access to dental care and costs back onto the national agenda.

National Oral Health Alliance

The VOHA's existence and apparent success was sufficient proof of concept for the Federal Council of the ADA to solicit support from many of the same organisations which had previously supported VOHA. The national bodies of these organisations[39] agreed to form a National Oral Health Alliance (NOHA) in 2010 in time to produce a pamphlet, *Stop the rot*, for the Federal election campaign of that year.

The NOHA and the VOHA, to a lesser extent, are like hibernating creatures who respond to the rise in political temperature at the approach of an election: facts are marshalled, questions posed, promises sought and media space and time are solicited, free where possible and paid when necessary.

Oral Health Tracker

The Oral Health Tracker (ADA, 2021) is an example of one good project sparking another into existence through the agency of friendship in a work-related network.

For a time, Rosemary Calder and Eithne Irving worked together in the Commonwealth Department of Health in Canberra. Eventually they both moved on; Calder to the Mitchell Institute (MI) at Victoria University in Melbourne and Irving to the ADA headquarters in Sydney. At MI, Calder's main interest was to advocate for an integrated approach to incorporating preventive strategies in health policy and she became the Head of the Australian Health Policy Collaboration. She established the Australian Health Tracker, which was a set of goals and metrics which could be used to inform and influence researchers and policy makers.

39 Initially these were ACOSS, ADA, Australian Dental and Oral Health Therapists Association, Australian Health Care Reform Association, Australian Healthcare and Hospitals Association, Australian Nursing Federation, ARCPOH, Dental Hygienists Association of Australia, Brotherhood of St Laurence, Health Issues Centre, National Rural Health Alliance and PHAA.

The Tracker was launched in 2013 (ADA, 2018). Eithne Irving was invited to attend and immediately saw the potential and utility for such a project related to oral health. The two colleagues assembled a group of experts to design and create a series of data sets and achievable goals relating to the social, behavioural and clinical measurement of oral health status. Much of the data was obtained from previous ARCPOH surveys, the National Oral Health Plan 2015–24 (COAG, 2015) and augmented by telephone surveys. Goals were reached by consensus of the participant experts. The completed Oral Health Tracker was funded by the ADA and is a joint venture with the Allied Health Professionals Council (AHPC). It was launched at Parliament House in Canberra on World Oral Health Day on 18 March 2018 (ADA, 2018). No other country had such a Tracker for prevention at the time and it won the Fédération Dentaire Internationale Media Prize for innovation that year. An ADA media release at the time said the Tracker was "consistent with the World Health Organization Action Plan to prevent chronic diseases across the globe, and updates will be issued on a regular basis through to 2025 to show how the nation is tracking in improving the state of its oral and general health" (ADA, 2018, para. 6).

Information from the Tracker can be presented and published more frequently than that of national surveys which, depending on funding, tend to take place once every five years, alternating between adults and children.[40] Data from the Tracker also reveal a broader social dimension to trends in diet and behaviours.

The tool can therefore both support evidence from national surveys and reinforce the need for them to provide accurate measurements and feedback. However, publication of the Tracker itself depends on funding and continued interest of the staff at MI and the ADA. There has been no publication since 2020, leaving questions about the long-term commitment to it.

Other alliances

Dentists for Cleaner Water was an initiative intended to encourage dentists to upgrade their waste systems, with the side benefit of showing that the profession was proactive and socially responsible. Initially set up to run from 2008 until 2011, it was extended to the end of 2012. Its partners were the ADAVB, the Victorian water industry and the Victorian Environmental Protection Authority (I. Crawford, Coordinator of Dentists for Cleaner Water, personal communication, July 22, 2020).

Mercury, a component of amalgam fillings, is an environmental contaminant. Dentists for Cleaner Water offered practices a subsidy of $1,000 to install dental amalgam separators to filter waste amalgam before it entered the sewage system. By around 2000 most Australian dentists had stopped or greatly reduced use of amalgam as a restorative material. However, they still had to remove it from teeth when replacing fillings. Prior to the program, amalgam was either rinsed into sewage systems or disposed of in landfill. Trapping amalgam at point of use meant that its constituents, mercury, silver and tin could be retrieved, processed and repurposed.

---

40 National surveys have been conducted in 1987-88 and most recently about every five years – National Survey of Adult Oral Health 2004-06, National Child Oral Health Survey 2012-14, and the National Study of Adult Oral Health 2017-18. A national child survey is planned for 2023-2024.

In October 2013 Australia joined the Minamata Convention on Mercury which had been finalised in January that year (Department of Agriculture Water and the Environment. Australia, no date) The Convention called for a phasing down of the use of dental amalgam but, by the time it came into force, Dentists for Cleaner Water had largely achieved that goal.

Summary

In this chapter we have seen how advocacy is needed initially to gain the notice of politicians in the welter of competing claims on their attention, then, having done that, to persuade them of the merits of the case advocated. For every issue advocated there is at least one counter-position. For water fluoridation it was a small number of prolific letter-writing "concerned citizens" while for proposals to limit the advertising and consumption of sugar-laden food and drink, there are the powerful commercial vested interests. Furthermore, although the scientific evidence or demonstrated benefit may support one side only, deeply held beliefs of the other side are often not susceptible to logic. This is why successful advocacy must use a variety of approaches to persuade policy makers and politicians.

These approaches may focus on the human rights of people who will benefit, for example, the right to have accessible and affordable dental care, or may emphasise the economic benefit to many versus the private profit of a few, as with a reduction in sugar consumption preventing non-communicable disease. Large rigorous epidemiology surveys can also sway an otherwise neutral politician, especially if the costs of not acting outweigh those of acting.

Advocacy can also harness the inchoate ideas of a large group of people who, individually, could not conceive of changing the status quo. Advocacy in relation to dental health has alerted policy makers to pent up frustrations around the lack of access to dental care. This is why timing can be critical and why advocacy efforts tend to build up before elections when politicians become more attuned to the issues dominating the minds and opinions of electorates (Chapter 4). The intersection of advocacy, evidence and timing is more likely to lead to success than one these elements alone.

References

Australian Council of Social Service (ACOSS) and Consumers' Health Forum (CHF). (1993). *Getting your teeth into health care*. Sydney, NSW: ACOSS and CHF.

Australian Dental Association. (ADA). (2018, March 20). *Launch of oral health tracker A world-first game change*r. <https://www.ada.org.au/News-Media/News-and-Release/Latest-News/Launch-of-Oral-Health-Tracker-a-game-changer-in-ta>

Australian Dental Association. (ADA). (2021). *Australia's oral health tracker*. <https://www.ada.org.au/Dental-Professionals/Australia-s-Oral-Health-Tracker>

Baum, F. (2015). *The new public health*. (4th ed.). South Melbourne: Oxford University Press.

Block, K. (2009). Deep structure and controversy: Re-reading the fluoridation debate. *Health Sociology Review, 18*(3), pp. 246-59.

Cancer Council Victoria. (CCV). (2021). *Rethink sugary drink*. <https://www.rethinksugarydrink.org.au/media/time-to-rethink-sugary-drinks.html>

COAG Health Council. (2015). *Healthy mouths, healthy lives: Australia's national oral health plan 2015–2024*. <https://www.health.gov.au/resources/publications/healthy-mouths-healthy-lives-australias-national-oral-health-plan-2015-2024?language=en>

Department of Agriculture Water and the Environment. Australia. (n.d.) *Minamata Convention on Mercury – A response to global concern*. <https://www.environment.gov.au/protection/chemicals-management/mercury>

Dooland, M. (1992). *Improving dental health in Australia*. Melbourne: National Health Strategy.

Health Department Victoria (HDV). (1986). *Ministerial review of dental services. Final report*. Melbourne: HDV.

Health Department Victoria (HDV). (1987). *District Health Councils Program. Annual review 1987*. <https://vgls.sdp.sirsidynix.net.au/client/search/asset/1299669/0>

Kefford, M. (1987). Health Issues Forum, occasional publication, p6.

Labonte, R. (1994). Health promotion and empowerment: Reflections on professional practice. *Health Educ Quarterly, Summer; 21*(2), 253-68, p. 255. <doi: 10.1177/109019819402100209>

PROV VPRS 8609. Sun News Pictorial (Sun). (1978, October 7). No author or page number given. Retrieved from Melbourne Metropolitan Board of Works 'Fluoride" clippings.

Quit. (2021). *Our story*. <https://www.quit.org.au/articles/our-story>

Slade, G. D., & Spencer, A. J., & Roberts-Thomson, K. F., AIHW, & Australian Research Centre for Population Oral Health. (2007). *Australia's dental generations. The national survey of adult oral health 2004-06*. Canberra: Australian Institute of Health and Welfare. <https://www.aihw.gov.au/reports/dental-oral-health/australias-dental-generations-survey-2004-06/summary>

World Health Organization. (WHO). (1978). *Declaration of Alma-Ata*. World Health Organization. (1978). Declaration of Alma-Ata. WHO Regional Office for Europe. <https://apps.who.int/iris/handle/10665/347879>

World Health Organization. (WHO). (1986). *Ottawa Charter for Health Promotion*. <https://www.euro.who.int/__data/assets/pdf_file/0004/129532/Ottawa_Charter.pdf>

Chapter 9
Financing of Dental Services – Who pays?

John Rogers

Introduction

The cost of dental care is a recurring theme whenever dentistry is discussed in Australia. When radio talk shows mention access to affordable care, the station switchboards light up. How much the next dental visit will take out of the bank account is a staple topic on social media.

In this chapter we review trends in expenditure on dental services over the past five decades and examine who pays, and how much. We look at how governments fund dental care compared with other health care, and whether dental fees have increased or decreased relative to the average weekly wage.

Total and per person dental expenditure

Total and per person dental expenditure in Victoria have increased since 1970.[41] For the years 1996–97 to 2018–19, Figure 9.1 shows per capita expenditure, while Figure 9.2 shows total expenditure (AIHW, 2020b).

Victoria has consistently ranked among the states with the highest per person dental expenditure. In 2018–19 state spending of $499 per person (Figure 9.1, Table 9.1) was 18% higher than the Australian average of $422. Only Western Australia ($596) and the Northern Territory ($516) spent more. In 1997 per person Victorian expenditure was $300 – higher than in any other state or territory, and 22% higher than the national average of $245 (Table 9.1).

Figure 9.1 Dental services expenditure per person, Victoria (constant prices), 1996 to 2019 ($)

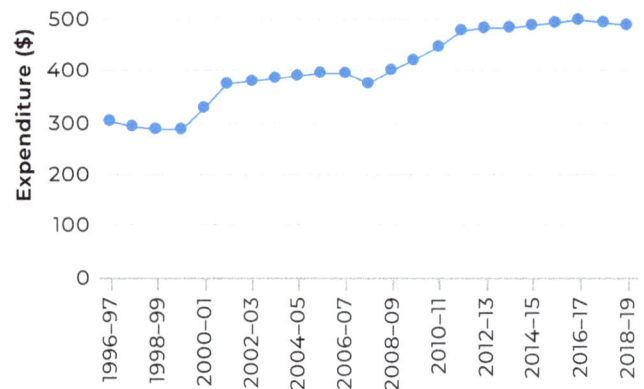

Source: Prepared using the AIHW data visualisation tool (AIHW, 2020b).

Access to private dental services can be influenced by the general state of the economy. The decrease in expenditure in 2007–08 shown in Figure 9.1 can be linked to the Global Financial Crisis (RBA, 2023).

In 2018–19 Victorian dental expenditure was $3.2 billion, more than double that of 1996–97 in constant prices (an increase of 227%) (Figure 9.2, Table 9.1), and represented 30% of total Australian spending of $10.6 billion (Table 9.1). That year, NSW spent the same amount on its larger population. Individuals were the major contributors, with governments and health insurers paying lesser amounts, as discussed in the next section. Sources of funding are shown in Figure 9.2.

41 Per person expenditure is calculated by dividing total dental expenditure by the population. It is different from individual expenditure which refers to out-of-pocket spending by individuals.

Figure 9.2 Total dental services expenditure by source of funds, Victoria (constant prices), 1996 to 2019 ($ millions)

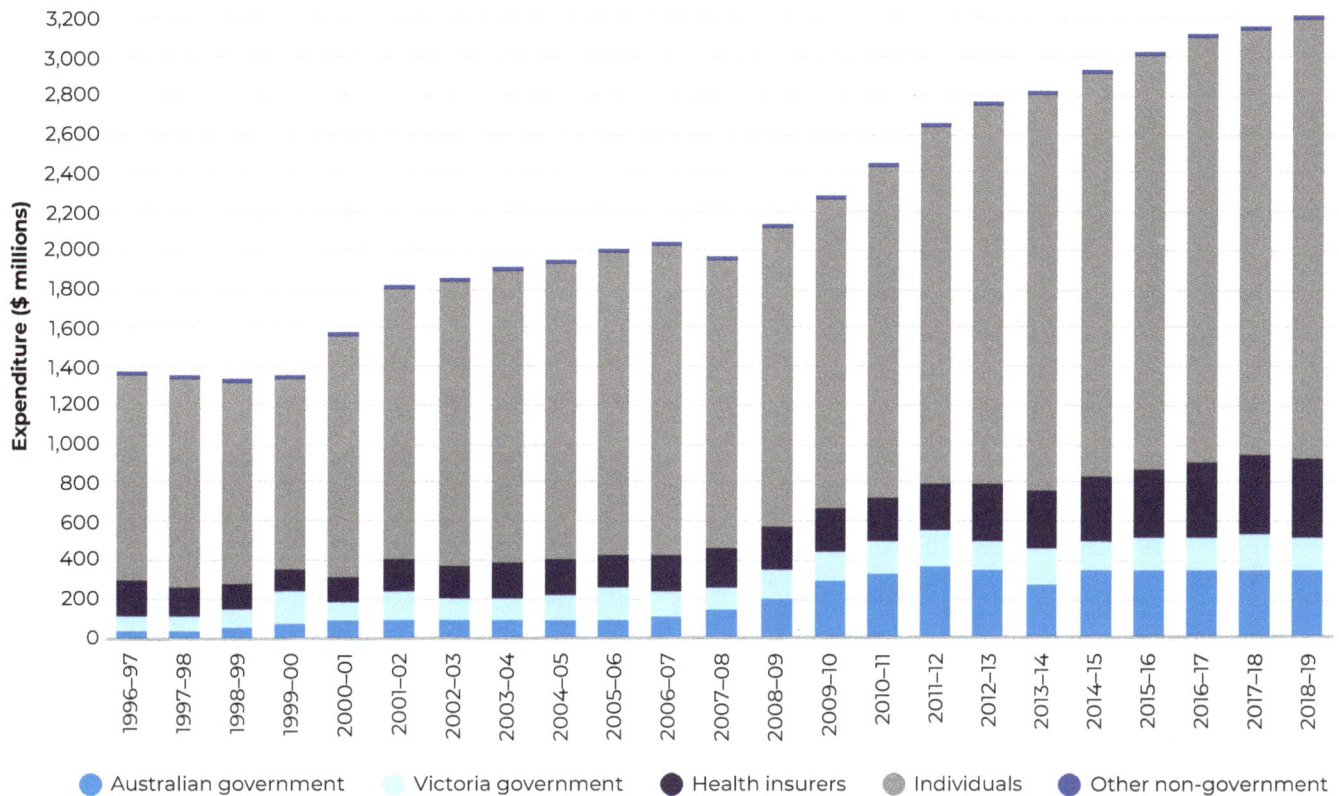

Source: Prepared using the AIHW data visualisation tool (AIHW, 2020b).

Table 9.1 Dental services expenditure, Victoria and Australia (constant prices), 1996–97 and 2018–19 ($)

	1996–97		2018–19	
	Victoria $	Australia $	Victoria $	Australia $
Total	1.368b	4.485b	3.203b	10.627b
Per person	300	245	499	422

Source: Prepared using the AIHW data visualisation tool (AIHW, 2020b).

Sources of funding

The four main sources of funding for dental services are individuals, health insurers, Australian governments and Victorian governments. In 2018-19 individual Victorians contributed the largest share of funding at 70%; health insurers contributed 13%; the Australian Government 11%, and the Victorian Government 5%. While relative contributions varied from state to state, Victorians contributed a larger share than all other Australians (70% compared with 57%). Other funders of dental services (governments and insurers) also contributed a smaller proportion of funding in Victoria than elsewhere (Figure 9.3) (AIHW, 2020b).

Figure 9.3 Sources of dental services expenditure, Victoria and Australia (constant prices), 2018–19 ($ millions and %)

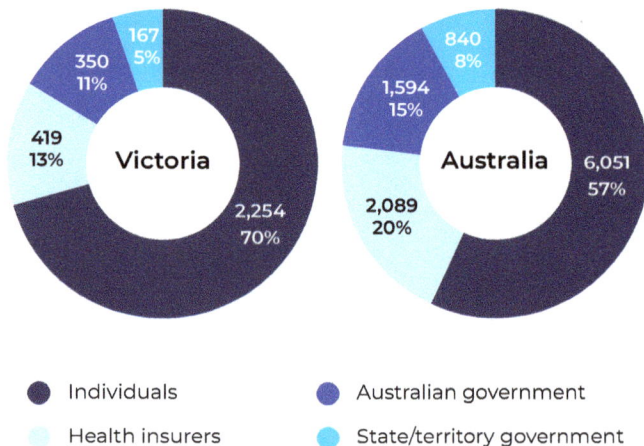

Source: Prepared using the AIHW data visualisation tool (AIHW, 2020b).

The proportion of expenditure contributed by each funding source has fluctuated over time with government contributions always minimal (Figure 9.3).[42] Between 1996–97 and 2018–19, the Australian Government share varied from 2–14%, the Victorian Government share from 5–12%; individuals' share from 69–81%, and that of health insurers from 8–13% (Table 9.2). The Victorian government contribution to dental expenditure increased from 2019–20 with the introduction of the Smile Squad school dental service, as discussed below and in Chapter 5.

Table 9.2 Sources of dental services expenditure in Victoria, 1996–97 to 2018–19

Source of funds	1996–97 %	2018–19 %	Range between 1996–97 & 2018–19 %
Victorian Government	6	5	5–12
Australian Government	3	11	2–14
Individuals	78	70	69–81
Health insurers	13	13	8–13
Other	0.2	0.4	0.1–0.7
Total	**100**	**100**	

Source: Data were prepared using the AIHW data visualisation tool (AIHW, 2020b).

42 Expenditure data by source for Victoria are only readily available from 1996–97.

Comparison with other health expenditure

Governments have always contributed a smaller proportion of total expenditure to dental services than to health expenditure overall. For example, in 2018–19, state and national governments contributed 65% of total Victorian health expenditure, while individuals and health insurers contributed 20% and 8%, respectively (Figure 9.4). The corresponding figures for dental expenditure were 16% (governments), 70% (individuals), and 13% (insurers) (Figure 9.3).

Figure 9.4 Total Victorian health expenditure by source of funds, 2018–19 (%)

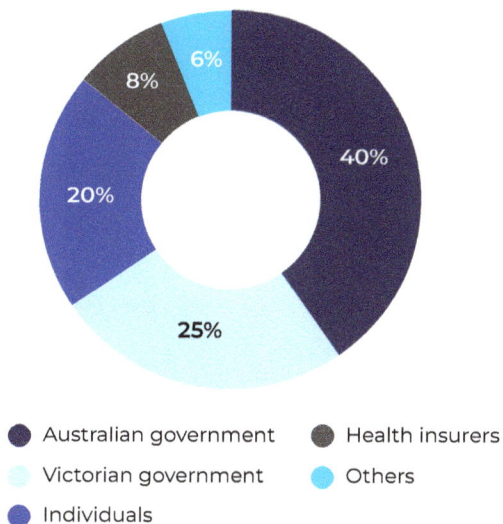

- Australian government
- Victorian government
- Individuals
- Health insurers
- Others

Source: Prepared using the AIHW data visualisation tool (AIHW, 2020b).

Between 1996–97 and 2018–19, total Victorian Government recurrent health expenditure increased by almost $8 billion (254%), from $3.4 to $11.3 billion (Table 9.3). The most marked change was a 3.5-fold increase in hospital expenditure. In that period, expenditure on community health increased 1.8-fold and on public health by 1.5 times.

The share of total recurrent health expenditure allocated to dental health decreased from 2.3% in 1996–97 to 1.5% in 2018–19, with a peak at 4.1% in 1999–00. These figures do not include the most recent AIHW data for 2019–20, which show that Victorian government expenditure on dental services increased significantly from $167 million to $190 million in that year (AIHW, 2021a).

Table 9.3 Victorian government dental services expenditure (constant prices) and increases compared with other areas of health expenditure, 1996–97 and 2018–19

Area	1996–97 ($ m)	2018–19 ($ m)	Increase x times	Increase %
Hospitals	2,553	9,043	x3.5	254
Dental	77	167	x2.2	117
Community health	474	857	x1.8	81
Public health	248	364	x1.5	47
Total recurrent expenditure	3,415	11,339	x3.3	232
Dental expenditure as a proportion of total recurrent health expenditure	2.3%	1.5%	–	–

Note: These data (AIHW, 2020b) show lower dental expenditure than that reported in the Victorian Government Budget papers for the corresponding years because the latter also include Australian government funds.

In Australia, dental treatment is one of the most expensive areas of health expenditure. At over $10 billion a year it is similar to the expenditure on General Practice services (AIHW, 2021b). Tooth decay on its own is one of the most expensive disease conditions to treat. At a total cost of $5 billion in 2018-19, treatment of tooth decay was more costly than falls (AIHW, 2021b).

More Victorians are facing cost barriers to accessing dental care: 29% of adults were unable to afford dental care in 2006, compared with 34% in 2017 (Chapter 10). There has been an increase in the amount of money withdrawn from superannuation to pay for dental care (Dalzell, 2022).

Australian government

A roller coaster of programs commenced by one government and closed by another has seen Australian government funding for dental health fluctuate from 1970 (Table 9.4).

Spending on dental health sank as low as 2% of national dental expenditure in the late 1980s and peaked at 18% between 2009–10 and 2013–14 (AIHW, 2020b). In 2018–19 the Australian government's share of dental health expenditure in Victoria was 11% (Figure 9.3).

Table 9.4 Major public dental programs funded by Australian and state/territory governments, 1970 to 2022

Financial year	Program (initiating government)	Focus	Status (Government)
1973–1981	Australian School Dental Scheme (ASDS) (*Whitlam Labor*)	Free school-based dental health service, largely provided by dental therapists.	Australian Government funding and responsibility ceased by *Fraser Coalition* in 1981.
1994–1996	Commonwealth Dental Health Program (CDHP) (*Keating Labor*)	Dental services for Health Care Card holders to reduce waiting lists and shift care from emergency to prevention and early management.	Commonwealth funding ceased by *Howard Coalition* in 1996
1997–current	Private Health Insurance Rebate (PHIR) scheme (*Howard Coalition*)	Income tested Commonwealth government rebate towards cost of private health insurance premiums.	Ongoing
2004–2013	Allied Health and Dental Care initiative which became the Chronic Disease Dental Scheme (CDDS) (*Howard Coalition*)	Medicare-subsidised private dental treatment for people with chronic illness impacting on their oral health or vice versa.	CDDS ceased by *Rudd Labor* in 2013.
2013–current	Dental National Partnership Agreements (NPA) (*Gillard Labor initiative implemented by Abbott Coalition*)	Commonwealth funding to states and territories for improving public dental services for adults on low incomes.	Ongoing
2014–current	Child Dental Benefits Schedule (CDBS) (*Gillard Labor initiative implemented by Abbott Coalition*)	Capped dental benefits covering a range of dental services for children who receive, or whose families receive, Government payments or benefits.	Ongoing

Note: These data (AIHW, 2020b) show lower dental expenditure than that reported in the Victorian Government Budget papers for the corresponding years because the latter also include Australian government funds.

Support for oral health has varied significantly among Australian governments. The story of the roller coaster of funding is outlined in Chapter 4. Policy on public dental care has been described as "being caught in a chilly stand-off between the Commonwealth and States or Territories, punctuated by warm outbursts of buck-passing and point-scoring" (Spencer, 2001, p. 50). Programs that fell victim to these policy swings included the Australian School Dental Scheme (ASDS), the Commonwealth Dental Health Program (CDHP), and the Chronic Disease Dental Scheme (CDDS). Other programs survived changes of government. These included the Private Health Insurance Rebate scheme (PHIR), the Commonwealth Child Dental Benefits Schedule (CDBS), and dental National Partnership Agreements (NPAs) (Table 9.4).

In general, Labor governments have tended to favour expanding public dental services (ASDS, CDHP and NPA), while Coalition governments have been more likely to support the individual to meet the costs of private care (PHIR and CDDS).

The Whitlam Labor Government introduced the ASDS in 1973 (DoHA, 1973). Under this scheme, jurisdictions could access new Australian government funds if they also contributed funding. Victoria and New South Wales were slower than other jurisdictions to participate. As a result, by the early 1980s when School Dental Program funds were absorbed into jurisdictional grants under the Fraser Coalition Government, these states were receiving less than $5 per primary school child, while South Australia, Western Australia and Tasmania were being paid more than $20 per child (Government bureaucrat, personal communication, 2006).

The CDHP introduced by the Keating Labor Government in 1993 was cancelled by the Howard Coalition in 1996 (Costello, 1996). The Howard Government introduced what became the CDDS in 2004 and increased its scope in 2007. This program was then replaced by the NPAs under the Gillard Government in 2013 and the CDBS announced by the Gillard Government and implemented under the Abbott Coalition Government 2014. The PHIR was introduced by the Howard Government in 1997 (Biggs, 2008). In 2018 rebates for people taking up private dental insurance under this scheme totalled $710 million, amounting to almost half (45%) of the Australian Government's total contribution to dental expenditure (Productivity Commission, 2020).

The health insurance rebate, which remains in place, results in a high proportion of funding being used to subsidise private health insurance, rather than providing dental care to the most disadvantaged. The benefits of subsidised private health insurance are more likely to flow to higher-income families who can afford the insurance premiums. Public health advocates have argued that the rebate increases inequality in oral health and have repeatedly called for these funds to be redirected to public dental services (PHAA, 2020; Menadue, 2021).

The CDBS and NPAs resulted from an accord between the Gillard Labor Government and Bob Brown's Greens in 2011 (Parliament of Australia, 2012). These programs were continued by the Abbott, Turnbull, and Morrison Coalition Governments. Despite various attempts on their parts to close them down and replace them with a Child and Adult Public Dental Scheme (caPDS), the legislation was blocked by the Senate. The first national partnership agreement, NPA1, ran from 2012–13 to 2014–15. The budgets of subsequent NPAs were 30% lower than that of NPA1.

Like the Whitlam Government school dental scheme, uptake of the Coalition's CDDS differed markedly by jurisdiction. Disproportionate distribution of Australian government funds to states and territories continued in the years 1996–97 to 2018–19. For example, in 2011–12, total per person expenditure from the Australian government was almost $99 in New South Wales, $67 in Victoria, and $26 in the Northern Territory (AIHW, 2020b).

The high point of Australian government dental funding to Victoria and New South Wales was in 2011–12, when the CDDS was at its peak. Since 2014–15 Australian government expenditure per person has remained stable (Figure 9.5). In 2018–19 Victoria ranked sixth among the eight jurisdictions, receiving $54 per person, while New South Wales ranked third at $69. South Australia received the highest per person contribution ($76), and the Northern Territory the lowest ($37) (AIHW, 2020b).

Figure 9.5 Australian government dental services expenditure per person (constant prices) in New South Wales and Victoria compared with the Australian average, 1996–2019 ($)

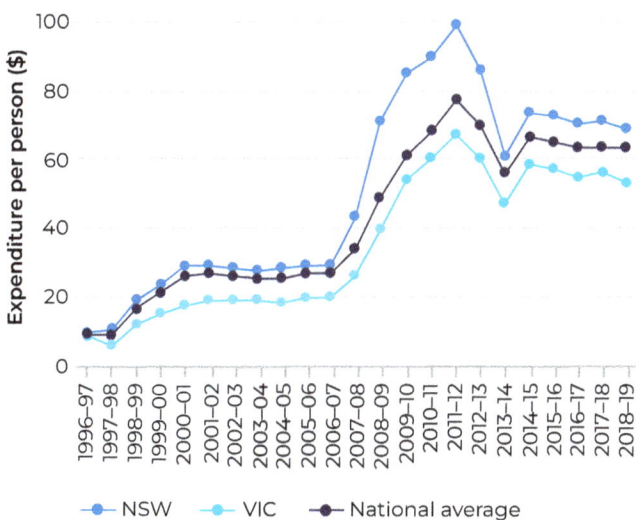

Source: Data were prepared using the AIHW data visualisation tool (AIHW, 2020b).

Victorian government

Detailed statistics are available for the years 1996–97 to 2018–19 (AIHW, 2020b), however, limited data exist for 1970 to 1996.

1970 to 1995

Analysis for the period 1970 to 1996 is further limited as the Victorian Government Budget papers did not separately itemise all public dental expenditure. Only some components of dental expenditure were identified, with remaining items included in general categories such as departmental salaries and global hospital budgets. This in itself is noteworthy because when expenditure was low (actually and relatively), there was less need for scrutiny than when amounts rose substantially: that is, it signifies low interest in dental health when minimal government money is used.

In the 1970s and 1980s Victorian governments paid subsidies for pre-school children's dental care to local governments that had dental clinics in their infant welfare centres. A subsidy was also paid to the Australian Dental Association (ADA) for providing lectures on dental public health to dental students. In 2020 dollars,[43] by 1988 the subsidy to infant welfare clinics was about $0.5 million and payments to the ADA were about $90,000 (Treasury, Victoria, 1988).

Only three references to total Victorian government dental budgets from 1970 to 1995 are on the public record. These sources detail Victorian government expenditure on dental services – total and per person – for the financial years ending 1985, 1991 and 1995 (Table 9.5).

43 Calculated using the Reserve Bank of Australia inflation calculator at <https://www.rba.gov.au/calculator/>

**Table 9.5 Victorian government expenditure on dental services
(current & constant prices) by total and per person 1984–85, 1990–91 and 1994–95 ($)**

Financial year	1984–85[2] $	1990–91 $	1994–95 $
Dental services (current $)	28.3m	40m	38.1m
Dental services (constant $)[1]	87.9m	85.6m	55.8m
Per person (constant $)	21	19	12

Sources: DHV, 1986; ADAVB, 1991; DH&CS, 1995; ABS, 2019.

Notes:

1 Constant prices are based on the 2019–20 financial year and were estimated using the Dental Deflator used
   by the AIHW for National health accounts analyses (J. Thomson, AIHW, personal communication, March 2, 2021).

2 As the constant price for 1984–85 pre-dates the AIHW deflator, the average for the following 3 years was used
   to estimate this figure.

The Ministerial Review of Dental Services (MRODS) in Victoria identified that $28.3 million was allocated for public dental services in 1985 (DHV, 1986). This represents $87.9 million and $21 per person in 2020 dollars. By 1991, total public dental expenditure had dropped to $86.5 million. Adjusting for population growth, this represented $19 per person in 2020 dollars (ADAVB, 1991; ABS, 2019). Following budget cuts by the Kennett Coalition Government, in 1995 the Victorian Government allocation for dental services was $38.1 million, equivalent to $55.8 million or $12 per person in 2020 dollars (DH&CS, 1995).

1996 to 2020

After adjustment for inflation, and despite peaks and troughs, overall, Victorian government spending on dental services increased between 1997 and 2020; from $77 million in 1996–97, to $190 million in 2019–20 (Table 9.6, Figure 9.6). The increase in 2019–20 was due to funding of the Smile Squad school dental initiative (Premier of Victoria, 2019).

Per person Victorian government dental expenditure (Figure 9.7) increased from $15 in 1997–98 to a peak of almost $40 in 1999–2000. Since 2005–06 it has fluctuated between $25 and $30 per person.

Most years, Victorian governments spent less per capita than other jurisdictions. Only recently has the advent of the Smile Squad improved Victoria's expenditure relative to the national average; an increase from 59% in 1996–97, to 82% in 2019–20 (Table 9.6).

Table 9.6 Victorian government dental expenditure compared with all states and territories (constant prices), 1996–97 and 2019–20 ($)

	1996–97		2019–2020	
	Victoria $	All jurisdictions $	Victoria $	All jurisdictions $
Total dental expenditure	$77m	$528m	$190m	$857m
Expenditure per person	$17	$29	$28	$34
% of national average	59%	–	82%	–

Source: Prepared using the AIHW data visualisation tool (AIHW, 2020b).

Figure 9.6 Victorian government dental expenditure (constant prices), 1996 to 2020 ($ millions)

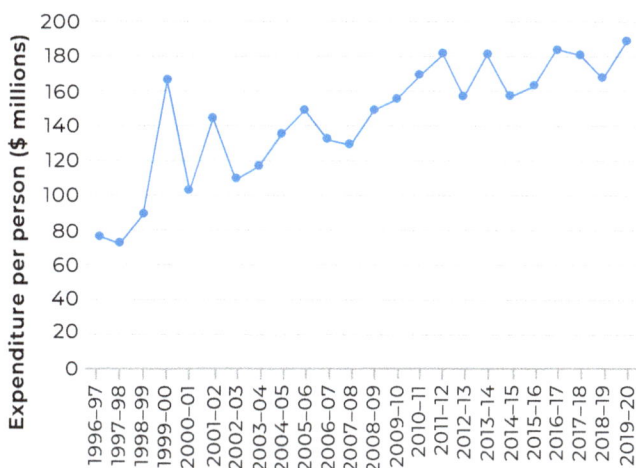

Source: Prepared using the AIHW data visualisation tool (AIHW, 2020b).

Figure 9.7 Victorian government dental expenditure per person (constant prices), 1996 to 2020 ($)

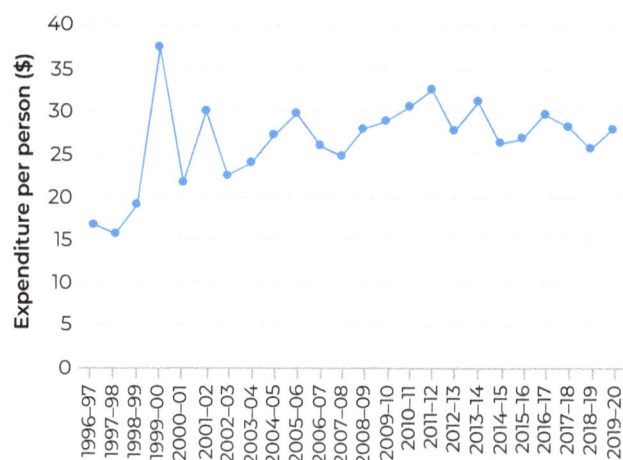

Source: Prepared using the AIHW data visualisation tool (AIHW, 2021a).

2021 and 2022

While detailed AIHW (Australian Institute of Health and Wellbeing) dental expenditure data for the financial years ending 2021 and 2022 have not been published at the time of writing, Victorian Government Budget papers for these years show increases in expenditure linked to implementation of the Smile Squad; from $250 million in 2019-20, to $297 million in 2020-21. An outcome of $294 million in 2021-22 was anticipated, and the target for 2022-23 is $328 million (Treasury & Finance, Victoria, 2022).

The COVID-19 pandemic has hampered implementation of the Smile Squad program. Only $294 million of $353 million budgeted for dental services in 2022 was able to be spent. As the Smile Squad program is rolled out, Victorian government per person dental expenditure will approach, and possibly surpass, the national average.

In December 2021, the Minister for Health, Martin Foley announced an additional $27 million to enable community dental agencies to catch up and meet increased demand for dental services from Victorians who had delayed or deferred treatment during the pandemic (Foley, 2021). As outlined in Chapter 5, the additional funding led to a reduction in the waiting time for general dental care to 17 months in December 2022 (ADAVB, 2023). Concern has been expressed that waiting times will increase unless the funding is recurrent (ADAVB, 2023).

Individuals

Out-of-pocket spending by individuals has always contributed the major share of total Victorian dental expenditure. Since routine recording commenced in 1996–97, individuals have contributed at least two thirds of total spending on dental services; for example, 78% in 1996–97 falling to 70% in 2018–19, with a range of 69–81% in the intervening years (Table 9.2).

At 70% of total Victorian dental expenditure in 2018–19, Victorians' out-of-pocket costs for dental care outstripped the national average of 57% (Figure 9.3). In that year, Victorians paid in excess of $100 more per person out-of-pocket than other Australians – $345 compared to $240. In total that year, Victorians spent $541 million more on dental services than residents of New South Wales (AIHW, 2020b).

Individual expenditure on dental care has also remained significantly higher than on other health services. In Victoria, just 20% of total health expenditure came from individuals in 2018–19, compared with 70% for dental care (Figure 9.3).

The high cost of dental services has long been a burden for many families, and the proportion of Victorians who have foregone treatment is increasing. In 2006, 29% of Victorian adults were unable to afford dental care, compared with 34% in 2017 (Chapter 10). This was a key reason that the Andrews Labor Government introduced the major new Victorian school dental program, the Smile Squad, in 2019. When fully implemented, the program will save families an estimated $400 a year per child in dental costs (Premier of Victoria, 2019).

Health insurers

Private health insurers' proportional contributions to dental expenditure in Australia decreased between 1981 and 1997, from around a third (32%) (DHV, 1986) to one seventh (15%) (AIHW, 2020b). In Victoria, the health insurers' share has generally been lower than the national average. It stood at 13% of total dental costs in both 1996–97 and 2018–19, ranging from 8–13% over this period (Table 9.2) (AIHW, 2020b).

As mentioned, a high proportion of Australian government funding for dental health is being used to subsidise private health insurance, rather than providing dental care to the most disadvantaged. Proponents of the rebate argue that it enhances individual choice, enables policy holders to bypass waiting times in the public sector, and reduces pressure on the public system. Nonetheless, the private health insurance rebate (PHIR) and the fact that higher income earners avoid paying the Medicare Levy surcharge (MLS) if they take out private health insurance, have led to calls from public health advocates for PHIR funds to be redirected to public dental services. These parties view the scheme as a form of middle-class welfare, that is, a transfer of public monies from government to people on higher incomes who can afford to take out private health insurance (with the bonus of minimising their tax obligations by avoiding the MLS), at the expense of those who do not have this option and are dependent on the public health system (PHAA, 2020; Menadue, 2021).

Changes in dental fees

Fees for private dental services are not regulated in Australia, and private dentists are free to set and adjust their fees as they wish. As a guide to members, the ADA publishes, and regularly updates, a schedule of dental services, in which each dental procedure is allocated an item number. The ADA has undertaken an annual survey of dental fees charged by its private practice members since 1966. Trend analysis of these survey results, shows that item costs for different dental procedures have increased at different rates over the past 50 years (Table 9.7 and Appendix 9).

Table 9.7 Dental procedure item costs and average weekly earnings, Australia, 1971 to 2020

Item	ADA item fee $[1]						Wage per week $[2]
	Oral exam	X-ray	Removal of tooth	Metallic filling	Adhesive (white) filling	Upper denture	
Item number[3]	011	022	311	511	521	711	
1971[4]	4[5]	2.4	4.6	5.2	6.6	64	96.4
2020	66	44	195	153	159	1400	1,711
Multiple of increase	x17	x18	x42	x29	x24	x22	x18

Source: The Barnard compilation is held at ADA headquarters in St Leonards, NSW (Barnard, 2012).
Fees in 2020 are from the ADA Bulletin.

Notes:
1. Item fees are derived from a summary of Australian Dental Association (ADA) fee surveys from 1966 to 2010 compiled by Peter Barnard (Barnard, 2012). Fees in 2020 are from the ADA Bulletin.
2. Average weekly wage (non-professional) data are from ABS (ABS, 2023).
3. The ADA assigns a three-digit code number to items or clinical procedures that are part of current dental practice.
4. Data for the years 1966 and 1974 have been used to estimate missing 1971 data for items 011 an 022.
5. 1971 items predate ADA item coding.

For the selection of items shown in Table 9.7, all items except oral exams increased at a rate higher than increases in Australian average weekly earnings between 1971 and 2020. While average weekly earnings increased by almost 18-fold over this period, ADA survey results show that fees either kept pace with average earnings or increased by up to 42 times. The largest increase was for the removal of a tooth. Why this has occurred is considered in Box 9.1. A complete picture of the changes in the intervening years is shown in Appendix 9.1.

While fees for oral exams (17-fold increase) and X-rays (18-fold) remained at a similar level to earnings, the cost of upper dentures (22-fold), adhesive (white) fillings (24-fold), and metallic fillings (29-fold) became relatively more costly. In general, dental fees have become less affordable when compared with average weekly earnings. This may explain why there has been an increase in the proportion of Victorian adults who report that they have avoided or delayed dental treatment because of cost (Chapter 10, Figure 10.15).

The substantial increase in fees for simple tooth extractions relative to other procedures since the 1970s (Table 9.7) prompts the question as to why this has occurred. Several factors come into play. A non-exhaustive summary follows.

Compared with simple extractions, restorative procedures such as fillings are now more advanced and have required substantial updating of equipment and materials. In contrast, the procedure and instruments for extracting a tooth from its socket have been remarkably constant for more than 100 years. While tooth elevators have been named after prominent surgeons, hinged forceps have hardly changed. The sudden and dramatic spread of HIV infection in the 1980s prompted great changes in infection control and sterilisation of equipment, as well as methods and protocols for the handling of all instruments, especially those penetrating body tissues such as forceps and elevators.

Over the past 50 years, the basic assumption of society and the dental profession has shifted from a norm of removable dentures, in favour of retaining the natural teeth for life, wherever possible. This, combined with fewer patients for each student or graduate clinician, has meant that dental extraction is now a less common procedure. As this has necessarily resulted in loss of an experience-based skill, clinical practitioners (and particularly young dentists) either refer more patients to specialists for extractions, or the procedure takes more time and effort. Extractions have become invested with more mystique, and contemporary clinicians perceive them to demand greater skills than did the dentists in earlier times, who possibly undervalued what they were so frequently doing.

Additional factors contribute to making the decision to extract a tooth more considered and less cavalier these days. Australians are living longer and the percentage of older people in the population is much higher than in the 1970s. Consequently, more people are living with chronic disorders stabilised by polypharmacy, including drugs that may compromise blood clotting and wound healing. Nowadays, when a tooth is deemed to be unsavable, careful investigation and planning of the extraction appointment, and a technique involving minimal trauma to the tissues, are essential. In addition, young people's teeth are healthier than ever before, and many have never had a dental procedure prior to undergoing a tooth extraction as part of orthodontic treatment. Their oral tissues may be robust, but the psychological impact of extractions can be distressing, which might necessitate extra support.

All these factors have driven up fees for the removal of teeth and led to the perception that it is a more complex procedure than it was believed to be in times past. Overall, tooth removal and the procedure itself were probably undervalued before.

Summary

After adjusting for inflation, spending on dental health services in Victoria has increased over the past 50 years. Individuals bear most costs (via out-of-pocket spending), and the smaller contributions of governments have fluctuated markedly. Private health insurers are the third contributor.[44]

There is a dearth of dental data prior to 1996 because there were no dis-aggregated dental figures in the health budgets.

In 2018–19, $3.2 billion was spent on dental services in Victoria out of a total of $10.6 billion spent nationally (AIHW, 2020a). More recently, with restricted access to dental care during the COVID-19 pandemic, national expenditure decreased to $9.5 billion in 2019–20 (AIHW, 2021a).

Australian and Victorian governments have contributed less than one fifth of dental spending. Conversely, governments currently pay two thirds of other health care costs (AIHW, 2020b). There has been a roller-coaster pattern in Australian oral health funding.

Victoria's total dental expenditure per person has generally been the highest of all Australian states and territories, with Victorians also paying the most out-of-pocket. In 2018-19 Victorians spent $100 more per person than other Australians ($345 compared to $240), and a total of $541 million more than New South Wales residents (AIHW, 2020b).

Successive Australian government contributions to Victorian dental expenditure have increased since the 1990s, rising from 3 to 11% of total dental expenditure in 2018–19 (AIHW, 2020b).

This represents a small proportion of dental expenditure and almost half of dental health funding has gone into subsidising private health insurance (45% in 2018), rather than providing dental care to the most disadvantaged (Productivity Commission, 2020).

Victorian governments' spending on dental services has fluctuated since 1970 but has always been less than 15% of total dental expenditure, and less than 5% of health expenditure overall (AIHW, 2020b). Since 2019, funding for the Smile Squad school dental program (Premier of Victoria, 2019) has represented a considerable increase in funding. After dropping to as low as 59% of the national per person average in the mid 1990s, by 2022 Victorian dental expenditure was expected to reach, and perhaps surpass, the national average (AIHW, 2020b).

Waiting times for general dental care (Chapter 5) indicate that government funding has not kept pace with demand for public dental care in Victoria since 1970. A key factor has been uncertain Australian government funding, due to programs being discontinued (Chapter 4).

Private health insurers' contributions to total Australian dental expenditure have decreased – from about 30% in the 1970s, to 20% in 2019 (DHV, 1986; AIHW, 2020b). The insurers' share has generally been lower in Victoria than in other jurisdictions, and was just 13% in 2018-19 (AIHW, 2020b).

Over the past 50 years, fees for most dental services have increased at a much higher rate than the Australian average weekly earnings' multiple of 18 times. While the cost of oral exams has increased 17-fold – in line with average weekly earnings – the cost of fillings, for example, has increased 24-fold.

---

44 Detailed dental expenditure data by these sources are available for the years from 1996–97, both in current and constant dollars (adjusted for inflation) (AIHW, 2020b). Some data about specific dental initiatives and from reviews are available prior to this time, but government budget papers bundled dental costs into general health expenditure.

In Australia, dental treatment is one of the most expensive areas of health expenditure. At over $10 billion a year it is similar to the expenditure on General Practice services (AIHW, 2021b). Tooth decay on its own is one of the most expensive disease conditions to treat. At a total cost of $5 billion in 2018-19, treatment of tooth decay was more costly than falls (AIHW, 2021b).

More Victorians are facing cost barriers to accessing dental care: 29% of adults were unable to afford dental care in 2006, compared with 34% in 2017 (Chapter 10). There has also been an increase in the amount of money withdrawn from superannuation to pay for dental care (Dalzell, 2022).

Appendix

Appendix 9 Dental procedure item costs and average weekly earnings, Australia, 1966 to 2020

	ADA item fee $[1]							Wage per week $[2]
Item	Oral exam	X-ray	Periodic exam or consultation	Removal of tooth	Metallic filling	Adhesive filling	Upper denture	
Item number[3]	011	022	112 or 114	311	511	521	711	
1971	4	2.4	na	4.6	5.2	6.6	64	96.4
1981	10.1	9.8	19.2	19	18.7	21.8	225	277
1991	26	21.2	42	52.6	45.6	51.8	478	579
2001	38	29	66	89	74	83	681	840
2010	59	41	102	157	123	133	1117	1,290
2020	66	44	120	195	153	159	1400	1,711
Multiple of increase	x16.5	x18.3	x33	x42.4	x29.4	x24.1	x21.9	x17.8

Source: The Barnard compilation is held at ADA headquarters in St Leonards, NSW (Barnard, 2012).
Fees in 2020 are from the ADA Bulletin.

Notes:
1. Item fees are derived from a summary of Australian Dental Association (ADA) fee surveys from 1966 to 2010 compiled by Peter Barnard (Barnard, 2012). Fees in 2020 are from the ADA Bulletin.
2. Average weekly wage (non-professional) data are from ABS (ABS, 2023).
3. The ADA assigns a three-digit code number to items or clinical procedures that are part of current dental practice.

References

Australian Bureau of Statistics. (ABS). (2019). *Australian historical population statistics* (3105.0.65.001), Population size and growth, Table 1.2 Population(a)(b)(c) by sex, states and territories, 30 June, 1901 onwards. <https://www.abs.gov.au/ausstats/abs@.nsf/Lookup/3105.0.65.001I-Note12014>

Australian Bureau of Statistics. (ABS). (2023). Average Weekly Earnings, Australia. <https://www.abs.gov.au/statistics/labour/earnings-and-working-conditions/average-weekly-earnings-australia>

Australian Dental Association Victorian Branch. (ADAVB). (1991). *Provision of dental care in the public sector*. ADAVB Newsletter.

Australian Dental Association Victorian Branch. (ADAVB). (2023, February 23). *Drop in waiting times for public dental care, but concerns remain over long-term access*. [Media release]. <https://adavb.org/news-media/media-releases/drop-in-waiting-times-for-public-dental-care--but-concerns-remain-over-long-term-access>

Australian Institute of Health and Welfare. (AIHW). (2020a). *Health expenditure Australia 2018-19*. <https://www.aihw.gov.au/reports/health-welfare-expenditure/health-expenditure-australia-2018-19/contents/summary>

Australian Institute of Health and Welfare. (AIHW). (2020b). *Health expenditure Australia 2018-19 data visualisation*. <https://www.aihw.gov.au/reports/health-welfare-expenditure/health-expenditure-australia-2018-19/contents/data-visualisation>

Australian Institute of Health and Welfare. (AIHW). (2021a). *Health expenditure Australia 2019–20*. <https://www.aihw.gov.au/reports/health-welfare-expenditure/health-expenditure-australia-2019-20/contents/summary>

Australian Institute of Health and Welfare. (AIHW). (2021b). *Disease expenditure in Australia, 2018-19*. <https://www.aihw.gov.au/reports/health-welfare-expenditure/disease-expenditure-australia/contents/about>

Barnard, P.D. (2012). *Australian dental fees surveys 1961 to 2011*. Australian Dental Association. <https://catalogue.nla.gov.au/Record/6002529>

Biggs, A. (2008). *Overview of Commonwealth involvement in funding dental care*. Parliamentary Research Publications, Research Paper no. 1, 2008-09. <https://apo.org.au/node/2696>

Costello, P. (1996). CPD HR No. 7, 20 August 1996:3274.

Dalzell, S. (2022, August 25). Australians raided $1.6 billion in superannuation savings to pay for health care. *ABC News*. <https://www.abc.net.au/news/2022-08-25/australians-using-super-retirement-savings-pay-health-costs/101368246?utm_campaign=abc_news_web&utm_content=mail&utm_medium=content_shared&utm_source=abc_news_web>

Department of Health, Australia. (DOHA). (1973). Annual Report of the Director-General of Health. <https://nla.gov.au/nla.obj-1745801827/view?sectionId=nla.obj-1847550851&partId=nla.obj-1751321551>

Department of Health, Victoria. (DHV). (1986). *Ministerial review of dental services: Final report*. Melbourne: Health Department of Victoria.

Department of Health and Community Services. (DH&CS). Victoria. (1995). *Future directions for dental health in Victoria*. Melbourne: VGPS.

Foley, M. (2021, December 22). *Boost for dental catch-up care*. [Media release]. <https://www.premier.vic.gov.au/sites/default/files/2021-12/211222%20-%20Boost%20For%20Dental%20Catch-Up%20Care.pdf?utm_source=miragenews&utm_medium=miragenews&utm_campaign=news>

Menadue, J. (2021). *Why dental care was excluded from Medicare and why it should now be included (an edited repost)*. <https://johnmenadue.com/why-dental-care-was-excluded-from-medicare-and-why-it-should-now-be-included-an-edited-repost>

Parliament of Australia. (2012). *Dental Benefits Amendment Bill 2012. 2012, Bills Digest No. 22, 2012–13*. <https://www.aph.gov.au/Parliamentary_Business/Bills_Legislation/bd/bd1213a/13bd022>

Premier of Victoria. (2019, May 26). *The Smile Squad – Free dental vans to hit schools soon*. [Media release]. <https://www.premier.vic.gov.au/smile-squad-free-dental-vans-hit-schools-soon>

Productivity Commission. (2020). *Report on government services.* <https://www.pc.gov.au/research/ongoing/report-on-government-services?id=141009&queries_year_query=2020&search_page_191702_submit_button=Submit&current_result_page=1&results_per_page=0&submitted_search_category=&mode=results>

Public Health Association of Australia. (PHAA). (2020). *Oral health policy position statement.* <https://www.phaa.net.au/documents/item/4565>

Reserve Bank of Australia. (RBA). (2023). *The global financial crisis.* <https://www.rba.gov.au/education/resources/explainers/the-global-financial-crisis.html>

Spencer, A. J. (2001). *What options do we have for organising, providing and funding better public dental care?* Australian Health Policy Institute Commissioned Paper Series 2001/02. Sydney: Australian Health Policy Institute. <https://catalogue.nla.gov.au/Record/989842>

Treasury, Victoria. (1988). *Finance 1987–88. The Treasurer's statement for the year ended 1988 and the report of the Auditor-General.* <https://www.parliament.vic.gov.au/papers/govpub/VPARL1988-92No4.pdf>

Treasury & Finance, Victoria. (2022). *Victorian budget 2022-23, Putting patients first, Service delivery, Budget paper no. 3.* <https://s3.ap-southeast-2.amazonaws.com/budgetfiles202223.budget.vic.gov.au/2022-23+State+Budget+-+Service+Delivery.pdf>

Chapter 10
Oral Health of Victorians 1970 to 2020 – Better or worse?

John Rogers

Introduction

Victorians' oral health has changed markedly in the 50 years since 1970. From a time when it was still common in some communities for a woman to be given a full set of dentures as a 21st birthday or wedding present, and most older people had full dentures, the majority of people are now keeping their natural teeth. There has been much progress, but it has been uneven and not shared equally by all.

In this chapter, we explore trends in the epidemiology of oral disease – the detective work of discovering the *who, what, when, where and how much* of oral health status. We examine the distribution and determinants of the three main oral diseases – tooth decay, gum disease and oral cancer – and explore changes in oral health behaviours, barriers to accessing dental care and patterns in oral health outcomes. These have all been shaped by the significant social and health system changes that have occurred over the past five decades.

Oral health indicators

There is reasonably good quality information to track the oral health of Australians and Victorians from the mid-1980s onwards. Australian population-wide oral health surveys were conducted for 1987–88, 2004–06, 2012–14 and 2017–18, and Victorian-specific surveys included oral health questions from 2011. Oral health data are also available from Australian Bureau of Statistics (ABS) and Australian Institute of Health and Welfare (AIHW) surveys. The indicators we look at are outlined in Box 1.

The oral health of adults and children will be considered in turn.

Adults

Oral health status

1 Number of teeth

More people are keeping more of their natural teeth.

Tooth loss affects the ability to eat, talk and smile. It impacts on confidence and a person's wellbeing. It is also associated with deteriorating diet and compromised nutrition, and so can adversely affect overall health (NACODH, 2012; Honeywell et al., 2021).

In 1979 only a third (34%) of Australians aged 65 years or older had retained some of their natural teeth, compared with 85% in 2018 (an increase of 250%) (Figure 10.1). The trend for Victorians would have been similar as population health surveys have generally shown no statistical difference between Victorians and Australians on this measure.

Figure 10. 1 Australian adults aged 65 years and over with some of their natural teeth, 1979 to 2018 (%)

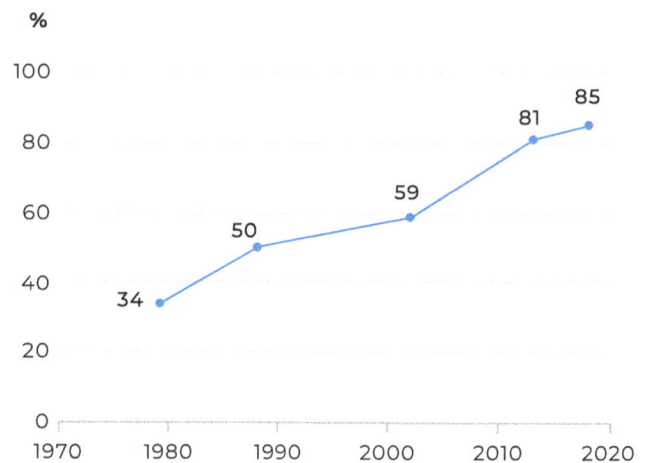

Sources: Sanders et al., 2004; NDTIS, 2013; ARCPOH, 2019.

Losing teeth is generally the result of tooth decay, gum disease or mouth trauma. However, cultural influences, medical beliefs and dental treatment options can also be important (Box 10. 2).

Box 10.2 Why have Victorians kept more of their natural teeth over the past 50 years?

Four main factors explain why Victorians have kept more of their natural teeth over the past 5 decades:

1 A decline in tooth decay

- Fluoride in water and toothpaste:
  Community water fluoridation (NHMRC, 2017) and fluoride toothpaste (Marinho et al., 2003) have been shown to reduce tooth decay in children and adults. While fluoride toothpaste has been available to Victorians since the mid-1970s, population access to fluoridated water has increased gradually over time. The first water supply to be fluoridated was the (then) small, semi-rural town of Bacchus Marsh in 1962. It was not until 1977 that Melbourne's water supplies were fluoridated. Extension into rural areas occurred in the 2000s. By 2017, 90% of Victorians had access to fluoridated water (NHMRC, 2017). The proportion increased to more than 96% by 2021, including 88% of rural and regional Victorians (DHV, 2021).

- Increased access to, and changes in, dental care:
  Preventive care in dental practice, facilitated by innovations such as dental sealants and topical fluoride has resulted in increased retention of natural teeth.

- There may have been some reductions in sugar consumption patterns since the 1970s but population-wide data are not available to confirm this. Consumption of sugar has found to be high in children with half of Australian children consuming four or more serves of sugar snacks a day (Do & Spencer, 2016); however, there may have been a relative reduction in families with higher levels of parental education and literacy.

2 Cultural changes

- Until the 1970s a full set of dentures, after extraction of all the teeth, was a common 21st birthday or wedding present for young women in some communities. The rationale was to reduce the future cost of dental care for the groom. From the 1970s community attitudes changed. Older family members, who had problems with their dentures, encouraged younger people to "hold on" to their teeth. Colour television in more homes encouraged the desire for nice smiles, and dentists became more reluctant to remove teeth.

3 Declining medical belief in focal sepsis

- In the first half of the 20th century, infection in and around the teeth was associated with a variety of systemic disorders and teeth were routinely removed as a possible cause. Belief in this theory of focal sepsis waned as health providers better understood the importance of retaining teeth.

4 Increased dental treatment options such as cheaper fillings, root canal treatment and dental crowns

- Filling, rather than extracting teeth became more popular in the 1970s because of the introduction of the high-speed handpiece (which cut down drilling time) and more frequent use of local anaesthetic.

2 Tooth decay

While tooth decay in Victorians overall has declined since the 1970s, the proportion of adults with untreated decay has risen over the past 20 years.

Since 1988 Victorian adults have experienced less tooth decay, as shown by the average number of teeth affected by decay (Figure 10.2).

Figure 10.2 Teeth affected by decay in Victorian adults by age, 1987–88, 2004–06 and 2017–18 (No.)

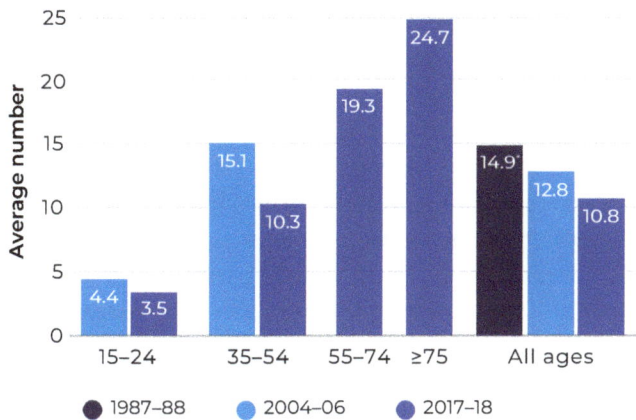

*Note: The 1987–88 data for all ages are Australian data.

Sources: Barnard, 1993; AIHW DSRU, 2008; AIHW, 2007; ARCPOH 2019.

In Victorian adults the number of teeth affected by decay has decreased by 28% since 1988 (from 14.9 teeth in that year [using the Australian average] to 10.8 in 2018) (Barnard, 1993; ARCPOH, 2019). Meanwhile, in the 15 years to 2018, the proportion of adults with untreated tooth decay increased from a quarter (24%) to a third (32%) (AIHW, 2007; ARCPOH, 2019).

3 Oral health inequality

3.1 Poorer people are increasingly more likely to lose their natural teeth than other Victorians

Oral health inequalities are caused by the conditions of daily living – the political, social and physical environments of modern societies. These shape the choices and options open to individuals (Watt & Sheiham, 2012).

While more people across all age groups are retaining more of their natural teeth, these improvements have not been shared equitably. As shown in Figure 10.3, the proportion of Victorian adults without any natural teeth varies markedly according to socioeconomic status.

Figure 10.3 Victorian adults without any natural teeth, 2004–06 and 2017–18 (%)

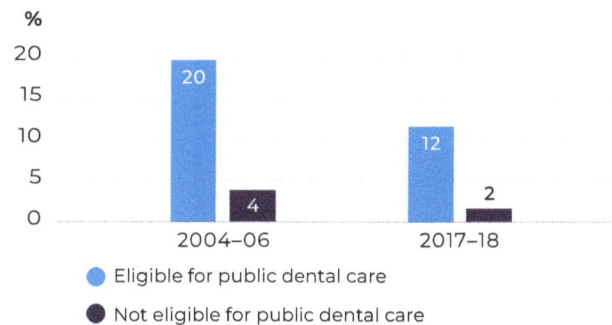

Note: In the 2004–06 survey classification was by pension and health card holders which is basically the criterion for eligibility for public dental care.

Sources: AIHW, 2007; ARCPOH 2019.

In 2018 people who were eligible for public dental care were six times more likely than non-card holders to have no natural teeth (an increase from five times more likely in 2004–2006) (AIHW, 2007; ARCPOH, 2019). This increase in the gap between richer and poorer is consistent with worldwide economic trends, which show a growing concentration of wealth among fewer people (Credit Suisse, 2020). Part of the difference is due to the older average age of card holders.

Rural residents were almost three times more likely than other Victorians to have no natural teeth in 2018 (8% of rural residents compared with 3% of other Victorians) (ARCPOH, 2019). In 1988 the disparity was just less than two-fold (23 compared with 13%) (HDV et al., 1988) – indicating an overall decrease in the prevalence of no natural teeth, but an increase in the inequality between rural and non-rural Victorians.

3.2 The tooth decay gap between card and non-card holders rose from 3 to 6 teeth from 2004–06 to 2017–18

Between 2004–06 and 2017–18 the number of teeth affected by decay remained the same (at 15) in those eligible for public dental care, while in other Victorians the number decreased by an average of 27% (from 12 to 9) (Figure 10. 4) (AIHW, 2007; ARCPOH 2019). Over this period, the "tooth decay gap" between card holders and non-card holders widened from three to six teeth.

Figure 10.4 Teeth affected by decay in Victorian adults, 2004–06 and 2017–18 (No.)

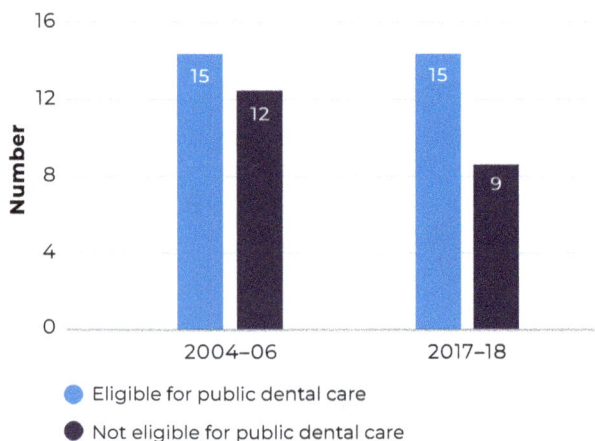

Sources: AIHW, 2007; ARCPOH 2019.

4 Gum disease

Victorian adults' understanding of gum disease is poor; the extent of gum disease has remained high, and the prevalence gap between card and non-card holders has doubled.

More than a quarter of all Victorian adults had moderate or severe gum disease in 2004–06 (26%) and 2017–18 (28%) (Figure 10.5) (AIHW, 2007; ARCPOH, 2019). This condition damages the soft tissue and bone surrounding the teeth, which can cause the teeth to become loose and lead to tooth loss. Rates increased with age, with half (51%) of those over 55–74 years old affected in 2018. Three quarters of women aged 75 years and older (77%) had gum disease in 2017–18 compared to two thirds of men (64%) (ARCPOH, 2019). While the difference was not statistically significant because of the relatively small number that were examined, there is a need to address these high rates of gum disease in older people. Further research is required to examine gender differences in oral health and develop initiatives to address them.

Figure 10.5 Victorian adults with gum disease, 2004–06 and 2017–18 (%)

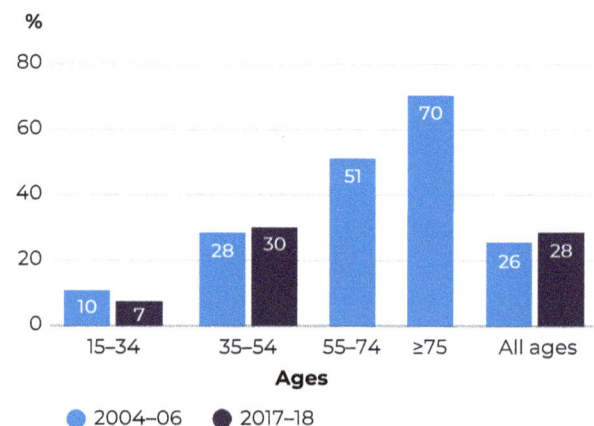

Sources: AIHW, 2007; ARCPOH 2019.

The difference in rates of gum disease in those eligible for public dental care and those not eligible, has doubled since 2004 (increasing from 9% higher in 2004–06 to 18% higher in 2017–18) (Figure 10.6). For those eligible for public dental care, rates of disease increased from 35 to 41% in this period, while the rates of disease for other Victorians were stable at 23 and 24% (AIHW, 2017; ARCPOH, 2019).

Figure 10.6 Gum disease in Victorians eligible and not eligible for public dental care, 2004–06 and 2017–18 (%)

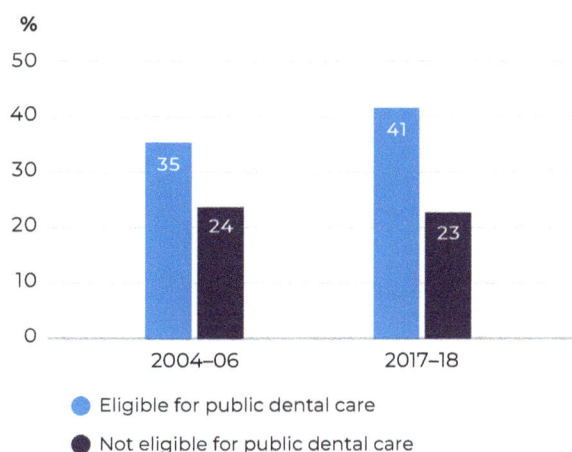

Sources: AIHW, 2007; ARCPOH 2019.

Understanding of gum disease among Victorians is poor. In the 2017 Victorian Population Health Survey (VAHI, n.d), the self-reported prevalence of gum disease was 11%, compared with the 28% reported for Victoria in the 2017–18 *National study of adult oral health* (ARCPOH, 2019). Given the potential for adverse systemic effects of gum disease on other parts of the body, such as the heart and joints, this sizeable gap underscores the need for better community understanding of gum disease as well as better access to treatment.

5 Oral cancer

Oral cancer mortality rates have decreased, but there have been recent increases in the incidence of tongue and oropharyngeal cancer.

Oral cancers affect the lips, tongue, floor of the mouth, salivary glands, oropharynx, and other parts of the oral cavity. Victorian age-standardised trend data on oral cancer incidence and mortality are available from 1982 to 2016 for all oral cancers except "other parts of the oral cavity" (AIHW, 2020a). These latter cancers comprise less than five per cent of all oral cancers.

Although total oral cancer presentations in Victoria increased from 1982 (which was the earliest date for consistent data) to 2016 (Figure 10.7), both incidence and mortality rates decreased (Figure 10.8) (AIHW, 2020a).

Figure 10.7 Oral cancer incidence and mortality, Victoria, 1982 to 2016

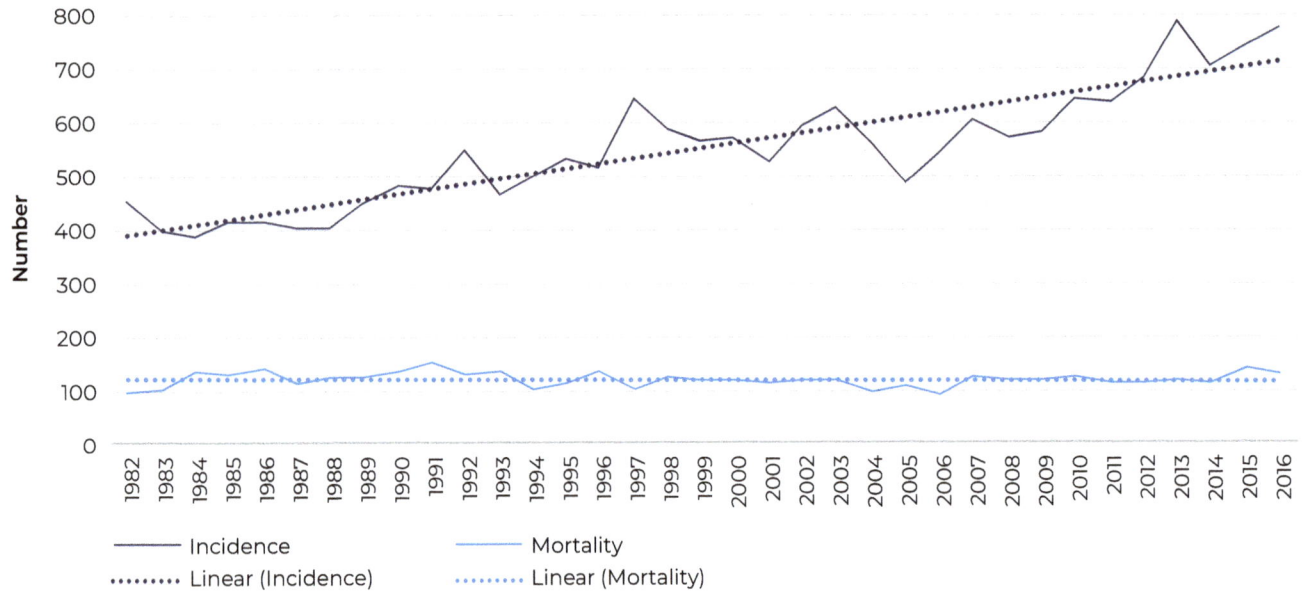

Legend:
— Incidence
— Mortality
······· Linear (Incidence)
······· Linear (Mortality)

Figure 10.8 Oral cancer incidence and mortality rates, Victoria, 1982 to 2016

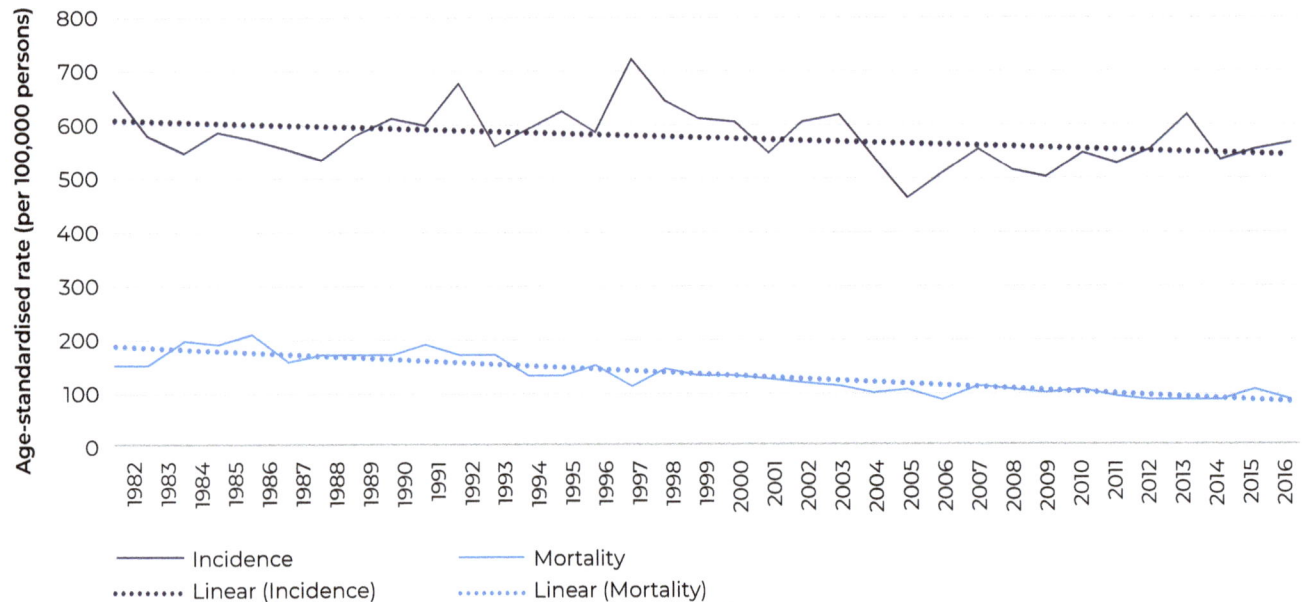

Legend:
— Incidence
— Mortality
······· Linear (Incidence)
······· Linear (Mortality)

Source: AIHW, 2020a.

Notes:

1. Figures 10.7 and 10.8 include cancers C00–C10: that is, Lip (C00), Tongue (C01–C02), Mouth, including Gum, Floor of mouth and Other mouth (C03–C06), Salivary glands (C07, C08) and Oropharynx (C09–C10).

2. "Other oral cancers" (C14) are excluded.

3. Rates based on counts less than 5 and greater than 0 have been suppressed.

Tables 10.1 and 10.2 summarise trends in oral cancer incidence and mortality in Victoria from 1982 to 2016

Table 10.1 Trends in oral cancer incidence, excluding "other oral", Victoria, 1982 to 2016, and cases in 2019

Age-standardised rate (per 100,000 persons)	Lip	Mouth	Tongue	Oropharyngeal	Salivary glands	Total*
1982	5.5	2.5	2.6	1.5	1.2	**12.1**
2016	2.4	2.1	3.2	2.5	1.1	**10.4**
% change	56%↓	16%↓	23%↑	67%↑	8%↓	**14%↓**
Cases in 2016	166	148	221	167	94	**702**
Cases in 2019	164	135	263	185	94	**841**

Table 10.2 Trends in oral cancer mortality, excluding "other oral", Victoria, 1982 to 2016, and cases in 2019

Age-standardised rate (per 100,000 persons)	Lip	Mouth	Tongue	Oropharyngeal	Salivary glands	Total*
1982	n.p.	0.8	1.0	0.8	0.3	**2.6**
2016	n.p.	0.4	0.6	0.4	0.2	**1.6**
% change	n.a.	50%↓	40%↓	50%↓	33%↓	**46%↓**
Cases in 2016	3	29	46	33	19	**111**
Cases in 2019	8	50	61	33	30	**182**

Sources: AIHW, 2020a; DHHS, 2021.

Notes:

1. *Tables 1 and 2 do not include "other oral cancers" (C014). To be consistent, cases in 2019 also do not include "other oral". The incidence was 12 per 100,00 and the mortality 8 per 100,00 for "other oral cancers" in 2019, taking the total incidence to 853 and the total mortality to 190.

2. n.a. not applicable.

3. n.p. not published due to small numbers, confidentiality, and/or reliability concerns.

Oral cancer incidence rates declined by 14% between 1982 and 2016 (Figure 10.7 and Table 10.1). Mortality rates declined by almost half (46%) over this time (Figure 10.8 and Table 10.2). However, the incidence of two oral cancers has increased. Oropharyngeal cancer increased by 67%, tongue cancer increased 23%, while the other three cancers decreased. Mortality rates have decreased in all sites since 1982.

Lip cancer has been associated with sun exposure while other cancers have traditionally been found in older men with a history of smoking or heavy drinking (Farah at al., 2014). Reductions in smoking and more sun protection are likely to explain the decreasing incidence of mouth, salivary gland and lip cancers (Wong & Wiesenfeld, 2018).

Tongue cancer has continued to have the highest mortality of oral cancer sites, although the mortality rate has decreased since 1982. From the early 2000s, the incidence has risen in people aged under 45 years without identifiable risk factors, particularly among women. More research is required.

The rise in incidence of oropharyngeal cancer from a relatively low base has been linked to infection by the human papillomavirus (HPV). Broad HPV vaccination of young people, which commenced in Victoria in 2007 for girls in Year 7 and in 2010 for boys in Year 7 (DHV, 2022), should progressively decrease oropharyngeal cancer rates.

Oral cancer is the 8th most common cancer in men and 14th most common in women (DHSV, 2023). In 2019, 853 Victorians were diagnosed with oral cancer and there were 190 deaths – an average of 16 people were diagnosed with oral cancer and three people died each week. This highlights the importance of oral health professionals undertaking screening and early detection of oral cancers, as has been identified in Victoria's Cancer Plan

(DHHS, 2020a). An Oral Cancer Screening and Prevention Program was established in 2019 with funding from the Victorian Government (DHSV, 2023). The program aims to increase the relative five-year survival rate for Victorians with oral cancer from a baseline of 66% in 2019 to 75% by 2030 (DHHS, 2020a).

6 Oral health problems

Self-reported oral health problems such as toothache, discomfort with appearance, and avoidance of eating food have increased particularly among low-income households.

Between 1994 and 2017 Victorians reported increased rates of oral health problems in the last 12 months (Figure 10.9).

Self-reported rates of

1. toothache almost doubled from 11 to 20 per cent (an increase of 82%);
2. discomfort with appearance increased from 21 to 35 per cent (an increase of 67%); and
3. avoidance of certain foods increased by 53 per cent (from 15 to 23%)

Figure 10.9 Victorian adults who self-reported oral health problems, 1994 to 2017 (%)

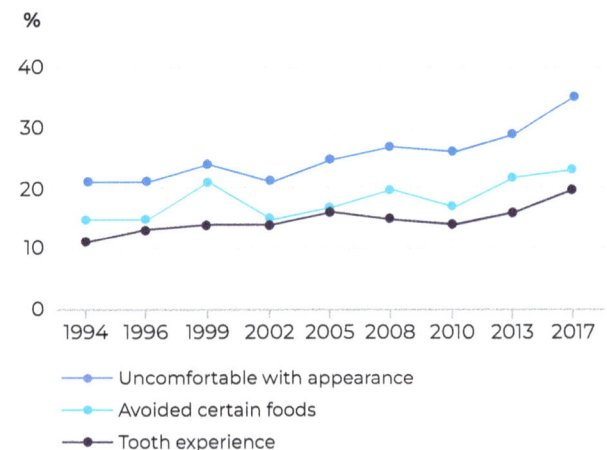

Sources: ARCPOH, 2020.

Measures of social impact give insight into the effect of oral health conditions on day-to-day living from the individual's perspective. Experience of social impact reflects both the level of oral disease experienced and whether that disease had been treated in a timely fashion.

Congruent with results for all Australians, Victorians living in lower income households reported these problems more often than those in high income households. In 2013 Australians living in households with less than $30,000 annual income, reported avoiding certain foods almost three times more often than those in households with annual incomes above $140,000. Those in poorer households also reported almost three times as much toothache and were almost twice as likely to be concerned about appearance due to dental health problems (Chrisopoulos et al., 2016).

7 Perceived oral health status

Perceived oral health status has worsened among low-income households

About a fifth of Victorian adults have rated their oral health as "fair" or "poor" since 1999 (Figure 10.10).

Figure 10.10 Victorian adults who self-reported fair or poor dental health, 1999 to 2017 (%)

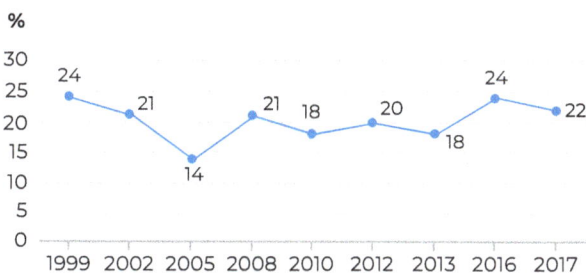

Sources: ARCPOH, 2020; DHHS, 2016; DHHS, 2018.

Perceived oral health varies markedly by socioeconomic status, with low-income groups more likely to report poorer oral health. In 2016 Victorians whose annual household income was more than $100,000, were almost three times more likely to report "excellent" or "very good" oral health compared with those living in low-income (less than $40,000 p.a.) households (48 compared to 17%). Conversely, those in low-income households were more likely to report having poorer oral health than those with high incomes (35 compared to 27%) (Figure 10.11).

Figure 10.11 Self-rated oral health by annual household income, Victoria, 2016 (%)

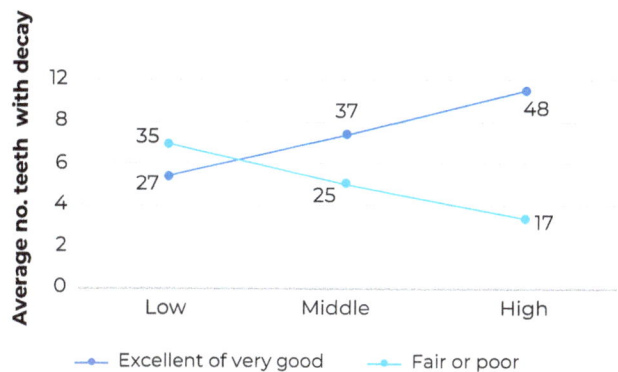

Sources: DHHS, 2018.

Perceived oral health status worsened between 2012 and 2016. In low-income groups reports of "excellent" or "very good" oral health declined over this period (from 30 to 27%) and, conversely, "fair" or "poorer" oral health increased (from 30 to 35%) (DHHS, 2016; DHHS, 2018).

Oral health behaviours

8 Toothbrushing frequency

The proportion of Victorian adults reporting toothbrushing once or more a day has

Toothbrushing frequency has increased slightly.

remained relatively constant since 1988, ranging from 96 to 98% (Figure 10.12). These are similar to Australian rates.

Figure 10.12 Victorian adults toothbrushing once a day or more, 1987–88, 2013 and 2017–18 (%)

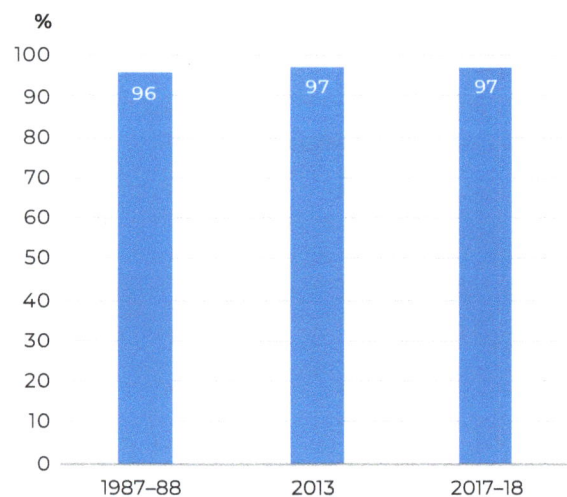

Sources: HDV et al., 1988; 2013 and 2017-18 data from AIHW, 2022.

Between 1987–88 and 2012, however, the proportion of adults reporting toothbrushing twice daily, as recommended, increased from 68 to 74% (Figure 10.13). In 2012, 23% of Victorian adults brushed once a day, while two per cent brushed less often. More recent data for brushing rates of twice or more a day were not available.

Figure 10.13 Victorian adults' toothbrushing frequency, 1988 and 2012 (%)

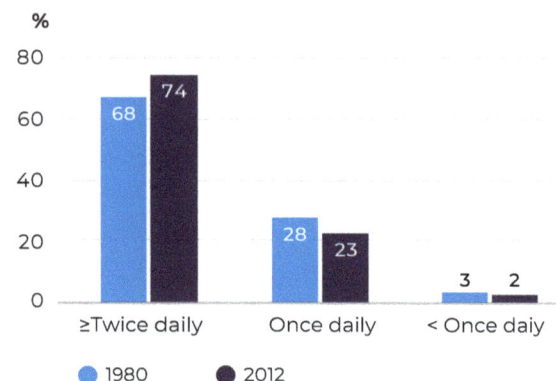

Sources: HDV et al., 1988; DHHS, 2016.

9 Dental visits

Dental visits by Victorian adults have been relatively stable over the past 40 years, with about half reporting a visit in the past 12 months across this period.

Consistent with Australian adults overall, since the 1980s just over half of Victorian adults have reported visiting a dental professional every 12 months (Figure 10.14). About three quarters of Victorian adults have reported dental visiting within a two-year interval – 77% in 2012 (DHHS, 2016) and 74% in 2016 (DHHS, 2018).

In 2012 and 2016, one in 10 Victorians reported that they had not visited a dental health professional for five years or more. The proportion doubled to one in five (22%) for those aged 65 years or older (DHHS, 2016).

Figure 10.14 Adults reporting dental attendance, 1987 to 2018 (%)

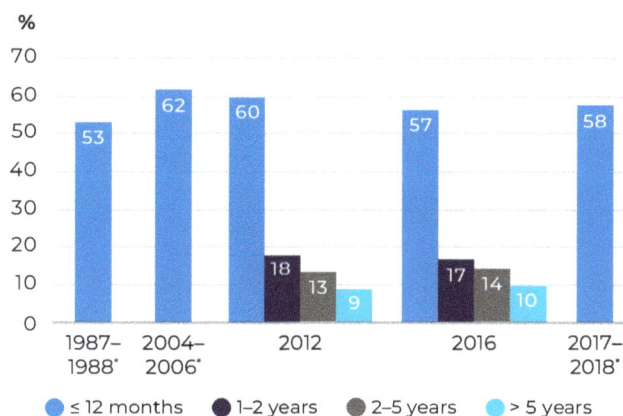

Legend:
● ≤ 12 months ● 1–2 years ● 2–5 years ● > 5 years

Sources: HDV et al., 1988; DHHS, 2016.

Notes:
1. *1987–88, 2004–06 and 2017–18 data are Australian data; 2012 and 2016 data are Victorian data.
2. Survey reports in some years have not included full dental attendance behaviour.

In 2016 a higher proportion of Victorian women (61%) reported visiting a dental health professional in the past 12 months, compared with 53% of men (DHHS, 2018). People on lower incomes and those without dental insurance were less likely to visit frequently. The inverse care law is evident in these data; people with higher dental needs were less likely to visit. The treatment provided also varied by socioeconomic status, with people on low incomes more likely to have teeth extracted as the affordable "choice", while those on higher incomes were more likely to have more complex care such as implants, root canal treatment and crowns.

In contrast to the figures presented in Figure 10.14, ABS surveys of health-related behaviours have recorded lower proportions of people who visit annually. Just under half of the respondents to recent ABS National Health Surveys reported that they saw a dental professional in the last 12 months: 48% in 2011–12 and 2014–15, and 49% in 2018-19 (ABS, 2012; ABS, 2015; ABS, 2019).

Annual dental visiting rates of just less than 50% are comparable to New Zealand and the United States of America, but lower than the over 70% reported in the United Kingdom, Germany and Scandinavian countries (Duckett et al., 2019).

Access to dental care

10 Avoiding or delaying dental treatment due to cost

More people are avoiding or delaying dental treatment due to cost.

In 2017 a third of Victorian adults avoided or delayed visiting a dentist due to cost (34%) – an increase of 17% compared with 2004–2006 (Figure 10.15).

Figure 10.15 Victorian adults who avoided or delayed visiting a dentist due to cost, 2006 to 2017 (%)

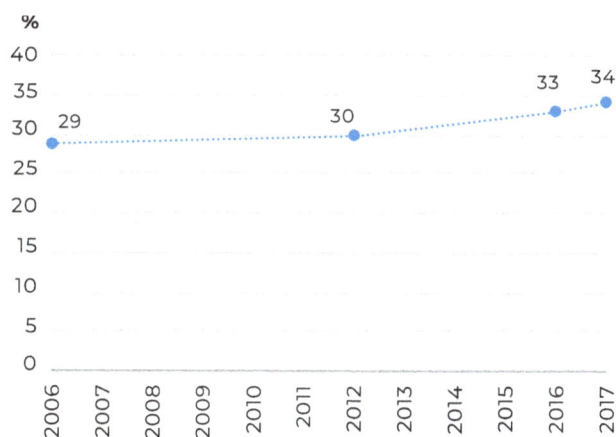

Sources: AIHW, 2007; Victorian Population Health Surveys, 2012 (DHHS, 2016), 2016 (DHHS, 2018) and 2017 (VHIA, n.d).

Avoidance and delayed visits varied with income and cultural and linguistic diversity (CALD). In 2016, 40% of Victorians on annual household incomes below $40,000 avoided or delayed visiting a dentist due to cost, compared with a quarter (26%) whose household incomes exceeded $100,000. The rise in delay in visiting may be associated with the flat lining of wages in 21st century Australia (ABS, 2020; Australian Government Treasury, 2017). People with CALD backgrounds also experienced greater difficulties in accessing dental care because of cost (Mejia et al., 2022).

11 Dental insurance

Around half of adults have held dental insurance since 1988.

Dental insurance is an enabling factor in visiting a private dentist. About half of Victorian and Australian adults have held dental insurance since 1988 (Figure 10.16). In Victoria the proportion has ranged between 46% in 1988 to 49% in 2012 (HDV et al., 1988; DHHS, 2016). Nationally, 52% of adults held dental insurance in 2017–2018 (ARCPOH, 2019). More people with some of their own teeth had insurance than those without any natural teeth – over half (53%) compared to less than a quarter (22%) (ARCPOH, 2019).

Figure 10.16 Victorians and Australians holding dental health insurance, 1988 to 2018 (%)

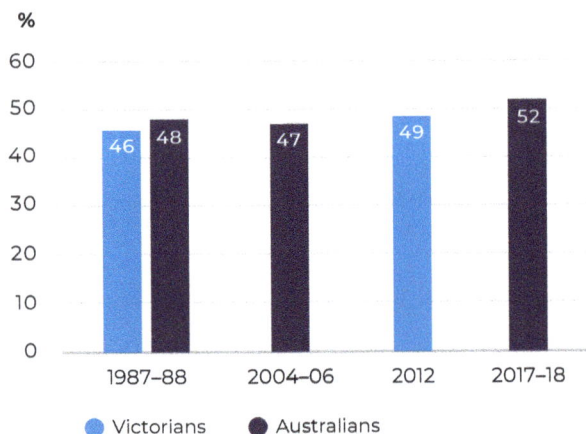

Sources: HDV et al., 1988; Barnard, 1993; AIHW, 2007; DHHS, 2016; ARCPOH, 2019.

In 2017–2018 Australian adults with insurance were almost twice as likely as uninsured people to have sought dental care within the past 12 months (70 compared with 43%) (ARCPOH, 2019). In the same year, uninsured people were almost four times more likely to have no natural teeth than insured Australians (7 compared to 2%) (ARCPOH, 2019).

Children

Oral health status

12 Tooth decay

While the prevalence of tooth decay in children has reduced markedly over the past 50 years, more than a third have this disease, with higher rates among disadvantaged children.

Pre-school children

Over half (57%) of Victorian pre-schoolers living in disadvantaged areas had tooth decay in 2015 (Graesser et al., 2022). Most of the decay (65%) was early stage "white spot" lesions that can be reversed with prevention interventions such as fluoride (in water, toothpaste and varnish) and reduced consumption of sugary food and drinks.

Children of non-English speaking backgrounds had higher rates of later-stage decay than other children (2.1 times). The corresponding figure for children of Aboriginal or Torres Strait Islander background was 1.9 times, and for those with parents who had pension or health care cards, 1.8 times higher (Graesser et al., 2022).

School children

Tooth decay in Australian children has declined considerably since 1970 when almost all children had tooth decay (Roder, 1971; Wright & Spencer, 1983) (Figures 10.17 to 10.20). The most recent population oral health survey of Australian children in 2012–2014 found that almost half (43%) of Victorian 5–10-year-olds had decay in their primary teeth, and a third (37%) of 12–14-year-olds had decay in their permanent teeth (Do & Spencer, 2016).

There is limited information about the extent of tooth decay in Australian children in the early 1970s. While there were studies of particular groups, there were no population-wide health surveys at this time (Roder, 1971; Wright & Spencer, 1983). Roder's research in South Australia showed extremely high decay rates. Victorian children are likely to have had similar rates.

In the early 1970s over 90% of children had tooth decay (Roder, 1971). By 2014 the proportion decreased to a third of children – 35% in 5–6-year-olds and 37% in 12–14-year-olds (Figure 10.17) (Do & Spencer, 2016). During this time, the average number of teeth affected by decay decreased from 6.5 and 10 to 1.3 and 0.9, respectively (Figure 10.18) (Do & Spencer, 2016). The decline in decay of the primary teeth of 5–6-year-olds has been levelling off from the late 1980s (Figure 10.17).

Figure 10.17 Decline in tooth decay in Victorian children aged 5–6 and 12–14 years, 1970 to 2014 (%)

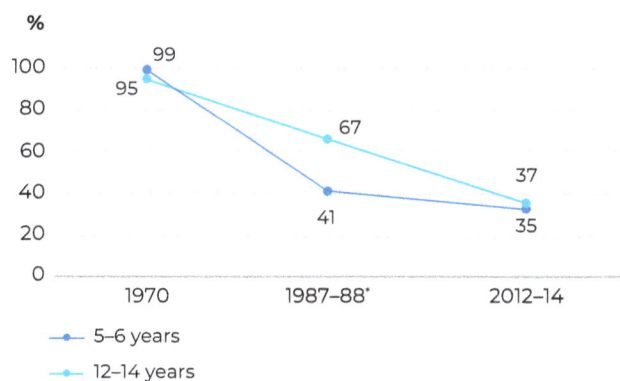

Sources: 1970 estimate from Roder, 1971; HDV et al., 1988; Do & Spencer, 2016.

Notes:

1. *Figures for 1997–98 are Australian, not Victorian.

2. Prevalence rates for tooth decay in children are commonly measured in 5–6 (or 6)-year-olds to show the proportion of children who have tooth decay in their primary teeth, and in 12–14 (or 12)-year-olds for the proportion affected with tooth decay in their permanent teeth.

Figure 10.18 Decline in the number of teeth with tooth decay in Victorian children aged 5–6 and 12–14 years, 1970 to 2012–14 (No.)

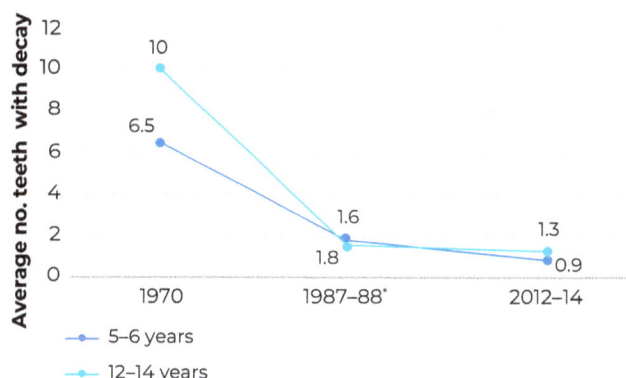

Sources: 1970 estimate from Roder, 1971; HDV et al., 1988; Do & Spencer, 2016.

*Note: Figures for 1987–88 are Australian, not Victorian.

Untreated tooth decay

The extent of both tooth decay and untreated tooth decay in children decreased between the population surveys of 1987–88 and 2012–14. Reductions were greater in the permanent teeth of the older children (Figure 10.19), compared with the primary teeth of the younger children (Figure 10.20) (Do & Spencer, 2016).

Figure 10.19 Primary teeth with decay and untreated decay in Victorian children ages 5–6 years, 1987–88 and 2012–14 (%)

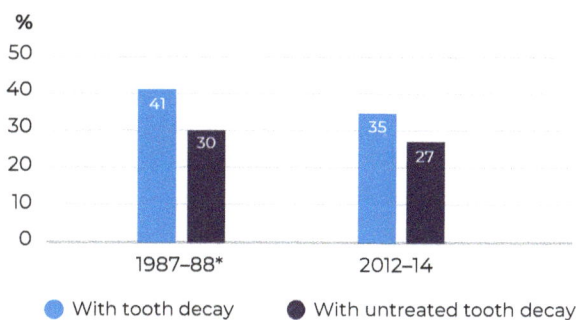

Sources: Barnard, 1993; Do & Spencer, 2016.

*Note: Figures for 1987–88 data are Australian, not Victorian.

Figure 10.20 Tooth decay and untreated decay in the permanent teeth in Victorian children aged 12–14 years, 1987–88 and 2012–2014 (%)

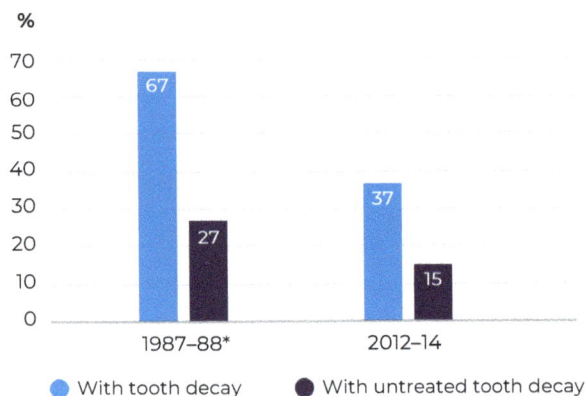

Sources: Barnard, 1993; Do & Spencer, 2016.

*Note: Figures for 1987–88 are Australian, not Victorian.

The proportion of children with dental fillings has decreased considerably over the past five decades. In 1970 most 12–14-year-olds (more than 90%) had fillings (Roder, 1971). In 1987–88 the corresponding figure was about half (56%) and, by 2012–14, a quarter (27%) of 12–14-year-old children had dental fillings (Do & Spencer, 2016).

Cavities at school entry

In 1970 only 5% of children had no cavities on school entry (5–6 years of age) (Figure 10.21) (Roder, 1971). By 1985 the proportion had risen to almost half (47%), and by 2012–14 to two thirds (65%) (Do & Spencer, 2016). The *Victorian action plan to prevent oral disease 2020–30* has set the state target for 2030 at 85% (DHHS, 2020b).

Figure 10.21 Victorian children with no dental cavities at school entry, 1970 to 2014 and 2030 target (%)

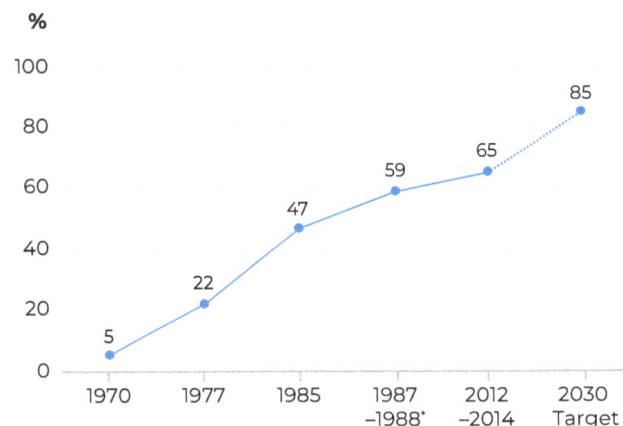

Sources: 1970 estimate from Roder, 1971; Victorian School Dental Service for 1977 and 1985; DHV, 1986; Barnard, 1993 for 1987-88 and Do & Spencer, 2016 for 2012-14;.

*Note: Figures for 1987–88 data are Australian, not Victorian.

Public dental clinic attendees

Recent improvements in the oral health of Victorian children and adolescents are evident in data from those attending public dental clinics. In the 11 years between 2009 and 2019, the proportion of young people visiting public clinics who were cavity free increased steadily (Figure 10.22) (DHV, 2023). For 0–5-year-olds, the increase was from about a half (54%) to three quarters. In 0–18-year-olds the increase was from about a third (36%) to a half (51%).

Figure 10.22 Public dental clients under 18 years old without cavities, Victoria, 2009 to 2019 (%)

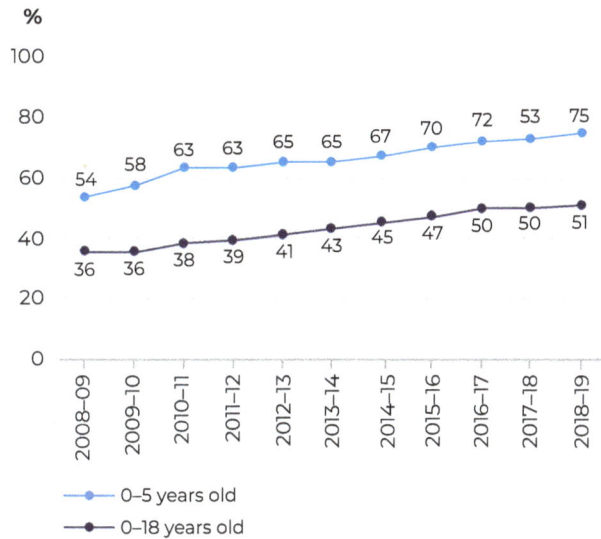

0–5 years old
0–18 years old

Source: DHV, 2023.
Note: These data are not representative of all Victorian children and adolescents as public dental clients are more likely to be from lower income families.

In spite of this, inequalities in tooth decay among children six years and under increased during the same period. Absolute and relative inequalities in prevalence and severity of tooth decay increased for children from CALD backgrounds and for children whose parents held concession cards (Lopez et al., 2022).

In children and adolescents identifying as Aboriginal or Torres Strait Islanders who accessed public dental services, the proportion who were cavity free increased from a quarter to almost half (23 to 44%) between 2009 and 2019 (Figure 10.23) (DHV, 2023). The gap in cavity-free status between those identifying as Indigenous and those who did not was 13% in 2009, and this decreased to 6% in 2019 (Figure 10.23).

Figure 10.23 Public dental clients under 18 years old without cavities by Aboriginal and Torres Strait Islander status, Victoria, 2009 to 2019 (%)

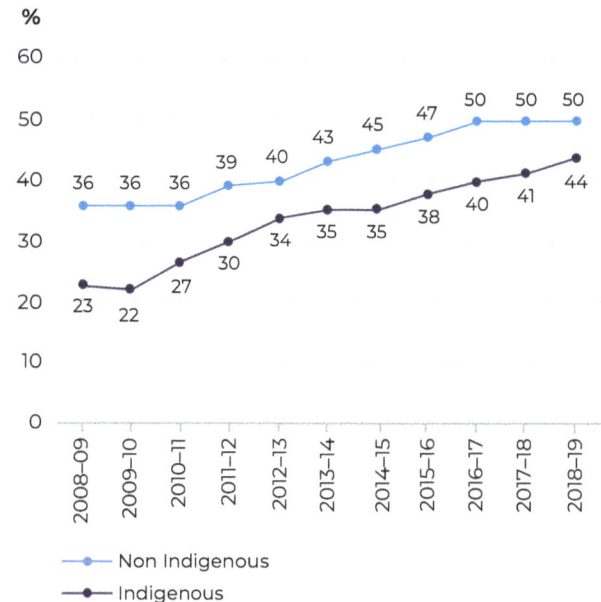

Non Indigenous
Indigenous

Source: DHV, 2023.

Distribution of tooth decay

While almost all Australian children had tooth decay in 1970, in the 2000s 20% of children suffered from 80% of all tooth decay.

As outlined earlier, in 1970 almost all Australian children had tooth decay (Figure 10.17). By 2014 the distribution of tooth decay was markedly skewed with a fifth (20%) of children aged 5–10 years having around 80% of all primary teeth surfaces with decay experience. In 11–14-year-olds, 17% had 80% of all permanent teeth surfaces with decay experience (Do & Spencer, 2016).

A social gradient of increased risk of tooth decay was evident in the 2012–14 survey (Do & Spencer, 2016). Children with more tooth decay were from households with lower incomes (Figures 10.24 and 10.25) and lower parental educational attainment.

In the primary teeth of 5–10-year-olds, half of the children from the poorest third of households had experience of tooth decay compared to a third of children from the highest income households (Figure 10.24). These children from poorer families were twice as likely to have untreated decay (36 compared to 18%).

Figure 10.24 Australian children aged 5–10 years with tooth decay in the primary teeth by household income, 2012–14 (%)

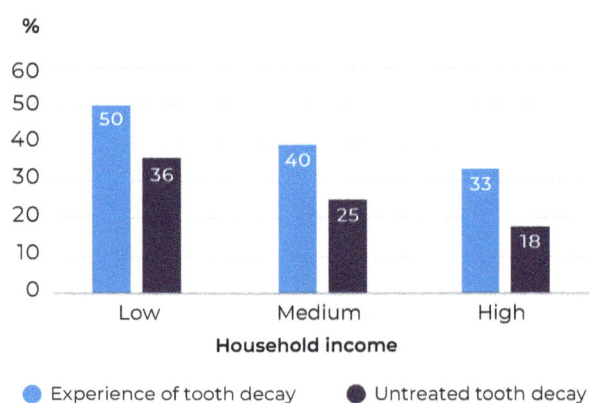

Source: Do & Spencer 2016.

There was a similar social gradient in the permanent teeth of 6–14-year-olds (Figure 10.25).

Figure 10.25 Australian children aged 6–14 years with tooth decay in the permanent teeth by household income, 2012–14 (%)

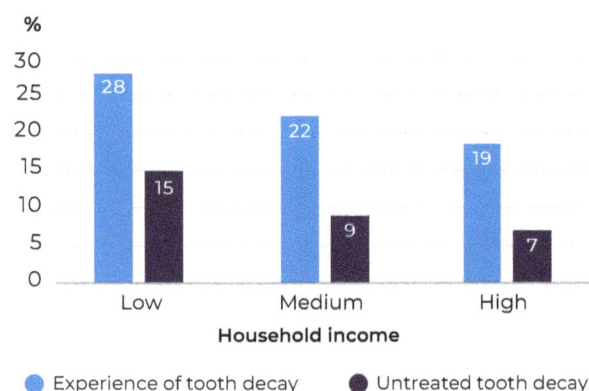

Source: Do & Spencer 2016.

Inequality was also evident in the number of primary tooth surfaces affected by tooth decay. Children aged 5–10 years from households with the lowest incomes had an average of 4.4 primary tooth surfaces affected by decay, compared to the 2.1 surfaces in children from the highest income group (Do & Spencer, 2016).

Oral health behaviours

13 Toothbrushing frequency

Children's toothbrushing frequency has improved, with scope for further improvement.

Limited available data suggest that it is likely that the proportion of children brushing the recommended twice a day increased between 1987–88 and 2012–14. Figure 10.26 shows toothbrushing frequency in children in two slightly different age groups, in Victoria and Australia, and in different time periods.

Figure 10.26 Children toothbrushing at least twice a day, 1987–88 and 2012–14 (%)

Sources: HDV, 1988; Do & Spencer, 2016.
Note: *Victorian children. **Australian children.

In spite of the increase in the proportion of children brushing the recommended twice a day, by 2014 almost a third of children were not brushing at this rate, suggesting a focus for future oral health promotion initiatives. Oral health promotion initiatives up to 2014, including 40 years of TV advertising, would appear not to have had a significant impact on changing toothbrushing habits. The next national oral health survey of children scheduled for 2024 will determine if there has been a recent increase in frequency.

The proportion of Australian children aged 5–9 years reported to be brushing once a day did not change significantly between 1987–88 and 2012–14 (from 94 to 95%) (HDV, 1988; ARCPOH NDTIS, 2013). In 2012–14 brushing frequency increased with age: 66% for 5–6-year-olds; 69% for 9–10-year-olds, and 71% for 13–14-year-olds (Do & Spencer, 2016).

14 Dental visits

Frequency of children's dental visits remained generally stable from the 1980s to the 2000s, with an increase for pre-school children.

For children, the reported frequency of dental visiting at 12- and 24-month intervals remained relatively stable between 1983 and 2017–18 (Figure 10.27). Twelve-monthly visiting declined slightly between 1983 (when 85% of children saw a dentist every year) and 2002 (when 79% visited yearly). Visiting every two years remained above 90% from 2002 to 2018.

Figure 10.27 Reported frequency of dental visits by Victorian children*, 1983 to 2018 (%)

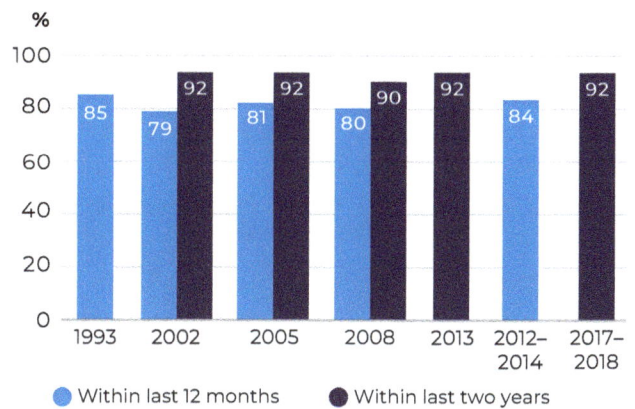

● Within last 12 months ● Within last two years

Sources: DHV, 1986 (Report 3, page 31); ARCPOH NDTIS 2002, 2005, 2008, 2013; Do & Spencer, 2016; AIHW, 2020a (KPI 14).
*Note: The age group to 2008 was 5–11-year-olds, and from 2013, 5–14-year-olds.

In 2012–14, 65% of Victorian children had a dental visit before five years of age, which was above the Australian average of 57% (Do & Spencer, 2016). This was also above the Australian average of 48% in 1983 (ABS, 1983 Children's Dental Health and Immunization Survey as reported in DHV, 1986, Report 3, page 31).

National comparisons

How does Victorians' oral health compare to other Australian states and territories and the national average?

Since 2012, Victoria has generally been above or close to the national average on six of the nine indicators of oral health shown in Table 10.3.[45] The state ranks in the top four jurisdictions for four indicators – the proportion of under five-year-olds who have had a dental visit, the proportion of children with fissure sealants, and the average number of teeth affected by tooth decay in both young and middle-aged adults. Compared with other jurisdictions, it ranks in fifth place or below on five of the indicators.

45 Determined by the National Child Oral Health Survey 2012-14 (Do & Spencer 2016) and the National Study of Adult Oral Health (NSAOH) 2017-18 (ARCPOH, 2019).

Its lowest ranking, in last place, is the percentage of 55–74-year-olds with no natural teeth. Children from states and territories with more developed school dental programs – such as South Australia and the Australian Capital Territory – have considerably less tooth decay than Victorian children. However, other socioeconomic and cultural variations also influence rates of tooth decay in these jurisdictions.

Table 10.3 Victorians' oral health compared with residents of other Australian states and territories, selected years

Oral health indicator	Australia (%)	Victoria (%)	Victoria's ranking (no.)	Best (%)	Worst (%)
Proportion of under 5-year-olds who have had a dental visit	57	65	4	75 Tas	50 Qld
Proportion of 6–14-year-olds with untreated tooth decay	27	29	6	17 SA	40 NT
Prevalence of untreated decay in secondary teeth, all ages	11	11	5	4 SA	20 NT
Average number of primary teeth affected by tooth decay in 5–10-year-olds	1.5	1.5	6	1 ACT	2.4 NT
Average number of adult teeth affected by tooth decay in 12–14-year-olds	0.9	0.8	5	0.3 ACT	1.6 Qld
Percentage of children with fissure sealants in at least one tooth	27	40	2	42 Tas	17 NSW
Average number of adult teeth affected by tooth decay in • 15–34-year-olds • 35–54-year-olds	4.1 10.3	3.5 10.3	3 equal 2	3.2 Tas 8.7 ACT	4.7 NSW 10.6 Qld, SA
Percentage of 55–74-year-olds with no natural teeth	8	11	8	1 ACT	11 Vic

Sources: Items 1–6 NCOHS 2012–14 & Do & Spencer, 2016; Items 7, 8 NSAOH, 2017–18 & ARCPOH, 2019.

Note: ACT = Australian Capital Territory; NSW = New South Wales; NT = Northern Territory; Qld = Queensland; SA = South Australia; Tas = Tasmania; Vic = Victoria.

Summary

The extent of changes in the oral health of Victorians since 1970 – that is, oral health status, oral health behaviours and inequality between groups – is shown in Table 10.4.

Table 10.4 Changes in Victorian's oral health 1970 to 2020 – better or worse?

Oral health status	Better	Same	Worse
People are keeping more of their natural teeth – from a third to 85% of older people.	●		
Tooth decay has declined, particularly in children, but it is still one of the most common health problems with over 80% of adults affected and over a third of 5–10-year-olds.	●		
The proportion of children attending public dental clinics who do not have cavities has increased and the gap between Indigenous and non-Indigenous children has narrowed.	●		
The proportion of adults with untreated decay has risen since 2000.			●
The extent of gum disease in adults is high – with over half of older people affected.			●
Oral cancer mortality rates have decreased, but the incidence of tongue and oropharyngeal cancer has risen recently.	●		●

Oral health behaviours, dental care and affordability, and oral health literacy	Better	Same	Worse
Toothbrushing frequency has increased slightly but a quarter of adults and a third of children do not brush twice a day.	●		
Adults' understanding of gum disease has remained poor.		●	
Adult dental visiting has been relatively stable with 50–60% visiting in the past 12 months, but with a reduction during the first two years of the COVID-19 pandemic.		●	
More people are avoiding or delaying dental treatment due to cost.			●
Children's dental visiting in the past 12 months has remained stable at around 85% since the 1980s. More pre-schoolers are making their first dental visit before 5 years of age.		●	
Self-reports of worsening oral health have increased overall – more people are reporting toothache, discomfort with appearance, and avoidance of certain foods.			●
Around half of all adults have held dental insurance since 1988.		●	
Oral health inequalities for some groups: low income, Indigenous, non-English speaking backgrounds compared with others			
Oral health inequality has increased: • Poorer people are increasingly more likely than others to lose their natural teeth. • The tooth decay gap between health care card holders and non-card holders rose from 3 to 6 teeth in the 12 years to 2018. • Inequalities in tooth decay among children aged six years and under have increased.			●
The gum disease gap between health care card holders and non-card holders doubled in the 2000s – from 9 to 18% higher.			●
Tooth decay has become more concentrated in particular populations with less than 20% of children experiencing 80% of all tooth decay – a higher proportion of which is in disadvantaged children.			●
Lower socioeconomic groups disproportionately self-report worsening oral health compared with others.			●

Gone are the days when a set of dentures was a twenty-first birthday or wedding gift for a woman, with reducing the future cost of dental care in mind. Most older people now retain their own teeth and tooth decay, particularly in children, has declined considerably since the 1970s.

Examining oral health in Victorian adults and children over the past 50 years, we have seen that decreases in tooth decay are likely due to several factors: the introduction of fluoride (in toothpaste and community water supplies); increased access to preventive dental care; an apparent increase in oral hygiene; a decrease in the use of tobacco; and possible changes in sugar consumption (Box 10.2).

We have reported on small improvements in oral health behaviours, including frequency of toothbrushing and regularity of dental visiting. The proportion of children attending public dental clinics who do not have cavities has increased and the cavity gap between Indigenous and non-Indigenous children has narrowed.

In spite of these improvements, tooth decay still affects a majority of adults and almost half of all children. As more people have retained their teeth, the prevalence of gum disease has also increased. More than half of older adults now have this condition.

While the overall incidence of oral cancers is decreasing, and fewer Victorians are dying from these diseases, oropharyngeal and tongue cancers are increasing.

We have described worsening perceptions of oral health and the consequences of poor oral health – such as toothache, concern with appearance and avoiding certain foods – for an increasing proportion of people since the 1990s.

This trend has occurred along with cultural shifts in attitudes to self-esteem, peer-pressure and health aspirations.

While levels of dental health insurance have remained stable, we have noted a concerning increase in the proportion of people avoiding or delaying dental treatment due to cost.

These issues disproportionately affect people from disadvantaged backgrounds. Oral diseases are socially patterned, and inequities are caused by the conditions of daily living: the political, social and physical environments of modern societies. These determinants shape the choices and options open to individuals (Watt & Sheiham, 2012).

When sugar first became available in medieval Europe, the prevalence of tooth decay was highest in the wealthy who could afford this new luxury (Carayon et al., 2016). Today, disadvantaged groups suffer most. People on low incomes, who are Indigenous, or from non-English speaking backgrounds are more likely to lose their natural teeth; have tooth decay and gum disease; avoid or delay treatment due to cost; and have more toothache, difficulty eating, and concern about the appearance of their teeth.

What can be done to address these inequities? Evidence-based interventions that have been proved to prevent oral disease are highlighted in Chapter 6: Prevention Interventions. Lessons from our review of the impact of sustained government funding on increasing access to dental care for the most disadvantaged are outlined in Chapters 4, 5, and 9. These, plus the likely contributions to better oral health of legislation and governance initiatives (described in Chapter 2) and workforce developments (Chapter 3) are brought together in our final chapter, *Future Tense*, in which we suggest a world's best-practice approach.

References

Australian Bureau of Statistics. (ABS). (2012). *Australian health survey first results, 2011–12.* (Released October 29, 2012). ABS. <https://www.abs.gov.au/ausstats/abs@.nsf/lookup/4364.0.55.001main+features12011-12>

Australian Bureau of Statistics. (ABS). (2015). *Australian health survey first results, 2014–15.* (Released December 8, 2015). ABS. <https://www.abs.gov.au/AUSSTATS/abs@.nsf/DetailsPage/4364.0.55.0012014-15>

Australian Bureau of Statistics. (ABS). (2019). *Experiences in Australia: Summary of findings 2018–19 financial year.* <https://www.abs.gov.au/statistics/health/health-services/patient-experiences-australia-summary-findings/2018-19#dental-professionals>

Australian Bureau of Statistics. (ABS). (2020). *Wage price index Australia.* ABS. <https://www.abs.gov.au/statistics/economy/price-indexes-and-inflation/wage-price-index-australia/latest-release>

Australian Government Treasury. (2017). *Analysis of wage growth.* Australia Government. <https://treasury.gov.au/sites/default/files/2019-03/p2017-t237966.pdf>

Australian Institute of Health and Welfare. (AIHW). (2007). *Australia's dental generations: the national survey of adult oral health 2004–06.* AIHW cat. No. DEN 165. Australian Institute of Health and Welfare (Dental Statistics and Research Series No. 34). <https://www.aihw.gov.au/reports/dental-oral-health/australias-dental-generations-survey-2004-06/contents/table-of-contents>

Australian Institute of Health and Welfare (AIHW). (2020a). *Cancer data in Australia.* This report was updated on October 4, 2022 by AIHW in a different format. <https://www.aihw.gov.au/reports/cancer/cancer-data-in-australia>

Australian Institute of Health and Welfare. (AIHW). (2020b). *National oral health plan 2015–2024: performance monitoring report.* AIHW. <https://www.aihw.gov.au/reports/dental-oral-health/national-oral-health-plan-2015-2024/contents/summary>

Australian Institute of Health and Welfare. (AIHW). (2022). *Oral health and dental care in Australia.* (Released March 17, 2022). AIHW. <https://www.aihw.gov.au/reports/dental-oral-health/oral-health-and-dental-care-in-australia/contents/preventative-strategies>

Australian Institute of Health and Welfare Dental Statistics and Research Unit (AIHW DSRU). (2008). *The national survey of adult oral health: 2004–06: Victoria.* Cat. no. DEN 181. Dental Statistics and Research Series no. 45. AIHW. <https://www.aihw.gov.au/reports/dental-oral-health/national-survey-adult-oral-health-vic-2004-06/contents/table-of-contents>

Australian Research Centre for Population Oral Health. (ARCPOH). (1994, 1996, 1999, 2002, 2005, 2008, 2010, 2012, 2013, 2016, & 2017). *National dental telephone interview surveys (NDTIS).* University of Adelaide.

Australian Research Centre for Population Oral Health (ARCPOH). (2019). *Australia's oral health: National study of adult oral health 2017–18.* University of Adelaide.

Australian Research Centre for Population Oral Health. (ARCPOH). (2020). Oral health impacts among Victorian adults from the National Study of Adult Oral Health (NSAOH) 2017–18. Victorian unpublished raw data separated from the Australian data cited in Brennan et al, 2020 cited below.

Barnard, P.D. (1993). *National oral health survey Australia 1987–88: A report of the first national oral health survey of Australia.* Australian Government Publishing Service.

Brennan, D.S., Luzzi, L., Chrisopoulos, S., & Haag, D.G. (2020). Oral health impacts among Australian adults in the National Study of Adult Oral Health (NSAOH) 2017–18. *Australian Dental Journal, 65*(S1), S59–S66. <https://onlinelibrary.wiley.com/doi/full/10.1111/adj.12766>

Carayon, D., Grimoud, A.M., Donat, R. & Catafau, A. & Esclassan, R. (2016). A history of caries in the Middle Ages: characteristics and cultural profiles. *Journal of the History of Dentistry 64*(2), 59–66. <https://pubmed.ncbi.nlm.nih.gov/28388022>

Credit Suisse Research Institute. (2020). *Global wealth report.* Credit Suisse Group. <https://www.credit-suisse.com/about-us/en/reports-research/global-wealth-report.html>

Chrisopoulos, S., Harford, J.E., & Ellershaw, A. (2016). *Oral health and dental care in Australia: key facts and figures 2015.* AIHW. <https://www.aihw.gov.au/reports/dental-oral-health/oral-health-dental-care-2015-key-facts-figures/summary>

Dental Health Services Victoria. (DHSV). (2023). *Oral cancer and screening program.* <https://www.dhsv.org.au/oral-health-programs/oral-cancer-screening-and-prevention.>

Department of Health, Victoria (DHV). (1986). *Ministerial review of dental services (MRODS) in Victoria, Final report.* State Government of Victoria.

Department of Health, Victoria. (DHV). (2021). *Annual report on drinking water quality in Victoria 2020–21.* State Government of Victoria. <https://www.health.vic.gov.au/sites/default/files/2022-03/annual-report-on-drinking-water-quality-in-Victoria-2020-21.pdf>

Department of Health, Victoria (DHV). (2022). *Vaccine history timeline.* <https://www2.health.vic.gov.au/public-health/immunisation/immunisation-schedule-vaccine-eligibility-criteria/vaccine-history-timeline>

Department of Health, Victoria. (DHV). (2023). Unpublished data used with permission from the Victorian Department of Health.

Department of Health and Human Services. (DHHS). (2016). *Victorian population health survey 2012. Selected survey findings.* State Government of Victoria. <https://content.health.vic.gov.au/sites/default/files/migrated/files/collections/research-and-reports/v/victorian-population-health-survey-2012.pdf>

Department of Health and Human Services. (DHHS). (2018). *Victorian population health survey 2016. Selected survey findings.* State Government of Victoria. <https://www.health.vic.gov.au/population-health-systems/victorian-population-health-survey-2016>

Department of Health and Human Services. Victoria. (DHHS). (2020a). V*ictorian cancer plan 2020–2024. Improving cancer outcomes for all Victorians.* State Government of Victoria. <https://www2.health.vic.gov.au/about/health-strategies/cancer-care/victorian-cancer-plan>

Department of Health and Human Services. Victoria. (DHHS). (2020b). *Victorian action plan to prevent oral disease 2020–30.* State Government of Victoria. <https://www2.health.vic.gov.au/public-health/preventive-health/oral-health-promotion/oral-health-planning>

Do, L.G., & Spencer, A.J. (Eds). (2016.). *Oral health of Australian children: the National child oral health study 2012–14.* University of Adelaide. <doi.org/10.20851/ncohs>

Duckett, S., Cowgill, M., & Swerissen, H. (2019). *Filling the gap: A universal dental care scheme for Australia.* Grattan Institute. <https://grattan.edu.au/report/filling-the-gap>

Farah, C.S., Simanovic, B., & Dost, F. (2014). Oral cancer in Australia 1982–2008: a growing need for opportunistic screening and prevention. *Australian Dental Journal, 59*(3), 349–59. <doi.org/10.1111/adj.12198>

Graesser, H., Sore, R., Rogers, J., Cole, D., & Hegde, S. (2022). Early childhood caries in Victorian preschoolers: A cross-sectional study. *International Dental Journal, 72*(3), 381–391. <doi.10.1016/j.identj.2021.05.013>

Health Department Victoria. (HDV), Royal Dental Hospital of Melbourne. (RDHM), Australian Dental Association Victorian Branch. (ADAVB) & Faculty of Science, University of Melbourne. (1988). *Australian national oral health survey 1987–88. First survey of oral health in Australia – Victorian sector. Report 1.*

Honeywell, S., Samavat, H., Hoskin, E., Touger-Decker, R.E., & Zelig, R. (2022). Associations between dentition status and nutritional status in community-dwelling older adults. *JDR Clinical & Translational Research, 8*(1), 93–101. <doi:10.1177/23800844211063859>

Lopez, D.J., Hegde, S., Whelan, M., Dashper, S., Tsakos, G., & Singh, A. (2022). Trends in social inequalities in early childhood caries using population-based clinical data. *Community Dentistry and Oral Epidemiology.* <doi.org/10.1111/cdoe.12816>

Marinho, V.C.C., Higgins, J.P., Logan, S., & Sheiham, A. (2003). Topical fluoride (toothpastes, mouthrinses, gels or varnishes) for preventing dental caries in children and adolescents. *Cochrane Database of Systematic Reviews*(4). <doi: 10.1002/14651858.CD002782.>

Mejia, G.C., Ju, X., Kumar, S., Soares, G.H., Balasubramanian, M., Sohn, W., & Jamieson, L. (2022). Immigrants experience oral health care inequity: findings from Australia's national study of adult oral health. *Australian Dental Journal.* <doi: 10.1111/adj.12942>

National Advisory Council on Dental Health. (NACODH). (2012). *Report of the National Advisory Council on Dental Health.* NACDH.

National Health and Medical Research Council. (NHMRC). (2017). *NHMRC Public statement 2017: water fluoridation and human health in Australia.* NHMRC. <https://www.nhmrc.gov.au/sites/default/files/documents/reports/fluoridation-public-statement.pdf>

Roder, D.M. (1971). The dental health and habits of South Australian children from different socio-economic environments. *Australian Dental Journal, 16*(1), 34–40. <doi.org/10.1111/j.1834-7819.1971.tb00978.x>

Sanders, A.E., Slade, G.D., Carter, K.D., & Stewart, J.F. (2004). Trends in prevalence of complete tooth loss among Australians, 1979–2002. *Australian and New Zealand Journal of Public Health, 28*(6), 549–554. <doi.10.1111/j.1467-842x.2004.tb00045.x>

Victorian Agency for Health Information. (VAHI). (n.d.). *Victorian population health survey 2017.* <https://www2.health.vic.gov.au/public-health/population-health-systems/health-status-of-victorians/survey-data-and-reports/victorian-population-health-survey/victorian-population-health-survey-2017>

Watt, R.G., & Sheiham, A. (2012). Integrating the common risk factor approach into a social determinants framework. *Community Dent Oral Epidemiol 40*(4), 289–96.<doi:10.1111/j.1600-0528.2012.00680.x>

Wong, T.S.C., & Wiesenfeld, D. (2018). Oral cancer. *Australian Dental Journal, 63*(S1), S91–S99. <doi.10.1111/adj.12594>

Wright, F.A.C., & Spencer, A.J. (Eds.). (1983). *Children's and community dental health: proceedings of a programme in continuing education conducted by the Faculty of Dental Science, University of Melbourne, November, 1982.* Department of Conservative Dentistry, University of Melbourne.

Chapter 11
And then came COVID-19

Jamie Robertson

Introduction

As in all other aspects of life, the impact of the COVID-19 pandemic on dental health and dental care has been profound and wide ranging. This chapter examines some of its effects in Victoria.

On 23 January, 2020 the city of Wuhan in China was put into a 76-day lockdown in a bid to stop the spread of a new coronavirus infection, later called COVID-19. That was the first major response to the disease and it was followed by a cascade of subsequent responses and actions around the world. The World Health Organization declared COVID-19 to be a pandemic on 11 March 2020 and the Victorian Government declared a state of emergency on 16 March. Other actions quickly followed; suddenly everyone knew about the virus called SARS-CoV-2, the genetic code of which was quickly identified.

The Australian Government closed international borders to all flights on 20 March except for a few carrying returning citizens and on 31 March Victoria went into its first lockdown. It was intended to last only four weeks but, in fact, it ended on 22 June 2020 after a series of gradual easings. In the few days between the announcement of a lockdown and its onset, there was panic buying of food and home necessities. One curious phenomenon, replicated elsewhere, was the sight of shoppers squabbling over toilet rolls. High-sugar foods and alcohol escaped such indignities.

A rationale for the lockdown was to flatten the curve of the expected wave of patients requiring hospital admission, outstripping the resources needed to cope with that. Over time, the idea of eliminating the virus gave way to the concept of its containment until society could develop herd immunity to COVID-19 through an enormous vaccination program, which, of course, depended on the creation of effective vaccines. These were developed in record time thanks to modification of protocols. All of that would take time, however, and Victoria would go through a series of six lockdowns which lasted until 22 October 2021. Overall, in the years 2020 and 2021, the city of Melbourne experienced 263 days of varying levels of restrictions. Some urban postcodes had an extra ten days of lockdown while regional Victoria escaped with a much lighter load.

In Australia each state made its own set of regulations for dealing with the pandemic but they were coordinated by meetings of a National Cabinet chaired by the Prime Minister. It first met on 13 March 2020 and replaced the Council of Australian Governments (COAG) in May 2020.

Regulations to minimise the risk of spreading COVID-19 were created to control the number of people in any setting and the minimum distance between any two people was set at 1.5 metres in Australia but two metres in Europe. This was considered the maximum range for droplet spread but it became evident that aerosol spread carried the virus further. In either case dental treatment necessitated much closer interpersonal distances and the aerosol from a high-speed drill potentiated the risk. For long periods of lockdowns, all private and public dental clinics had to stop all treatment except for brief emergency care. Infection control procedures were heightened and the use of personal protection equipment (PPE) (meaning N95-grade masks, eye shields, gloves, hair covers and disposable gowns) became mandatory for all clinical workers.

The result was that all surgeries were closed for most of the week and staff were rostered for the few hours of emergency care, if any. Across the whole economy, employees were retained under a federal government scheme called JobKeeper which paid $1,500 per employee each fortnight. This was a huge cost to the nation but an economic lifeline for families. This scheme ended in October 2020 and was replaced for the 2021 lockdowns by the COVID-19 Disaster Emergency fund for people who were forced to work less than 20 hours per week.

Dental health outcomes

Existing and potential dental patients

The entire experience of the pandemic has affected people across society and in the dental workforce as well as dental health delivery systems and the education of the future dental workforce. Some impacts have been immediate, such as catching COVID-19 itself, while other impacts may take a long time to end or even be revealed, such as Long COVID and mental health issues.

During lockdowns all elective dental services were stopped. This meant that courses of care, regardless of the type and branch of dentistry, and any outreach preventive services were suspended and routine examinations were postponed. Waiting lists naturally grew longer and the uncertainty of when lockdowns might end made practices hesitant to plan a return to full service. The situation was worse for patients hoping to attend public community clinics. Lower socioeconomic status (SES) patients and migrants had less access to health information. They had often only attended due to episodes of pain in normal circumstances, but now the reduced hours and staff at clinics drove many to seek relief of pain at medical practices, which were themselves operating minimally.

One question which pervaded society during the height of lockdowns and the pandemic was, when would it all end and normality return? Indeed, what would normality look like at the other end? The mindset during an emergency is entirely different from that enjoyed in a post-emergency situation. An emergency may heighten anxiety but it also prompts actions to find solutions to problems. It has been noted that higher SES groups negotiated their way to solutions to their emergencies better than lower SES groups trying to find public sector clinics (Stennett & Tsakis, 2022). At the start of 2022 the average waiting period for general care in Victorian public dental clinics was 24.7 months and eight of the 51 clinics had waiting periods of over three years (ADAVB, 2022). With such long waiting times, minor problems can become major to the point of non-restorability. In comparison, waiting times at private clinics, where about 80% of services are provided, have not been so long, but, this notwithstanding, the sustained improvement in oral health indices since 1970 may worsen for a short period due to the COVID-19 pandemic.

Compounding the lack of available dental treatment has been the observed change in the diets of many people during lockdown episodes. While stories of increased weight-gain and higher alcohol consumption during lockdowns have been anecdotal in Australia, an English survey of buying habits during lockdowns has verified these unhealthy developments (Stennett & Tsakis, 2022). Surveys of supermarket sales across all SES groups are regularly conducted. Three surveys were compared: one on the day before the onset of the first lockdown; one from the year preceding that; and one 12 weeks after the onset. The lockdown-associated surveys showed high rises in the sales of "free sugar" food and drink across society with the last survey showing a more modest rise. Sales of oral hygiene products rose only slightly and even declined for the lowest SES group at the third survey. While a different survey of alcohol sales at the same time showed no overall increase in sales, it revealed that heavy drinkers bought much more, meaning that other people bought less.

The implication is that cariogenic "comfort" foods were consumed in greater quantities at a time when dental care was largely unavailable, and less attention was paid to the social grooming aspects of oral hygiene. It is too early to tell what effects this phenomenon may yet have on caries rates wherever it occurred. Again, anecdotally, dentists have reported seeing more fractures of ceramic restorations and broken teeth subsequent to the pandemic constraints on dental care, perhaps due to additional stressors, or to the reduced ability to seek regular dental examinations. Further, the increased consumption of alcohol among heavy drinkers may lead to a rise in the incidence of oral cancers in the coming years. Long-term outcomes will depend on how soon, if at all, eating and drinking behaviours return to the mean.

When lockdowns began in Victoria in 2020, Dental Health Services Victoria (DHSV) took the opportunity to set up and test a telehealth screening project to give dental advice to, or arrange emergency appointments for people using public dental clinics. For the 12 months of May 2020 until April 2021, 2,942 people used the service, which was reviewed and adjusted throughout (Lin et al, in press). People accessed the program either through the DHSV website or by being referred to it when they phoned or presented at the Royal Dental Hospital Melbourne (RDHM) for treatment. The questions were designed to be easy for people with low health literacy and poor command of English and interpreters were readily available. It was assessed by patients as being helpful and simple to use but when clinics re-opened, its utility subsided because staff who were trained

to operate the service were needed to work through the heavy backlog of patients that had built up during the pandemic and to cover for staff who were themselves falling ill with COVID-19.

An enduring benefit has been that clinicians are now more comfortable doing telehealth follow-ups to treatment rather than having patients present for a few minutes. In addition, telehealth is now used more frequently for clinician-to-clinician discussions regarding the interpretation of images or lesions or for simply providing advice.

Dental practice staff

Throughout the pandemic, the entire dental workforce has been subject to the same strictures as the rest of the population, except that they were given the status of essential workers for the few hours each week that clinics were open (Aphra, 2020). The intimate environment of a dental surgery heightened the awareness of possible contagion of the SARS-CoV-2 virus. Infection control procedures were adhered to with more attention to detail as was donning and doffing of PPE, all of which made some activities more time-consuming and cumbersome even though patient contact was briefer than usual. When N95 face masks became available and the preferred option for protection from aerosols, they were found to be tighter fitting than the older surgical masks and, when combined with face visors, they restricted visibility causing frequent stops during procedures. In addition, clear plastic visors could interfere with magnifying loupes on glasses.

Dental education

From a dental perspective, apart from people with illness or in pain, perhaps the most affected group during the lockdowns was the body of dental students who found their whole courses of study suspended. Face-to-face lectures stopped, as did all clinical practice at the two Victorian dental schools and any institutions running Oral Hygiene, Dental Prosthetics and Dental Assisting courses.

It was relatively easy to arrange remote lectures through Zoom or Microsoft Teams and students probably took to it with more alacrity than their lecturers. However, it was also easier for students to miss lectures and a sense of interaction was lost, particularly with tutorials. As for practical and clinical sessions, they were stopped entirely. This had enormous ramifications for students in the final year of whatever course they were studying because they could not graduate without gaining certain clinical skills.

A survey in 2021 reviewed the attitudes of dental students at many dental schools, mainly in the USA and Middle East, concerning the impact of the pandemic on their education (Farrokhi et al., 2021). The authors found common themes in students' concerns, namely, the interruption to, or drop in quality of practical learning; the uncertainty about their career prospects; infection control as it related to the coronavirus; the inability to complete their courses; and, finally, the mental stress which all these placed on them. On the positive side, the pandemic forced students to learn new skills in distance learning and to use virtual computerised patients as well as deepening their understanding of infection spread and control.

At the University of Melbourne Dental School (MDS) and at La Trobe University's Department of Dentistry all patient clinics stopped at the end of March 2020. In the case of La Trobe no warning was given by Bendigo Base Hospital.[46] This affected all students in every course and year level. A major problem at the outset was the uncertainty of when a return to normal might occur and, in the case of overseas students, when Australia's borders might re-open to allow students back into the country. The Australian Government had closed all border entry points on Friday, 20 March 2020 and had urged all overseas students to return to their own countries. Earlier, on 12 February, the Victorian Government had offered assistance packages to all overseas students but the national government measures overrode these.

By the end of May 2020 operative technique clinics with "phantom heads" were re-opened with modified spacing to comply with distancing mandates. This was fine for the domestic cohort but not the banished overseas students. At MDS, clinics with real patients only re-opened in November and for final year students the teaching period was extended until March 2021 to allow more supervised practice. As happened in all medical services, there was an initial scramble for N95 face masks which were in short supply. At La Trobe, the Department of Dentistry rued donating clinical gowns to Bendigo Base Hospital when its own clinics closed. When they re-opened, the price of gowns had increased dramatically, causing further budgetary strain.

When patient-treating clinics reopened, clinic times at MDS and La Trobe were extended in 2021 to provide catch-up practice. La Trobe dental students were most inconvenienced because they practise at six external community clinics. This did not help any overseas students who were locked out of Australia.

---

46 A/Prof Rebecca Wong, Deputy Head of School, MDS, University of Melbourne, personal communication, April 4, 2022, and A/Prof Rachel Martin, former Head of Department of Dentistry, La Trobe University, personal communication, April 12, 2022.

As there are many Canadian dental students in Australian dental schools, the National Dental Examining Board of Canada (NDEB) has been setting practical exams for them annually in Sydney before they return to their home provinces. This is a necessary step to permit them to register in Canada and it has been convenient for the students to assemble in one place. Due to the pandemic, the NDEB did not visit Australia in 2020 and in 2021 had to change the venue to Griffith University in Brisbane because Queensland had fewer pandemic restrictions than Sydney. University teaching timetables were adjusted to allow the Canadian students to attend the Brisbane exams.

Summary

Though unwelcome, the COVID-19 pandemic and its consequent restrictions prompted resourcefulness and invention at dental schools and in health institutions. Unfortunately for some prospective patients, minor oral health problems deteriorated into unrestorability. However, provisional covers saved many more teeth than would have been lost without them. Infection control protocols were tested and strengthened, patient management was improved even though waiting lists grew longer, and clinical staff came to a deeper understanding of their own links to public health, which was something many had never thought about before. Further, in DHSV and in some private sector clinics, teledentistry trials were undertaken for later addition to communication protocols with prospective and existing patients. In the first six months, the whole experience was underwritten by the national government's JobKeeper program, without which many employed dental workers, clinical and administrative, would have lost their jobs.

References

Australian Dental Association Victorian Branch. (ADAVB). (2022, February 2). *Public dental waiting lists balloon as impacts of COVID-19 bite*. [Media release]. <https://adavb.org/news-media/media-releases/public-dental-waiting-lists-balloon-as-the-impacts-of-covid-19-bite>

Australian Health Practitioner Regulation Authority. (Aphra). (2020). Dental Board of Australia. (2020/03/24). COVID-19-update-to-dental-practitioners.

Lin, C., Goncalves, N., Scully B., Heredia, R., & Hegde, S. (in press). Supporting patient-centred care and access to public dental services through Telehealth during COVID-19, J*ournal of Telehealth and Telecare*, Draft. Viewed 1 April, 2022.

Farrokhi, Farid, Mohebbi, S.Z., Farrokhi, Farzaneh, & Khami, M.R. (2021). Impact of COVID-19 on dental education – a scoping review. *BMC Medical Education 21*(1), 587.

Stennett, M., Tsakis, G. (2022). The impact of the COVID-19 pandemic and oral health inequalities and access to oral healthcare in England. *British Dental Journal 232*(2), 109–114.

Chapter 12
Future Tense – So what?

John Rogers and Jamie Robertson

Introduction

This chapter considers the many changes which have occurred since 1970 and notes that not everyone has benefitted equally. Challenges lie ahead. Possible future developments are measured against the six guiding principles set out in the World Health Organization's (WHO) Global Strategy on Oral Health (WHO, 2022a).

Our look back at developments in dental public health in Victoria and Australia from 1970 to 2022 begs the question of what might be the lessons for the future? What are possible future directions based on the findings of our research? This chapter looks at the current state of oral health and the dental system, and explores a way forward.

Victoria and Australia have been through a revolution in dental legislation and governance (Chapter 2), in dental workforce developments and education (Chapter 3), in the oral health care system (Chapters 4, 5 and 8) and oral disease prevention and oral health promotion (Chapter 6), in the evolution of clinical services with considerable technological innovation (Chapter 7) and in their financing (Chapter 9). Clearly there has been great progress, but it has been uneven and not shared by all (Chapter 10). And then along came COVID-19 (Chapter 11) with myriad complications and consequences, some still indeterminate.

Developments in the state of oral health and the dental system

Positive developments

There have undoubtedly been significant improvements in the oral health of Victorians since 1970. The extent of tooth decay in children has decreased, from more than 90% experiencing decay to less than half today (Chapter 10). The gap between decay rates in Aboriginal and Torres Strait Islander and non-Indigenous children is closing. Adults are keeping their teeth longer. From a time when it was still common in some communities to be gifted a full set of dentures on the threshold of adult life, and two-thirds of people over 65 years had full dentures, that proportion is now less than a fifth.

These improvements have been the result of a range of prevention interventions (Chapter 6). Most significant has been the introduction of community water fluoridation and increased use of fluoride toothpaste. There has been some, but not universal, development of more orally-healthy environments in health, childcare and school settings. Programs to support other health and childcare workers to promote oral health have been successfully implemented. On a population level there have been some improvements in oral hygiene. And while consumption of sugar is high with half of Australian children consuming four or more serves of snacks containing sugar each day (Do & Spencer, 2016), there may have been a relative reduction in families with higher levels of parental education and literacy (Chapter 10). The frequency of dental visits has been relatively stable across the population.

Further positive developments have been a partial shift to more preventive dental care (Chapter 7), a tripling of the number of Victorian public dental clinics and, when additional Australian government funds have been available, successful public dental programs (Chapter 4; Chapter 5).

There has also been an evolution in the composition of the oral health workforce which has enhanced access to dental care. The dentist workforce has been supplemented by oral and dental health therapists, hygienists and prosthetists who are now legislated to provide clinical dental services in addition to dentists.

Governance of dentistry has been democratised in keeping with other health professions. The all-dentist, mostly male, seven-member Dental Board of Victoria has been replaced, after several iterations, by a dental board membership that is more representative of the community. The 12-member Dental Board of Australia (DBA) that now oversees dental practice has a majority of women, five dentists, two oral health therapists, a prosthetist, and four community members.

Expectations about oral health have also changed. Aspirations have increased, with more people wanting to have an attractive, functioning natural dentition for most of their adult lives. At the same time, there has been less consumer participation in the oral health sector perhaps than in other parts of the health system. Although Dental Health Services Victoria (DSHV) has a Community Advisory Committee and community health services have similar mechanisms across their broad range of services, not just for oral health, there are almost no consumer or community groups specifically representing and advocating around the oral health consumers' needs and perspectives.

On the other hand – The challenges ahead

The less positive side of the developments of the past five decades is that a large, unequal burden of preventable oral disease remains. In fact, oral health inequity has increased recently. People who are socially disadvantaged or on low incomes, who live in regional areas, or have additional health care needs remain at higher risk of poor oral health. Further, some Aboriginal and Torres Strait Islander people also experience poorer oral health than other population groups. The boxes below reveal the mixed picture of oral health status (Box 12.1) and access to dental care (Box 12.2) since 1970.

Box 12.1 Ups and downs in the oral health of Victorians from 1970

- Significant improvements in the oral health of Victorians notwithstanding, a large, unequal burden of preventable oral disease remains (Chapter 10).
- Inequality has increased. The tooth decay gap between health care card holders and non-card holders rose from three to six teeth in the 12 years to 2018.
- More people are retaining their natural teeth for longer (up from a third of older people to 85%) but more people are consequently prone to gum disease and tooth decay. More than half of all older people have moderate or severe gum disease.
- While tooth decay has declined, it is still one of the most common health problems, with more than 80% of adults affected and more than 40% of 5–10-year-olds.
- Tooth decay is one of the most expensive disease conditions to treat. Costing $5 billion in Australia in 2018–19, the treatment of tooth decay was more costly than the treatment of falls (Chapter 9).
- Victorians have more untreated tooth decay than most other Australians.
- Tooth decay is the leading cause of preventable hospitalisations in children aged under 10.
- Although oral cancer mortality rates have decreased, the incidence of tongue and oropharyngeal cancer has increased since 2010.

Box 12.2 Access to dental care from 1970

- Cost as a barrier to seeking dental care has increased (Chapter 10). Historically, per capita spending on dental care in Victoria has exceeded that of any other state or territory, with Victorians also paying more in out-of-pocket costs than other Australians. Fees for most dental services have increased at a higher rate than average weekly earnings (Chapter 9). There has been an increase in the amount of money withdrawn from superannuation to pay for dental care (Chapter 9).
- Dental visits by Victorian adults have been relatively stable over the past 40 years, with about half reporting a visit in the previous 12 months (Chapter 10). Since 2020 the COVID-19 pandemic has interrupted this pattern with fewer people making dental visits.
- Although access to public emergency dental care has improved, concession card holders face long waiting times for general care and their oral health needs have not been met. In 2019, prior to the COVID-19 pandemic, the Victorian dental budget was sufficient to treat about 400,000 of the 2.2 million eligible Victorians each year; less than 20% a year (Chapter 5).
- Governments cover less than 20% of dental costs, compared with around 65% of other health care costs and more for general practitioners (Chapter 9).
- Australian government funding has followed a roller-coaster trajectory, with many programs initiated but not maintained. While Victorian government dental funding per person has generally been lower than in other states and territories, recent *Smile Squad* funding, which provides free dental care for all Victorian government school students, will bring expenditure close to parity (Chapter 9).
- In 2019 Victoria's ratio of dentists to population ranked third lowest in the country, with its public dentist rate ranking lowest. Rates of non-dentist dental practitioners were the second lowest in Australia. Dental public sector salaries in Victoria remain the lowest in Australia (Chapter 3).
- Australian government funding has been found to be the most important factor in addressing the oral health needs of the most disadvantaged (Chapter 5).

In summary developments since 1970 have created both winners and losers. High standards of oral health are enjoyed by many sectors of the community while poor oral health remains a key indicator of disadvantage. Dental care has simply not been managed in the same way as general health care. The mouth has been left out of the body.

A judgement could be made that Hubert Humphrey's moral test of government has not been met in relation to oral health. With the exception of primary school-aged children, Australian governments have fallen short in how they "treat those who are in the dawn of life, the children; those who are in the twilight of life, the elderly; and those who are in shadows of life, the sick, the needy, and the handicapped" (Humphrey, 1977). While community support for a national scheme within or beside Medicare has been constant (Cresswell, 2011), the current public dental system could be seen as little more than a tattered safety net.

The way forward

Oral health in the future

Looking forward, what are the pressing oral health issues of the future likely to be? What needs should be planned for as we look towards the two decades? Box 12.3 summarises the likely picture based on the trends observed since 1970. Many variables, some unanticipated, could have an impact on this picture, not least financial and technological changes and immigration levels and sources.

Box 12.3 Oral health issues in the future

- The prevalence of tooth decay at the population level in children may plateau or decrease. However, the concentration of disease is likely to increase. Much will depend on whether the seemingly inexorable increase in the marketing, relative affordability and availability of unhealthy food continues. Other factors will include children's diets; access to fluoride in water, toothpaste and professionally applied varnish; oral hygiene; and dental care.
- More adults are likely to keep more of their teeth, resulting in fewer full dentures but also more gum disease. Gum disease rates would also be affected with increases in obesity and associated diabetes.
- Older adults will require more dental care as the exposed roots of retained teeth will increase the risk of tooth decay. Old fillings, crowns and bridges will require repair.
- The impact of poor oral health on poor general health will intensify as the population ages, resulting in increased demand for health services and rising health care costs.
- Expectations about oral health will continue to increase, leading to greater demand for bleaching of teeth, orthodontic treatment, veneers, crowns and implants, as well as for further public dental programs and possibly an expansion of the services that they provide.
- Access to dental care will depend on the cost of private care, the availability of public dental funding, and the size and composition of the oral health workforce.
- Disparities in oral health are likely to increase if inequity in the community increases. Oral diseases are likely to continue to be diseases of people with low incomes.

Enablers and barriers for getting oral health on the crowded policy agenda

Before we propose a way forward, we need to consider how the significant oral health policy changes of the past were engineered. What were the enablers or drivers of increased government funding and system improvements?

The 14 significant government-funded initiatives implemented between 1970 and 2020 occurred in cycles – every 20 to 25 years for national programs, and every 10 to 15 years for Victorian government programs (Chapter 4). The analyses of our case studies of three of these significant government-funded initiatives found that oral health moved up the political policy agenda and that oral health policy changes occurred when Kingdon's three policy streams – problem, proposal, and politics – connected and a "policy window", or favourable confluence of events, brought increased attention to dental health issues (Kingdon, 2010) (Chapter 4, Figure 4.5).

In each of our case studies, the problem was well defined and perceived as serious. The proposal was compatible with government values and vision; plausible; technically feasible; and the cost was reasonable. Political motivation and opportunity were evident and it was important that decision makers heard a loud community voice. In general, strong, and vocal support from a coalition of community and advocacy organisations has been influential in achieving change (Chapter 8). In two of the case studies presented, pending elections opened the policy window. In the third case, a government budget provided the policy opportunity.

When devising an advocacy strategy, it is also necessary to consider the barriers to policy change. The perception that oral health has a low political profile has been a key barrier to reform (Chapter 4). This may be because oral disease is not usually life-threatening and is not as emotionally "marketable" as other health concerns such as cancer in children. Moreover, oral conditions are predominantly episodic, and most people are usually only concerned when they experience symptoms of pain or discomfort. The lack of a persistent, well-organised consumer voice, the high cost of dental care, and the isolation of dentistry from other health programs may also have been barriers to significant policy change.

From time to time these barriers have been overcome. As noted above, since 1970 there have been 14 significant initiatives at state and national levels (Chapter 4). Oral health advocates have continued to carefully articulate the problems and put forward proposals to fix them. They have managed the politics, while waiting for a policy window. Ultimately many factors, including fortunate timing and favourable budget circumstances, must also exist for policy success (Chapter 4).

A world's best practice approach

It is timely to consider how the *Global strategy on oral health* adopted by the WHO in May 2022 could provide a framework for action in Victoria and Australia (WHO, 2022a). This strategy espouses a bold vision of universal oral health coverage for all individuals and communities by 2030. It sets out four overarching goals to guide Member States (Box 12.4), while six guiding principles and six strategic objectives underpin and direct the path for governments towards realisation of the vision.

Box 12.4 WHO Global Strategy on Oral Health, 2022

Vision – universal health coverage (UHC) in oral health for all individuals and communities by 2030.

Four overarching goals guide Member States:

1. Develop ambitious national responses to promote oral health
2. Reduce oral diseases, other oral conditions, and oral health inequalities
3. Strengthen efforts to address oral diseases and conditions as part of UHC
4. Consider the development of targets and indicators

Six guiding principles underpin and direct the path for governments:

1. A public health approach to oral health
2. Integration of oral health into primary health care
3. Innovative workforce models to respond to population needs for oral health
4. People-centred oral health care
5. Tailored oral health interventions across the life course
6. Optimising digital technologies for oral health

Six strategic objectives for governments have been identified:

1. Oral health governance
2. Oral health promotion and oral disease prevention
3. Health workforce
4. Oral health care
5. Oral health information systems
6. Oral health research agendas

Source: WHO, 2022a.

The WHO is well aware that the world's nation states vary in their political economies and capacities and that concepts and ideas will be interpreted and enacted in a variety of ways according to existing health systems.

Current Victorian and national health and oral health plans are based on principles and strategies that are broadly consistent with the WHO global strategy on oral health. Their focus is on a population approach with emphasis on prevention and oral health promotion; a reduction in health inequity; enhanced access to services; multisector collaboration; enabling the workforce; improving information systems; and undertaking relevant research. These plans include *Australia's National preventive health strategy 2021–2030* (DH-A, 2021); *Healthy mouths healthy lives. Australia's national oral health plan 2015–2024* (COAG, 2016); *Victorian action plan to prevent oral disease 2020–30* (DHHS, 2020); and Dental Health Services Victoria's *Our strategic direction 2022* (DHSV, 2022). They are summarised in Appendix 1.

Having looked at how Victoria's oral health status and care systems have developed over the past 50 years, and with current Victorian and Australian plans in mind, we now draw on the six WHO strategic objectives to consider possible future directions. We propose a set of high-level recommendations for broad discussion. These suggestions offer a starting point for more detailed development of proposals. Priorities, timelines, funding and implementation responsibilities all need to be determined. We appreciate that this requires making difficult choices among the many options for using resources.

Strategic objectives

1 Oral health governance

The first of the WHO strategic objectives is to improve the political and resource commitment to oral health, strengthen leadership and create partnerships. Three actions, all relevant to Victoria and Australia, are proposed: namely, integrate oral health into all relevant policies and public health programs, strengthen the capacity of the national oral health unit and create sustainable partnerships within and outside the health sector. The governance of the workforce is also relevant.

Integrate oral health into all relevant policies and public health programs

In Victoria the history of integration of oral health into all relevant policies and public health programs has had mixed results. The case studies on inclusion of oral health in the Victorian Public Health and Wellbeing Plans and in the *National preventive health strategy 2021–2030* show that more needs to be done to raise the profile of oral health (Chapters 4 and 6).

Strengthen the capacity of the national oral health unit

The need to strengthen leadership to guide the development of national oral health programs is highlighted in the current national oral health plan (COAG, 2015). Better coordination of programs across jurisdictions and government departments will assist in providing effective and efficient oral health programs. Notably, the national plan recommended the appointment of an Australian Chief Dental Officer who would be supported by a National Oral Health Advisory Committee, but this has not yet been acted on.

Leadership for good public health policy would also be strengthened by inclusion of oral health control and prevention in the remit of the Australian Centre for Disease Control that is currently being established.

Create sustainable partnerships within and outside the health sector

Regarding partnerships within and outside the health sector there has been some limited progress in Victoria and Australia. Alliances such as the National Oral Health Alliance and the Victorian Oral Health Alliance should continue to bring together key professional, welfare and consumer organisations, university dental schools and research institutes that are committed to improving Victorians' oral health status and access to dental care (Chapter 8). However, the sector remains poorly resourced in terms of research and advocacy organisations, compared to other areas of the health system.

Governance of the workforce – Ahpra

All types of dental clinician come under the one category of dental practitioner governed by the Dental Board of Australia (DBA). Like all other national health boards, the DBA is required to have a health profession agreement with the Australian Health Practitioner Registration Agency (Ahpra) that sets out fees, budget and the range of services provided by the DBA to regulate the profession. It is through such agreements with all 15 boards that Ahpra administers the National Registration and Accreditation Scheme which is the practical manifestation of the National Law.[47]

---

47 See <https://www.ahpra.gov.au/~/link.aspx?_id=D4E5EF420D3C4EAB8B247FDB72CA6E0A&_z=z>

Policies related to the oral health workforce are now predominantly made at the national rather than the state level. Now that all health professions are governed by the same national law, it is more difficult for states to make unilateral policy choices. To some extent the states must now all travel like a convoy of ships, moving at the speed of the slowest. After the radical changes in 2009–10, when the national law introduced one scheme for registered health professionals in Australia (Chapters 3 and 4), further workforce changes are likely to be incremental until a future government decides that the public is not being well served.

From time to time, an issue relating to a health professional, usually a medical practitioner, hits the media headlines. Such stories highlight the slow and reactive nature of professional governance and regulation. An enquiry may say to a board "must do better", but it would be better if the whole apparatus of the National Scheme and Ahpra were to have mandated reviews at nominated intervals. Reviews which imply possible structural or procedural shake-ups might prod Ahpra into a more proactive role.

In summary, the way forward to improve oral health governance and leadership in Victoria and Australia would include the following actions:

- Further integrate oral health into all relevant policies and public health programs.
- Enhance population oral health skills and experience in the Australian Department of Health to improve national planning.
- Include the prevention of oral disease and oral health promotion in the remit of the Australian Centre for Disease Control that is currently being established.[48]
- Subject Ahpra to triennial or quinquennial reviews but give it more resources to respond faster to notifications about oral health practitioners who place the public at risk of harm.

2 Oral health promotion and oral disease prevention

The WHO call under this strategic objective is for evidence-based, cost-effective and sustainable interventions to promote oral health and prevent oral diseases.

As explored in Chapter 6, it is apparent that while there have been successful prevention programs in Victoria over the last 50 years, often they have been at a relatively small scale. Community water fluoridation has been a standout example but broader opportunities for prevention of oral disease and reduction of inequity have not been realised. Indeed, inequity has increased (Chapter 10). Budgets for prevention have been small and successful pilot programs have often not been funded more broadly. From a macro perspective, funding for oral health care is considerably misaligned in favour of post disease treatment, rather than prevention.

A public health approach, the first of the WHO Global Strategy's guiding principles, requires an emphasis on preventing disease by analysing its distribution and determinants; establishing health promoting environments; enabling people to increase control over, and to improve their health; and reducing inequities in access to care. There must be upstream action on important factors, including legislation and improving social, economic, educational and environmental determinants. The more conducive to good health these factors are, the easier it is to live a healthy life – making the healthy choices the easier choices. This approach has delivered proven benefits in other aspects of health policy, including in reticulated water supplies, sanitation, inoculations, road trauma and smoking cessation (Chapter 1).

48 <https://www.health.gov.au/our-work/Australian-CDC>

There have been some successful prevention interventions in Victoria since 1970 that we have reviewed in Chapter 6 and below we propose actions from the lessons learned. Such programs as a whole reflect the five broad actions areas of the Ottawa Charter for Health Promotion (WHO, 1986), namely: develop healthy public policy; create supportive health promoting environments; develop personal skills; strengthen community action; and re-orient health care services toward prevention.

As discussed in Chapter 6, the social, economic, political and environmental determinants of poor oral health – "the causes of the causes" such as income, education and housing – largely lie outside the health system but can be influenced by health policy and practice. Health policy can help to promote healthy environments, influence early childhood development and provide access to affordable health services of decent quality. These are all social determinants of health (PAHO & WHO, 2023).

Victorian initiatives to build public oral health policy are discussed in depth in Chapters 2, 4, 5 and 6. Legislation to implement community water fluoridation in Victoria in the 1970s has had a significant impact on preventing tooth decay and has saved an estimated one billion dollars over 30 years in dental costs and time off from work (Jaguar Consulting, 2016). Policies, regulations and guidelines have also been used to create health promoting environments in childcare settings, schools and aged-care facilities. Government funding (Chapters 2, 4, 5 and 9) and workforce changes (Chapter 3) have enhanced access to dental care.

One key shortfall has been the lack of use of fiscal measures such as a sugar levy to reduce consumption of sweetened drinks. Such fiscal measures have been successful in reducing the consumption of tobacco and alcohol and have proven effective in reducing sugar consumption internationally (Park & Yu, 2019; WHO, 2022b). It has been estimated that a 20% tax on sugar-sweetened beverages in Australia would prevent 3.9 million decayed-missing-filled teeth over 10 years and save $666 million over that time (Sowa et al., 2019).

There are successful oral health promotion programs in Victoria that are integrated with health promotion programs using a common risk factor approach. However, they are being implemented on a relatively small scale (Chapter 6). Also, not all prevention interventions have been sufficiently funded to allow for robust economic evaluation, thereby limiting their utility in terms of informing policy.

The way forward for prevention of oral health problems in Victoria and Australia would include these actions:

1. Expand community water fluoridation to meet or exceed the target of providing 95% of rural and regional Victorians access to fluoridated drinking water by 2030 (DHHS, 2020).

2. Scale-up Victorian prevention programs that have been evaluated to be cost effective. For example:

- Collaborate with health, education and welfare professionals who interact with young children and their families (Chapter 6, Section 2.1).
- Create oral health promoting environments in pre-school, school, and aged care settings (Chapter 6, Section 2.2).

- Extend preventive value-based dental care by employing minimal intervention approaches such as fissure sealants, Hall crowns, silver diamine fluoride and community-based fluoride varnish programs (Chapter 6, Section 5.2).
- Trial the involvement of other health professionals in applying fluoride varnish (Chapter 6, Section 1.2).
- Support peer-led oral health promotion programs (Chapter 6, Section 4.2).
- Mandate oral health assessment on entry into residential care such as aged care and disability facilities; develop oral health care plans and provide support to residents in these settings.

3. Enhance access to preventive and value-based dental care (Chapter 6, Section 5.2) through secure, ongoing national government funding (Chapter 12, WHO Strategic Objective 4).

4. Advocate for inclusion of oral health in all health plans, including in local government Public Health and Wellbeing plans and in the implementation of the *National preventive health strategy 2020-2030* (Chapter 6, Section 1.4).

5. Consider implementing evidence-based interventions that have not yet been tried in Victoria and

- further restrict advertising of sugar-rich foods to children: for example, remove the advertising of unhealthy food from government-owned property;
- introduce a national sugar levy; and
- include oral health prompts in routine health checks.

6. Implement a national oral health literacy campaign.

7. Include the prevention of oral disease and oral health promotion in the remit of the Australian Centre for Disease Control that is currently being established (WHO Strategic objective 1).

8. Include a focus on prevention in oral health information systems (Chapter 12, WHO Strategic Objective 5).

9. Undertake prevention research, monitoring and evaluation (Chapter 12, WHO Strategic Objective 6) focussing on addressing oral health inequalities (Tsakos et al., 2022), economic evaluation, community-based participatory research, and interdisciplinary research.

3 Health workforce

The WHO health workforce strategic objective is to develop innovative workforce models to respond to population oral health needs. Three main actions have been proposed: to develop the appropriate composition and size of the dental workforce; to work with other relevant health professionals; and to expand workforce education to respond to population oral health needs.

Composition and size of the dental team

Had we the luxury of starting over, it would make sense to plan for a dental workforce pyramid in Australia. At the base, a large number of practitioners would treat the most common, simple problems; fewer professionals would treat complex problems; while at the apex, a few specialists would manage the most complex problems. This is the basis of a cost-effective and efficient approach. As it is, the dental pyramid is almost inverted as 70% of practitioners are dentists (Chapter 3).

Australia is more advanced than most countries in the dental workforce area as there is a mix of dental clinicians with varied scopes of practice and length of training. Dental specialists, dentists, oral and dental health therapists, hygienists and prosthetists provide oral health care supported by dental assistants.

Arguments about who could, or should, do what for whom have raged since long before 1970. Contentious issues have remained unresolved, even after dental therapists and prosthetists came into being. The addition of hygienists and dental assistants with enhanced skills has further muddied these waters – that is to say, does the dental workforce act as an orchestra, and if so, who holds the baton? Or does it perform as an ensemble, with each worker knowing when and how to perform? Overlying all these debates are questions of political philosophy concerning *laissez-faire* versus government planning.

It is more likely that the scope of practice of the various practitioner groups will be varied by regulation, either amicably or through contest. Such change will probably occur in response to innovations in technology or materials, or as a logical measure to optimise use of time and skill. There is scope for dental assistants - the Cinderellas of the dental workforce – to gain more formal recognition and recompense for the contribution they can make to service provision and productivity. The topical application of fluoride varnish to the teeth of young children is a simple, current example. Varnish can now be applied by dentists, therapists, hygienists and, more recently, by Certificate IV dental assistants (Chapter 6). Another possibility is for dental assistants to scan and record children's mouths with intraoral cameras, either as a triage or surveillance measure. Artificial intelligence may then be used to analyse and flag damaged or vulnerable dentitions and soft tissues.

In a school dental service, teachers could also perform the scanning before any dental personnel become involved.

Technological innovation, together with a growing number of dental specialists on one hand and oral health therapists on the other, make it quite possible that the ranks of the "Jack of all trades" general dentist will be hollowed out in coming years. Biomedical knowledge continues to grow exponentially, both in relation to the genetic and environmental understanding of disease and how to better prevent or manage it. New knowledge will require the whole panoply of specialties, and any new varieties, to work collegially with other dental and medical practitioners. Concurrently – through regulation, technological advancement or both – opportunities will increase for therapists and hygienists to prevent or treat the more common problems in a greater proportion of the population.

As well as determining the appropriate mix of the dental workforce there is a need to tackle the size of the workforce. We have noted Victorian population growth from about 3.4 million in 1970 to 6.7 million in mid-2022.[49] While the COVID-19 pandemic has stalled the upward trend since 2020, and other factors may also affect immigration and birth rates, it is probable that Victoria's population will continue to grow. The proportion of people over 65 years of age will rise and other population groups – whether defined by ethnicity, place of residence, comorbidities or level of income – will be more vulnerable to disease and the lack of access to care. Other factors are evolving treatment concepts and materials, and shifting cultural norms (Birch et al., 2020).

49 See <https://www.population.net.au/population-of-victoria/>

If the different dental professions are to grow, collaborate and complement each other, more research into skill mixes and team functioning is required. There have only been a few investigations to date such as Nguyen and colleagues' review of how to make public dental services more efficient (Nguyen et al., 2019). Only when teaching institutions understand the optimal size and mix of the oral health workforce will they be able to enrol appropriate numbers of trainees on a national basis.

However, while it is easy to talk about educating appropriate numbers, in the absence of a national oral health workforce plan, in practice each tertiary institution seeks to maximise its student numbers and associated income.

Action is also required to address the difficulties of recruitment and retention in the public sector in Victoria. As outlined in Box 12.2, Victoria's ratio of public oral health professionals to population and its public dental salaries are among the lowest in Australia. Sustained Australian government funding for public dental care is needed to address this (WHO Strategic Objective 4).

Work with other relevant health professionals

Non-dental professionals are already helping to promote oral health in Victoria as outlined in Chapter 6. Nevertheless, more can be done. The *Healthy families, healthy smiles* preventive program builds the knowledge, skills and confidence of health- and early education professionals to promote oral health when they interact with young children and families. Aboriginal Health Practitioners can now apply fluoride varnish to teeth. These programs could be scaled up and further engage pharmacists, nutritionists, general practitioners and paediatricians.

Expand workforce education to respond to population oral health needs

Curricula and training programs need to adequately prepare health workers to manage and respond to the public health aspects of oral health and address the environmental impact of oral health services. The immediate challenge in Australia is that workforce training courses and their curricula have developed historically in uncoordinated, or even mutually antagonistic, ways. University curricula are routinely reviewed for content innovation and priority but seldom with national needs as the overarching principle.

Oral health professionals need an understanding of the basic epidemiology of oral health and how to reduce the burden of oral disease through prevention and oral health promotion interventions. Health promotion competencies for dental professionals are outlined in the recently released *Professional competencies of the newly qualified dental professional* (ADC, 2022). Knowledge is required of the challenges faced by groups and populations at greater risk of oral disease and theories of behavioural change. Intra- and inter-professional education and collaborative practice are also important to allow the integration of oral health services in health systems at the primary care level.

To ready the oral health workforce for the future, the following steps need to be taken:

- Develop and test workforce models of the optimal mix of practitioner types to meet community needs, and refine these for population subgroups in private, public and corporate environments.
- Scale up the two most promising candidates for trial across Australia, recognising that more than one model may be needed.
- Reduce the pay gap between Victorian public dental staff and their peers in other states.

- Maximise the use of all members of the dental team.
- Develop and strengthen partnerships with other health and welfare workers to enhance oral health promotion as part of their practice (WHO Strategic objective 2).
- Prepare health workers to manage and respond to the public health aspects of oral health and address the environmental impact of oral health services.

4 Oral health care

This strategic objective is aimed at increasing access to essential oral health care – safe, effective and affordable – for the whole population. Action is required in Victoria and Australia to enhance access to value-based oral health care that is integrated into general primary health care.

Enhance access to oral health care

In a blame game between the states and Australian governments, public funding for dental services has often fallen between the cracks. Governments have covered less than 20% of dental costs, compared with 65% of other health care costs (Chapter 9). Public dental performance has fluctuated subject to the ebb and flow of budgets, most markedly in Australian government funding (Chapter 5). While access to public emergency dental care has improved in Victoria, disadvantaged groups have historically faced long waiting times for general care. Considerable additional recurrent resources from the Australian government would be required if Australia is to meet the WHO vision of UHC in oral health for all individuals and communities by 2030.

Value-based oral health care

As discussed in Chapter 6, value-based oral health care is a person-centred and preventive approach that has the potential to deliver the outcomes that matter most to people at a lower cost (Porter, 2010). In the public sector, DHSV is developing a model that is to be extended to community dental agencies. The intention is to provide high-value care (that contributes to patient oral health outcomes, and is cost effective), while eliminating low-value care (that does not improve health outcomes and is less cost effective) (Hegde & Haddock, 2019).

A key aspect of a value-based care model that can provide a more preventive approach in the delivery of public dental services is having a funding model that rewards optimal client outcomes rather than treatment outputs. Blended funding models with a risk-adjusted capitation base and outcome-based components have been proposed (Hegde & Haddock, 2019). The Department of Health and DHSV are reviewing funding models. It is likely that a shift to a more preventive and value-based focus will require additional funding, at least in the short term, if the high demand on public programs continues (Chapter 5).

The ideal preventive approach is to focus on early childhood, with screening to identify oral disease in its early stages, intervention to arrest its progression, and maintenance of oral health in the future through oral health promotion activities. Promotion of oral health should be part of the broader health promotion role that other health professionals, who see children more regularly than oral health practitioners, carry out.

Integrating oral health care into primary health care

The association between oral health status, in particular gum disease, and certain systemic disorders has been known for many years. This is especially the case when the oral signs and symptoms were effects of the disorder – for example, vitamin C deficiency and leukaemia both cause oral soft tissue lesions. Causal or adverse associations of poor oral health with systemic disorders such as diabetes and heart disease took longer to demonstrate. However, just as oral health practitioners must now be alert to their patients' general health and medications, so must medical practitioners take account of the oral health status of those under their care. If optimal health care is to be provided, health promotion and disease prevention policies everywhere need to encourage investigation for cross linkages.

The likelihood of comorbidities rises with age. In future there is likely to be greater interdisciplinary cooperation to increase oral health literacy among people with comorbidities, both as a good in itself and as a means to ameliorate any adverse impacts of poor oral health. This is already happening for patients with Types 1 and 2 Diabetes Mellitus but there is scope to extend it to people with cardiovascular disease, renal transplants, gestational Diabetes Mellitus, and disorders causing xerostomia (dry mouth), as well as in general antenatal clinics and palliative care settings. Such developments may need changes to scope of practice and different funding arrangements under Medicare and private health insurance schemes.

Dental health technology

Currently, neither private nor public dental clinic information technology (IT) systems interact with the Medicare IT system. While there is much to do to achieve this, it is a work in progress. The more fully integrated dental and general health care provision becomes, the greater the possibility for early detection of disease, cross-referral of patients and joint management of disorders. Developments to enhance the utility of the individual My Health Record will hopefully facilitate integration.

For enhanced access to people-centred oral health care for all, the following are needed:

- Sustained Australian government funding for public dental services to improve access to preventively focused value-based care.
- Phased integration of basic dental care into Medicare, starting with a Seniors Dental Benefit Scheme as recommended by the Royal Commission into Aged Care Quality and Safety (RCACQ&S, 2021). With monitoring, evaluation and adjustments this could subsequently be extended, for example, to people with certain chronic health conditions such as endocrine and cardiovascular disorders and to people who are currently eligible for public dental services (Duckett et al., 2019; Maskell-Knight, 2022).
- Funding systems that focus on oral health outcomes that matter to people.
- A new public–private partnership model that includes value-based care with strong governance, monitoring and evaluation arrangements.
- More compatible dental and medical record systems which bring together health information and are linked to Medicare.
- Innovation in modalities and programs to take dental care to people who are unable to travel to clinics either because of infirmity or remote geographical location.

5 Oral health information systems

Planning for provision of whole-of-life care requires surveys of oral health status at regular intervals and, if oral health status and disease trends in populations are to be understood, reliably assured funding to conduct these surveys will be needed. Such knowledge is essential for strategic planning of disease management and associated workforce requirements. To date, the conduct of oral health surveys in Australia has been erratic because state and national governments have not resolved funding and frequency issues. Amit Chattopadhyay and co-authors have noted the *ad hoc* nature of oral health surveillance in Australia (Chattopadhyay et al., 2021). Notwithstanding the excellent work of the Australian Institute of Health and Wellbeing (AIHW), they consider the lack of formal structures set up specifically to collect and collate data to be far from ideal, also that funding is arbitrary and irregular, and that variables can differ in their definition and inclusion from survey to survey, or in other data collections.

Teledentistry already permits remote consultations and transfer of images and photographs to facilitate diagnosis and treatment. In future this mode of care will play an increasing role in education and disease prevention. The WHO has developed a comprehensive program called mOralHealth (WHO & ITU, 2021) in which the "m" stands for mobile devices. In rural or urban settings where there are no resident professionals, mOralHealth will bring information both to primary health workers and patients. Furthermore, if database compatibility levels are not considered and do not allow for data sharing as competing internet programs and mobile apps are developed and used, their effectiveness will be compromised.

Digital technologies provide the opportunity to amass metadata for research and strategic planning purposes which can subsequently be quarried for a range of uses. The addition of data from the private sector would add more power to any inquiry but problems of ethics and compatibility need to be overcome. Access to demographic and economic data already supports planning, however, de-identified clinical data from the whole range of practices would contribute better and more comprehensive evidence for decision making.

To improve policy planning for care and workforce deployment there is a need to:

- Enhance the surveillance and information capability of oral health information systems to support evidence-based policy development: in particular, to establish a system to measure and monitor oral health equity, use data from private dental practices and dental insurers, and enable linkages with broader health data systems.
- Progress and further utilise ehealth (for example, teledentistry) as a means to overcome lack of access to services, promote oral health education to disparate groups, and as an additional modality for professional education.
- Conduct national oral health surveys regularly, every five years at a minimum, alternating between child and adult oral health, as proposed in the *National oral health plan 2015–2024* (COAG, 2015); also ensure that qualitative surveys supplement existing quantitative surveys to gain more information for policy development.

6 Oral health research agenda

Oral health research is inadequately funded in Australia. Less than 1% of National Health and Medical Research Council research funds are provided for oral health research (Chapter 4).

Necessary improvements include:

- Research addressing the public health aspects of oral health, such as investigations of upstream interventions; oral health inequalities (Tsakos et al., 2022); primary health care interventions including community-based participatory research; the impact of oral health on general health; minimally invasive interventions; learning health systems; workforce models; digital technologies, and environmentally sustainable practice.
- Economic analyses to identify targeted cost-effective interventions.
- Increased funding for oral health research.
- Research into the barriers and enablers for the translation of research into policy and practice.

Conclusion

Improving oral health and reducing longstanding inequities requires action at all levels of government and in all sectors of civil society. The WHO *Global strategy on oral health*, adopted by the World Health Assembly in May 2022, provides a useful framework for identifying actions required to achieve the WHO vision in Victoria and Australia. The overall vision is universal health coverage in oral health for all individuals and communities by 2030.

Based on the findings of our look back to 1970, we have recommended areas for action on oral health under each of the six strategic objectives of the WHO global strategy. To progress this ambitious reform agenda, substantial discussion and policy attention are needed to determine priorities, timelines, funding and implementation responsibilities.

Universal oral health care for all individuals and communities would enable Australians to enjoy the highest attainable state of oral health and contribute to healthy and productive lives. The tattered safety net needs repair. The mouth should be brought back into the body.

We must consider every option carefully and, if the path to UHC is a long one, along the way we must tackle the unequal burden of poor oral health experienced by those who already bear the burden of social and economic inequality.

We hope that the findings of this study and the proposals put forward will contribute to an important national conversation about how to achieve the WHO vision.

Appendix

Appendix 12 Key recent national and Victorian oral health and general health plans

Initiative	Intent/Principles	Strategic focus areas
National preventive health strategy 2021–2030 (DH-A, 2021)	**Aims** 1. All Australians have the best start in life 2. All Australians live in good health & wellbeing for as long as possible 3. Health equity is achieved for priority populations 4. Investment in prevention is increased **Principles** 1. Multi-sector collaboration 2. Enabling the workforce 3. Community participation 4. Empowering & supporting Australians 5. Adapting to emerging threats & evidence 6. Equity lens 7. Embracing the digital revolution	1. Reducing tobacco use 2. Improving access to and the consumption of a healthy diet 3. Increasing physical activity 4. Increasing cancer screening and prevention 5. Improving immunisation coverage 6. Reducing alcohol and other drug harm 7. Promoting and protecting mental health
Healthy mouths healthy lives: Australia's national oral health plan 2015–2024 (COAG, 2015)	**National goals** 1. Improve oral health status by reducing incidence, prevalence and effects of oral disease 2. Reduce inequalities in oral health status across Australian population **Principles** 1. Population health approach 2. Proportionate universalism 3. Appropriate & accessible services 4. Integrated oral & general health	1. Oral health promotion 2. Accessible oral health services 3. System alignment and integration 4. Safety & quality 5. Workforce development 6. Research & evaluation

Initiative	Intent/Principles	Strategic focus areas
Victorian action plan to prevent oral disease 2020–30 (DHHS, 2020)	**Vision** 1. Good oral health for all Victorians by 2030 2. Reduce the gap in oral health for people who are at higher risk of oral disease **Principles** 1. Evidence-informed oral disease prevention policy, programs & services 2. Well-understood oral health status of Victorians 3. Enhanced evaluation to inform evidence base & future activity 4. Quality data for population & service level planning, monitoring & evaluation	1. Improve the oral health of children 2. Promote healthy environments 3. Improve oral health literacy 4. Improve oral health promotion programs, screening, early detection & prevention services
Dental Health Services Victoria Strategic Direction, 2022 (DHSV, 2022)	**Vision** 1. A future where every Victorian is disease and cavity-free 2. Creating change – Improving access, changing behaviour and eliminating disease 3. Improving the oral and dental health of pregnant people, infants, children and adolescents, adults 18–64, and adults 65 plus	1. Empower – Focus on prevention and early intervention 2. Care – Deliver world-class oral and dental healthcare 3. Lead - Reform, build and improve oral healthcare through key partnerships

References

Australian Dental Council. (ADC). (2022). *Professional competencies of the newly qualified dental practitioner.* Melbourne, Australia: ADC. <https://adc.org.au/files/accreditation/competencies/ADC_Professional_Competencies_of_the_Newly_Qualified_Practitioner.pdf>

Birch, S., Ahern, S., Brocklehurst, P., Chikte, U., Gallagher, J., Listl, S., Lalloo, R., O'Malley, L., Rigby, J., Tickle, M., Tomblin Murphy, G., & Woods, N. (2020). Planning the oral health workforce: Time for innovation. *Community Dent Oral Epidemiol, 49*(1), 17–22. <doi.org/10.1111/cdoe.12604>

COAG Health Council. (2015). *Healthy mouths, healthy lives: Australia's national oral health plan 2015–2024.* <https://www.health.gov.au/resources/publications/healthy-mouths-healthy-lives-australias-national-oral-health-plan-2015-2024?language=en>

Chattopadhyay, A., Christian, B., Gussy, M., Masood, M., Hegde, S., Raichur, A., Martin, R., & Kenny, A., (2021). Oral health surveillance in Australia: The need for ongoing data to inform public health decision-making. *Australian Journal of Primary Health, 28*, 18–22. <https://www.publish.csiro.au/PY/PY21001>

Cresswell, A. (2011, August 20–21). Health of the nation [chart], *Weekend Australian*, p. 6.

Dental Health Services Victoria. (DHSV). (2022). *Our strategic direction 2022. A future where every Victorian is disease and cavity-free.* <https://www.dhsv.org.au/about-us/our-organisation/news/dhsv-shares-bold-new-vision-to-improve-victorias-oral-health>

Department of Health. Australia. (DH-A). (2021). *National preventive health strategy 2021–2030.* <https://www.health.gov.au/resources/publications/national-preventive-health-strategy-2021-2030#:~:text=National%20Preventive%20Health%20Strategy%202021–2030%20–%20Glossary&text=Description%3A,over%20a%2010%2Dyear%20period.>

Department of Health and Human Services. Victoria. (DHHS). (2020). *Victorian action plan to prevent oral disease 2020–30.* <https://www2.health.vic.gov.au/public-health/preventive-health/oral-health-promotion/oral-health-planning>

Do, L.G., & Spencer, A.J. (Eds). (2016.). *Oral health of Australian children: the National child oral health study 2012–14.* University of Adelaide. <doi.org/10.20851/ncohs>

Duckett, S., Cowgill, M., & Swerrisen, H. (2019). *Filling the gap: A universal dental care scheme for Australia.* <https://grattan.edu.au/wp-content/uploads/2019/03/915-Filling-the-gap-A-universal-dental-scheme-for-Australia.pdf>

Hegde, S., & Haddock, R. (2019). *Re-orienting funding from volume to value in public dental services. Issues brief 32.* Deeble Institute for Health Policy Research. <https://ahha.asn.au/system/files/docs/publications/deeble_issues_brief_no_32_reorienting_funding_from_volume_to_value__0.pdf>

Humphrey, H. H. (1977). *Congressional record remarks at the dedication of the Hubert H. Humphrey Building, November 1, 1977,* vol. *123*, p. 37287. Washington: USA.

Jaguar Consulting. (2016). *Impact analysis: Expanding water fluoridation in Victoria. 2016.* [Unpublished data]. Melbourne: Department of Health and Human Services Victoria.

Kingdon, J.W. (2010). *Agendas, alternatives, and public policies.* (Updated edition, with an epilogue on health care). New York: Longman.

Maskell-Knight, C. (2022). *Priorities for a new health minister.* John Menadue's Public Policy Journal. <https://johnmenadue.com/priorities-for-a-new-health-minister/>

Nguyen, T. M., Tonmukayakul, U., & Calache, H. (2019). *A dental workforce strategy to make Australian public dental services more efficient. Human resources for health, 17*(1), 1-9.

Pan American Health Organization. (PAHO) & World Health Organization. (WHO). (2023). *Social determinants of health.* <https://www.paho.org/en/topics/social-determinants-health>

Park, H. & Yu, S. (2019). *Policy review: Implication of tax on sugar-sweetened beverages for reducing obesity and improving heart health. Health Policy and Technology, 8*(1), 92–95. <https://www.sciencedirect.com/science/article/abs/pii/S2211883718301862>

Porter, M. E. (2010). What is value in health care. *N Engl J Med, 363*(26), 2477–2481.

Royal Commission into Aged Care Quality and Safety. (RCACQ&S). (2021). *Final report.* <https://agedcare.royalcommission.gov.au/sites/default/files/2021-03/final-report-volume-1_0.pdf>

Sowa, P. M., Keller, E., Stormon, N., Lalloo, R., & Ford, P. J. (2019). The impact of a sugar-sweetened beverages tax on oral health and costs of dental care in Australia. *European journal of public health, 29*(1), 173–177.

Tsakos, G., Watt, R. G., & Guarnizo-Herreño, C. C. (2023). Reflections on oral health inequalities: Theories, pathways and next steps for research priorities. *Community Dentistry and Oral Epidemiology.*

World Health Organization. (WHO). (1986). *The Ottawa charter for health promotion.* <https://www.who.int/publications/i/item/ottawa-charter-for-health-promotion>

World Health Organization. (WHO). (2022a). *Global strategy on oral health.* <https://apps.who.int/gb/ebwha/pdf_files/WHA75/A75_10Add1-en.pdf>

World Health Organization. (WHO). (2022b). *WHO manual on sugar-sweetened beverage taxation policies to promote health diets.* <https://www.who.int/publications/i/item/9789240056299>

World Health Organization (WHO) & International Telecommunications Union (ITU). (2021). *Mobile technologies for oral health: An implementation guide.* Geneva: WHO & International Telecommunications Union. <https://www.who.int/publications/i/item/9789240035225>

Abbreviations

Note that the terms "Australian, Federal, Commonwealth and National" are all interchangeable when applied to the Government of Australia.

ABS	Australian Bureau of Statistics
ACOSS	Australian Council of Social Service
ACSQHC	Australian Commission on Safety and Quality in Health Care
ADA	Australian Dental Association
ADAVB	Australian Dental Association Victorian Branch
ADC	Australian Dental Council
ADOHTA	Australian Dental and Oral Health Therapists Association
ADT	Advanced Dental Technician
AHMAC	Australian Health Ministers Advisory Council
AHMC	Australian Health Ministers' Conference
AHPRA or Ahpra	Australian Health Practitioner Regulation Agency
AHWMC	Australian Health Workforce Ministerial Council
AIHW	Australian Institute of Health and Welfare
ALP	Australian Labor Party
ANPHA	Australian National Preventive Health Agency
ARCPOH	Australian Research Centre for Population Oral Health
ASDS	Australian School Dental Scheme
CCV	Cancer Council Victoria
CDBS	Child Dental Benefits Schedule (Commonwealth)

CDC	Centers for Disease Control and Prevention
CDDS	Chronic Disease Dental Scheme (Commonwealth)
CDHP	Commonwealth Dental Health Program
CDP	Community Dental Program (Victoria)
CHC	Community Health Centre
COAG	Council of Australian Governments
DA	Dental Assistant
DAC	Dental Advisory Committee
DBA	Dental Board of Australia
DBV	Dental Board of Victoria
DH	Dental Hygienist
DHHS	Department of Health and Human Services (Victoria)
DHS	Department of Human Services (Victoria)
DHSV	Dental Health Services Victoria
DPBV	Dental Practice Board of Victoria
DPH	dental public health
DSRU	Dental Statistics and Research Unit, University of Adelaide
DT	Dental Therapist
FTE	full-time equivalent
GDC	General Dental Council (British)
H&CS	Department of Health and Community Services (Victoria)
HCV	Health Commission of Victoria
HDV	Health Department Victoria
HIC	Health Issues Centre
IRSD	Index of Relative Socioeconomic Disadvantage

LP	Liberal Party	**NPA**	National Partnership Agreement (on Public Dental Services)
LTU	La Trobe University	**OHMG**	Oral Health Monitoring Group (national)
MCH	Maternal and Child Health		
MIOH	Midwifery initiated oral health education program	**OHSC**	Office of the Health Services Commissioner (Victoria)
MDS	Melbourne Dental School	**OHT**	Oral Health Therapist
MRDAW	Ministerial Review of the Dental Auxiliary Workforce (Victoria)	**OMS**	Oral and Maxillofacial Surgery
		PHIR	Private Health Insurance Rebate (Commonwealth)
MRODS	Ministerial Review of Dental Services (Victoria)	**RDHM**	Royal Dental Hospital of Melbourne
NACODH	National Advisory Council on Dental Health	**RMIT**	Royal Melbourne Institute of Technology
NACOH	National Advisory Committee on Oral Health	**SDS**	School Dental Service (Victoria)
NCOHS	National Child Oral Health Survey 2012-14	**UHC**	Universal Health Care
		VACCHO	Victorian Aboriginal Community Controlled Health Organisation
NCP	National Competition Policy		
NDIS	National Disability Insurance Scheme	**VAGO**	Victorian Auditor General's Office
NDTIS	National Dental Telephone Interview Survey	**VCOSS**	Victorian Council of Social Service
		VDS	Victorian Denture Scheme
NHHRC	National Health and Hospital Reform Commission	**VOHA**	Victorian Oral Health Alliance
NHMRC	National Health and Medical Research Council		
NOHA	National Oral Health Alliance		
NOHP	National Oral Health Plan		
NOHPSG	National Oral Health Promotion Steering Group		
NOHS	National Oral Health Survey 1987-88		
NSAOH 2004-06	National Survey of Adult Oral Health 2004-06		
NSAOH 2017-18	National Study of Adult Oral Health 2017-18		
NP	National Party		

www.ingramcontent.com/pod-product-compliance
Lightning Source LLC
Chambersburg PA
CBHW051555030426

42334CB00034B/3447